Current Topics in Microbiology and Immunology

210

Editors

Springer
Berlin
Heidelberg
New York
Barcelona
Budapest
Hong Kong
London
Milan
Paris
Santa Clara
Singapore
Tokyo

Immunology of Silicones

Edited by M. Potter and N. R. Rose

With 136 Figures and 132 Tables

Springer

MICHAEL POTTER, M.D.
Chief
Laboratory of Genetics
Bldg. 37, Rm. 2B04
National Cancer Institute
National Institutes of Health
37 Convent Drive MSC 4255
Bethesda, MD 20892-4255
USA

NOEL R. ROSE, M.D. PH.D.
Professor of Pathology and Molecular
Microbiology and Immunology
Departments of Pathology and of Molecular Microbiology
and Immunology
John Hopkins University
615 N. Wolfe Street, Rm. 4027
Baltimore, MD 21205
USA

Cover illustration:
INFLAMMATORY SILICONE GEL GRANULOMA: The early response to silicone gels is characterized by a dense cellular infiltration of different cell types. This figure shows stages in the formation of giant cells around the silicone gel vacuoles.

Cover design: Künkel+Lopka, Ilvesheim

ISBN-13: 978-3-642-85228-2 **e-ISBN-13: 978-3-642-85226-8**
DOI: 10.1007/978-3-642-85226-8

Softcover reprint of the hardcover 1st edition 1996
Library of Congress Catalog Card Number 15-12910

Typesetting: Camera-ready by authors
SPIN: 10497576 27/3020 – 5 4 3 2 1 0 – Printed on acid-free paper

Preface

This issue of *Current Topics in Microbiology and Immunology* records the proceedings of a Workshop on the Immunology of Silicones held at the Natcher Conference Center, National Institutes of Health, Bethesda, Maryland, March 13 and 14, 1995. A large number of investigators from North America and Europe met to discuss available data on how the immune system responds to silicones and related materials. Some aspects of this field are controversial. Nonetheless, the meeting was marked by a civil and open exchange of scientific information and divergent interpretations, reflecting the traditions of scientific communication.

Each invited participant was asked to submit an article summarizing his/her presentation. Most of the papers are published as submitted, with only editorial changes to conform with the guidelines given to each contributor or revisions to clarify aspects of the paper. The papers should not be regarded as peer-reviewed publications. This preface will attempt to outline some of the immunological areas of investigation relating to silicones.

GENERAL

The great range of viscosity of liquid and cross-linked silicone polymers and the elasticity of silicone rubbers made it possible to fabricate materials that mimic the consistency of tissues ranging from bone to mammary tissue. This has brought silicones into wide usage, and probably the largest group of persons involved are the recipients of silicone gel-filled breast implants (SBIs). It has been estimated that at least 800,000 women in the U.S. alone have been implanted with SBIs over the last two decades [see COOK]. Implants are not stable indefinitely, and after a period of years silicone materials will ultimately leak into tissues. An issue of considerable controversy is whether implants evoke disease. Although the issue of silicone-related disease remains a major clinical concern, it was not the primary subject of this meeting, rather the discussions focused on evidence about how the immune system responds to silicones.

CHEMISTRY OF SILICONES

Silicones are synthetic chemicals that do not occur naturally, thus the Si-O backbones in these long polymers are not directly (if at all) attacked by the enzymatic machinery of the body. The commonly used mammary implants contain two physically different forms of silicone polymers, the highly crosslinked elastomeric shell or casing (elastomer) and the silicone gel contained within. Both contain multiple molecular species of silicones.

Elastomer

The elastomer casing is made of highly crosslinked silicones, and also contains fumed silica. It is not impermeable, and liquid silicones within can slowly escape. The elastomer interfaces with connective tissues. There is probably a considerable quantitative range of tissue reactions to the elastomer in a genetically heterogeneous population, reflected in the extent of interfacial fibrous capsule formation [SHANKLIN *et al.*]. Such reactions are not specific for silicone elastomers but might be induced by other polymers which have a similar consistency. As pointed out by WOLF *et al.*, all materials 'age', and silicone elastomers are no exception. Gradually with time (averaging 10 years or more), the elastomer casing may erode and permit silicone gel to enter the surrounding fibrous tissue capsule and tissue beyond.

Because of the presence of fumed silica in the elastomer, it is relevant to discuss the immunology of SiO_2 (silica). It has been known for many years that certain forms of SiO_2 are strongly fibrogenic [see ALLISON]. This initiates a process that involves the ingestion of the silica particle by macrophages which then secrete fibrogenic cytokines, e.g., TNF-α, TGF-β. Components of the elastomer shell then may stimulate an inflammatory response via macrophages.

Silicone Gel

To produce the desired viscosity, the silicone gel is only partially crosslinked and much of the 'gel' is composed of filler, i.e., long chain linear polymers usually 1000 centistoke (cs) polydimethylsiloxane (PDMS). Gels also contain lower molecular weight unpolymerized silicones that are derived from the polymerization reactions [see LANE and BURNS]. The latter include a series of linear and cyclic compounds ranging from 3 to 300^+ siloxy units (1000 cs PDMS has about 330 siloxy units). A frequently discussed low molecular weight compound is octamethylcyclotetrasiloxane which is called D4. The crosslinking step is carried out inside the elastomeric casing. Some silicone gel material, including liquids escape through the elastomer shell may migrate in tissues and may even be transported to regional lymph nodes.

A critical question is whether silicone materials in the body can be degraded and give rise to new silicone – related species of molecules, or even silica. Chemical changes also can hypothetically take place in the gel itself [see BATICH *et al.*, WOLF *et al.*] with the formation of degradation products such as silanols. Only fragmentary data are available on the chemistry and kinetics of this degradation process and on the reactivity of these putative silanols. The fate of low molecular weight silicones with 3 to 10 siloxy units is also not known. There is some early evidence that certain low molecular weight siloxanes are toxic to cells in tissue cultures [FELIX *et al.*]. GARRIDO *et al.* discussed their evidence obtained by nuclear magnetic resonance spectroscopy that the silicone gel itself can be degraded *in vivo* into products that appear in blood plasma. The chemical identity of such intermediate compounds awaits further analytical data. This area of investigation is not clearly defined, and many more data are essential to determine if biologically active materials are formed from the degradation of the high molecular weight polymers.

REACTIVE CAPSULES AND T-CELLS

The character and generation of capsules vary with the individual, but, importantly, in some persons the capsule may also contain cells of immune system origin, e.g., lymphocytes, plasma cells and macrophages [see SHANKLIN *et al.*, HARDT *et al.*, YOUNG *et al.*, O'HANLEN *et al.*]. These interactive tissues may show varying degrees of inflammation. The capsule around a mammary implant is not just a simple fibrous wall between implant and host, but also a tissue buffer zone into which some of liquid materials from the implant gel contents can enter and become organized as silicone granuloma tissue. These are chiefly liquids that are loosely incorporated in the silicone gel itself during its preparation that slowly bleed through the elastomeric shell. It is difficult to directly quantitate silicones in tissues by chemical methods, but this can be achieved indirectly by oxidizing silicones to silicon. Using this approach PETERS *et al.* have shown the capsules around implants contain high amounts of extractable silicon.

An important aspect of immunological reactivity to SBIs concerns the role of T-lymphocytes. Silica has been implicated as a possible proximal agonist from the studies of SHANKLIN *et al.* who have observed SiO_2 crystals in capsules. They have provided indirect evidence that peripheral blood lymphocytes from SBI recipients are hyperreactive in *in vitro* cell proliferation assays to SiO_2 [SHANKLIN, SMALLEY *et al.*]. Further, anti IL-2 inhibited the incorporation of [^{3}H] thymidine into DNA of SiO_2 – stimulated lymphocytes. More direct evidence of specific T-cell activity in capsules is provided in the immunohistopathological studies of

O'Hanlon *et al.* They typed the TCR V-gene families expressed in capsular tissues and suggest local immune responses occur in capsules. Young *et al.* HLA typed and found a statistically significant overrepresentation of HLA-DR53 in symptomatic patients. In the course of this study they discovered the intriguing finding that 81 % of their symptomatic patients had autoantibodies to B-cells. McDonald *et al.* have provided additional evidence that the intraperitoneal injection of silicone gels in selected strains of inbred mice primes peritoneal cells to induce proliferation in splenic T-cells. Wilson and Munson found a suppression in NK cell activity following subcutaneous implantation of silicone gels.

ADJUVANCY

One of the important questions discussed at the workshop concerns the immunological adjuvancy of silicones and the specific conditions under which silicones can act as adjuvants. An early publication by Naim, Lanzafame and Van Oss (Immunol. Invest. 22:151, 1993) indicated that the *in vitro* emulsification of silicone gels with aqueous solutions of bovine serum albumin (BSA) provides mixtures that give a strong enhancement of the humoral immune responses to BSA in rats even exceeding those obtained with the classical complete Freund's adjuvants (CFA). An important finding in the study by Naim was the striking difference between silicone oils and gels. The (20 cs PDMS) silicone oil was inactive. In a follow-up study (Naim *et al.* Immunol. Invest. 24:537, 1995), silicone oils of higher viscosity were tested (100, 350, 1000 and 12,500 cs). The high viscosity (12,500 cs) oil gave a significant increase in the humoral response 79–98 days later, approaching that of the gel, suggesting increased viscosity and polymer chain lengths are critical factors. The adjuvant properties of silicone gels have been confirmed in other laboratories [see Klykken and White, Nicholson *et al.*]. Octamethylcyclotetrasiloxane (D4), a lower molecular weight silicone precursor found in gels, was also found to have an adjuvant effect [Nicholson *et al.*, Klykken and White]. This was ascribed to its inflammatory properties.

One of the conventional functions of some immunological adjuvants is to capture and slowly release protein antigen. This provides an artificial but nonetheless persistent source of antigen for antigen processing and presenting cells, and sustains immune responses. The high molecular weight silicone oils and gels may vary in efficiency in this respect. While the experiments with silicone gel/protein mixtures provide convincing evidence of adjuvancy when subjected to a manipulated *in vitro* emulsification procedure, they do not demonstrate that silicone gels which contact tissues produce a similar effect in vivo, particularly in subcutaneous sites. It is premature to draw such a conclusion at this time.

ASPECIFIC BINDING OF SILICONES TO IMMUNOGLOBULINS AND PROTEINS AND THE QUESTION OF ANTIBODIES TO SILICONE

VAN OSS and NAIM have discussed and defined the nature of aspecific binding of proteins, in particular immunoglobins (Ig), to hydrophobic surfaces, such as provided by silicones, and showed that IgG in aqueous solution binds to silicone with a high binding energy. They point out that hydrophobic molecules, e.g., silicones "do not fear or repel water. They attract water molecules with considerable energy". Thus, an Ig molecule can bind to a silicone surface via almost any of its solvent surfaces. This property complicates and obscures "the emergence of any paratope that is specific for a given low-energy epitope". In view of these physiochemical considerations, it is not surprising that most studies have failed to identify silicone-specific antibodies [see ROSENAU *et al.*, BUTLER *et al.*, ROSE *et al.*].

AUTOANTIBODIES

The adsorption of proteins to silicone surfaces may denature the protein and hypothetically generate protein-silicone particles that can be taken up by antigen-processing and -presenting cells. The silicones involved in particle formation may be derived from the silicones that bleed through the elastomer shell or from silicone gel materials that escape through larger tears into the subcutaneous spaces. Such immunogenic particles have not been made, but fragmentary evidence suggests that silicone gel material may be more effective than oils [see NAIM *et al.*, POTTER *et al.*]. The likely available antigens would include proteins in connective tissues, tissue breakdown products such as cell membranes, or proteins that are found in inflammatory tissues, e.g., collagens, fibrinogen, fibronective components of cell membranes (e.g., glycolipids), and cytoplasmic or nuclear nucleoproteins [see KOSSOVSKY *et al.*, ROWLEY *et al.*, ALVING *et al.*]. Many of the clinical studies depend upon comparing levels of autoantibodies to such tissue protein in symptomatic versus asymptomatic SBI recipients. Because the symptomatic SBI recipients may have other independently arising conditions, a cause-and-effect relationship between the presence of silicones and antibodies of various specificities cannot be proven. Here, animal studies could be of considerable help. In this connection it is of interest that the i.p. injection of silicone oils (1000 cS DMPS) or silicone gels in mice is associated with the appearance of antibodies to cholesterol [ALVING *et al.*]. The intraperitoneal and subcutaneous sites, however, are very different, as peristalsis and the movement of the intestines could potentially have a physical emulsifying effect. Further, the peritoneal space is associated with a large resident macrophage population.

It is known from independent studies on natural antibodies that many of these are polyreactive with binding activity for chemically diverse antigenic specificities, including a variety of autoantigens [see CASALI and SCHETTINO]. These antibodies may arise in an independent way that does not require obvious specific antigenic stimulation. The precursor cells that give rise to these antibodies may be non-specifically stimulated by the presence of silicones. Further research in this intriguing immunological problem may be useful in understanding the immunology of silicones.

ANTINUCLEAR ANTIBODIES IN SBI RECIPIENTS

Antinuclear antibodies (ANAs) in SBI recipients have been extensively utilized in clinical studies [CLAMAN and ROBERTSON, BRIDGES *et al.*, SILVERMAN *et al.*, TAN *et al.*, and LEWY] using the HEp-2 assay to detect ANAs. The range of positive reactions in healthy controls varied from 0–8 %; in healthy SBI recipients, 3–35 %; in symptomatic SBI recipients, 30–35 %; and in fibromyalgia patients, 25–28 % [CLAMAN and ROBERTSON, BRIDGES *et al.*, SILVERMAN *et al.*]. These data indicate that antinuclear antibody titers are increased in women with SBIs. It remains to be established whether the specificity of these antibodies to various nucleoproteins differs in SBI individuals compared with patients with idiopathic autoimmune disease.

Differences in the specificities of antibodies to collagen have been described [ROWLEY *et al.*]. Further work in this area is needed to determine if there is a unique profile of autoantibodies in SBI recipients.

SILICONE GELS IN MOUSE PLASMACYTOMA FORMATION

The i.p. injection of silicone gels, like paraffin oils, triggers or sets in motion the formation of plasma cell tumors in the BALB/c strain of mice that is genetically susceptible to peritoneal plasmacytoma induction. In contrast, the high viscosity 1000 cs and 12,500 cs oils have not proven to be effective. In these induction experiments free silicone gel is injected into the peritoneal cavity. Much of the gel remains in a single mass that lies unattached in the peritoneal space; however, small fragments and liquids can break away and become incorporated into a silicone granuloma that forms chiefly on mesenteric surfaces. This mobile gel material appears as vacuoles in histological sections. The connective tissues that form around these gel fragments contain numerous inflammatory cells including lymphocytes and plasma cells. The tissue response to 1000 cs silicone oils is strikingly different. Though scattered lymphocytes and plasma cells can be seen, the vacuoles are much more tightly packed together and the striking intervacuolar inflammatory component seen with gels is much diminished or absent.

The inflammatory microenvironment generated by the gel persists for many months and the surrounding tissue appears to be a permissive tissue site for plasmacytoma development. This may depend upon the local production of various cytokines, e.g., IL-6, and other constituents by inflammatory cells.

COINCIDENCE OF MULTIPLE MYELOMA AND MGUS IN SBI RECIPIENTS

A clinical question that was much discussed at the meeting was the finding of an M-component (a monoclonal band of Ig) in the serum of SBI recipients. When M-components persist over a period of many months they are called monoclonal gammopathy of undetermined significance (MGUS). Unrelated to the silicone question it is well known that MGUS is quite frequently encountered in individuals in the 6th decade and beyond and has approached approximately 1 % in the various studies reported [see HERRINTON and KYLE]. KYLE has followed 241 MGUS patients that were diagnosed in non-SBI recipients over a period of 29 years and found that 25 % subsequently develop into a more serious disease.

The coincidence of MGUS in an SBI recipient is to be expected based on the independent prevalences of both states. There are at this time no properly age-matched controlled studies available that permit evaluation of the significance of MGUS in 4th, 5th or 6th decade SBI recipients or whether there is an excess of MGUS in SBI recipients. It is firmly hoped that unbiased data can be ascertained on this point. One technical difficulty in any such study will be defining MGUS, and this concern relates to the sensitivity of the serum electrophoretic methods employed. When highly sensitive methods of detection are used, they may detect M-components that are produced by B-cell clones that are hyperreacting to some kinds of antigenic stimulus. These M-components may not be persistent. Examples of disappearance of the M-component following explantation were reported [SILVERMAN *et al.*].

A similar epidemiological problem relates to the occurrence of multiple myeloma (MM) in SBI recipients [TRICOT *et al.*, GARLAND *et al.*, SILVERMAN *et al.*] but the incidence of MM is much less than MGUS. For example, the American Cancer Society estimated there would be 12,700 new cases of MM in the US in 1994 (American Cancer Society Facts and Figures 1994). This is sufficient, however, to again anticipate the coincidence of MM in an SBI recipient. Several physicians who specialize in treating MM have reported the coincidental occurrence of SBIs in MM [TRICOT *et al.*, GARLAND *et al.*, SILVERMAN *et al.*].

There is no trend in existing independent epidemiological studies of MM to indicate that the incidence of this disease has undergone an increase in recent years. KYLE, for example, has seen no matches in his Olmstead County epidemiological study of reported cases of MM in SBI recipients. To begin to explore this relationship, a registry of cases of MM in SBI recipients has been established at the NCI [see RABKIN and POTTER], but this can be no substitute for an appropriately controlled study. It is relevant to quote Henry Claman's article in this connection: "One hopes that the current climate of medicolegal activity will calm down so that such studies can be done" [CLAMAN and ROBERTSON].

The organizers believe that this collection of papers will be of use to immunologists in formulating approaches to solving these problems.

MICHAEL POTTER
NOEL R. ROSE

Acknowledgements

We thank Dr. Alan Rabson for his support, enthusiasm and encouragement in developing the Immunology of Silicones Workshop. We are indebted to Ms. Victoria Rogers for her many contributions to the organization of the Workshop and for her expertise in preparing this book.

Table of Contents

Silicon, Silica, Silicones: Chemistry and Degradation

Interaction of Silicones with Proteins and Tissues

Cellular Reactions to Silicone Implants

Autoimmune Antibodies

MGUS, Myeloma, Plasmacytoma

Epidemiology

List of Contributors

(Their addresses can be found at the beginning of their respective chapters.)

ACKERMAN, J.L. 49
ALLISON, A.C. 147
ALTMAN, C. 323
ALVING, C.R. 181
ANDERSON, J.D. 277
BAINES, C. 39
BALLESTER, O.F. 361, 385
BARLOGIE, B. 357
BATICH, C. 13, 245
BENSON, K. 361
BERENSON, J. 367
BOGDANOVA, A. 49
BONA, C. 299
BORNKAMM, G.W. 93
BRADY, T.J. 49
BRANDON, H.J. 25
BRIDGES, A.J. 277, 283
BRUCKER, R.F. 59
BURNS, D.E. 277
BURNS, S.A. 3
BUTLER, J.E. 75
CASALI, P. 167
CHENG, L.L. 49
CHRISTIANSEN, B. 75
CLAMAN, H.N. 265
CONTE, V. 59
CONWAY, D. 327
COOK, A.D. 307
COOK, R.R. 419
CUELLAR, M.L. 291
DEPALMA, D. 13
DICK, G. 237
EMERY, J.A. 245
ESPINOZA, L.R. 291
EZRAILSON 337
FARMELO, M.J. 361
FELIX, K. 93
FIELD, T. 283
FREUNDLICH, B. 323
FRONDOZA, C.G. 139, 299
GARLAND, L.L. 361, 385
GARRIDO, L. 49
GERSHWIN, M.E. 59, 307
GLUCK, O. 317
GOLDMAN, B.D. 59
HALL, M.F. 227
HALPERN, G.M. 59
HARDT, N.S. 13, 245
HERRINTON, L.J. 389
HILL, S.L. 123
HOCHBERG, M.C. 411
HOMBURGER, H.A. 427
HOTEKAYAMA, R. 299
IPPOLITO, K.M.L. 103
JAGANNATH, S. 357
JANZ, S. 93
JERINA, K.L. 25
JONES, L. 299
KAPLAN, J.D. 277
KEMPLE, K. 277
KLYKKEN, P.C. 113
KOSSOVSKY, N. 327
KOSSOWSKY, R. 327
KUMAGAI, Y. 291
KUPPERS, R.C. 269
KURLAND, L.T. 427
KYLE, R.A. 375
LANDAVERE, M.G. 123, 269

Silicon, Silica, Silicones: Chemistry and Degradation

Silica, Silicon and Silicones...Unraveling the Mystery

T. H. Lane, Ph. D., FRSC and S. A. Burns[1], Ph. D.
Dow Corning Corporation, Midland, MI
[1] Expert witness in breast implant litigation

History

Silicon is an element - the second most abundant element in terrestrial earth. However, silicon is never found in nature as the raw element, but rather in combination with oxygen to yield various forms of silicas, silicates, glasses, and sand. Silicon in this combination with oxygen, makes up 75% of the Earth's crust. The name for the element, silicium from the Latin, silex, meaning rock was suggested by Davy to reflect the sources of silicon [1]. The name was later changed by Thompson to silicon to draw attention to the relationship to the elements carbon and boron [2]. Whatever you call it, it has been serving the occupants of this planet since the appearance of grasping mammals and utilitarian application of the naturally occurring forms of silicon as tools, weapons, glasses, and gems predates recorded history [3].

Berzelius proposed the chemical symbol for Si in 1819 [4] and in 1824 was the first to isolate the element from a silicate [5]. Some thirty years later, just as Mark Twain was beginning his literary career and our country was engaged in a civil war, Friedel and Crafts determined the atomic weight of Si to be 28 and generated the first silicon-carbon bond and determined it to be stable [6]. Since silicon-carbon bonds do not occur in nature, this discovery created a new branch of silicon chemistry and the basis for silicones and their related chemistries.

The growth of organosilicon chemistry parallels the history of organometallic chemistry largely because of the need to find flexible and efficient methods for the formation of silicon-carbon bonds. Friedel and Crafts' dialkylzinc route demonstrated the feasibility and stability of a silicon-carbon bond, but was neither easy nor was it controllable. In 1900, Grignard published his discovery of the reagent named after him and shortly thereafter Kipping had reacted silicon tetrachloride with ethylmagnesiumiodide to obtain a mixture of ethylchlorosilanes [7]. This observation directed Kipping and his work for nearly fifty years yielding discoveries and insights into the preparation of both organosilicon compounds and silicones. His work also served as the basis for the first industrial preparation of dimethyldichlorosilane and its conversion into commercially viable silicones in the early 1940s. However, this Grignard route to the precursor to silicones was costly and very inefficient. If large scale production was to continue to be viable, a new route to dimethyldichlorosilanes was required.

Initial experiments carried out in 1940 and later published in 1945 [8] by Rochow provided the solution to the problems of large scale manufacture of dimthyldichlorosilane and therefore, commercial silicones. The direct reaction of methyl chloride with silicon, in the presence of copper and other catalysts yields the desired methylchlorosilanes in good yields with a substantially reduced waste stream. Since the initial publication of this discovery, thousands of papers have been published demonstrating the flexibility of this process to give a host of industrially important organosilicon compounds. The major monomer from this process, dimethyldichlorosilane, is produced in well over a billion pounds per year by several basic producers of silicones. Along with other organo-chlorosilanes, dimethyldichlorosilane forms the basic building block for dozens of different siloxanes, which are formulated into hundreds of materials for thousands of applications in nearly every industry around the world.

Definitions and Nomenclature

Silicon

Silicon is an element which does not occur in its simplest form in nature. The element, silicon, must be reclaimed from the natural silicas which make up the Earth's crust, see Table I for relative abundance of selected elements in the crust.

Table I. Terrestrial Abundance of Selected Elements in the Earth's Crust (PPM)

Element	PPM	Element	PPM
H	8,700	Na	26,000
C	800	Si	257,000
N	300	S	600
O	495,000	K	24,000
Ag (silver)	0.10	Au (gold)	0.005

The atomic symbol for silicon is Si and its atomic mass is 28. Silicon is found in Group IV of the periodic table of elements as is carbon. Historically, this close family relationship to carbon has led many scientists to undertake the investigation of organosilicon chemistry in the belief that a realm of chemistry awaited discovery wherein silicon would freely replace carbon. A new realm of chemistry was revealed; however, silicon was not a replacement for carbon. Silicon is a very unique element. Some comparisons between carbon and silicon are given in Table II.

There are several properties that distinguish carbon from silicon. For example, silicon atoms are larger than carbon and this increase in size has many ramifications on the chemistry of silicon. Bonds involving silicon are longer than comparable bonds to carbon as illustrated in Table III. Longer bonds to silicon are derived directly from the larger atomic size of the elements. This larger size of silicon also reduces the possibility of stable, multi-bonded compounds. That is to say, pi-type bonding (Si=O) is very limited in silicon compounds and seen only under extreme conditions, if at all.

Table II. A Comparison of Si and C

	Carbon (C)	Silicon (Si)
Atomic Weight	12.011	29.0855
Electronic Structure	[He]2s22p2	[Ne]3s23p2
Melting Point	3500 C (sublimes)	1410 C
Electronegativity	2.55	1.80
Atomic Radius	1.53 A	1.93 A (9)
Atom Volume (cm3/mole)	4.58	12.1
First Ionization Potential	11.264 eV	8.149 eV

Table III. Comparative Bond Lengths (A)

	H	C	O	N	Cl	F
C	1.09	1.53	1.42	1.47	1.77	1.32
Si	1.48	1.89	1.63	1.74	2.01	1.54

The lower electronegativity of silicon results in more polar Si-element bonds when compared to carbon. This bond polarity also contributes to strong silicon bonding and often provides the thermodynamic driving force for some reactions involving silicon compounds. A comparison of bond strengths for silicon and carbon is shown in Tabel IV.

Table IV. Bond Strengths of Bond (kcal/mol)

	C	Si	H	O	N	Cl	F
C	82.6	89.4	92.0	91.0	80	81.0	104
Si	89.4	80.5	90.3	128	100	97.2	142

Carbon and silicon share a tetrahedral geometry and have a valence of four. However, silicon is capable of forming stable compounds with an expanded valence state of five or even six, carbon cannot. This ability to expand its valence state opens a host of reaction pathways that carbon cannot participate in, adding to the uniqueness of the silicon.

Silica

The term silica denotes the compound silicon dioxide, SiO_2. Silica is an ubiquitous chemical substance with rich chemical, geological, and commercial importance. Commercially, it is the sole source of elemental silicon and silica is used in large quantities as a constituent of building materials, ceramics, concretes and glasses. In its various amorphous forms, it is used as a desiccant, adsorbent, reinforcing agent, binder, builder for detergents and as a catalyst component for support.

The basic structural unit of silica is a tetrahedral arrangement of four oxygen atoms around a central silicon atom. Structurally, silica represents an infinite three dimensional network by sharing the oxygen atoms of a given tetrahedron with a neighboring silicon. The majority of naturally occurring silicas are crystalline. Common examples of crystalline silica include quartz, cristobalite and tridymite.

Amorphous silica has the same basic atomic structure as crystalline silica, but lacks a highly ordered geometry. Fumed silicas, which are amorphous, are generated by burning silanes and are used as reinforcing agents in many elastomeric and rubber silicone products.

Silicates and Silicic Acid

Silicates are metal terminated lower molecular weight forms of silica. These materials can be water soluble if the number of silicon atoms in the molecule is eight or less. Chemically, silicic acid is $Si(OH)_4$, but it exists only in aqueous environments and generally in one of its oligomeric forms, poly(silicic acid).

Silanes

Silane is a discrete molecule whose structure is SiH_4. However, Silane is also used to describe derivatives of SiH_4. For example CH_3SiCl_3 is often referred to as methyltrichlorosilane.

Substituents on Silicon

There are a variety of functional groups which can appear on silicon. Some of the more important examples are summarized in Table V.

Table V. A List of Common Substituents on Silicon

Silanol	Si-OH
Silylamine	$Si\text{-}NH_2$
Methoxysilane	$Si\text{-}OCH_3$
Vinylsilane	$Si\text{-}CH{=}CH_2$
Acetoxysilane	$Si\text{-}O(CO)CH_3$
Chlorosilane	Si-Cl
Disilane	Si-Si
Disiloxane	Si-O-Si

Silicone

Silicone is the generic description for an entirely synthetic polymer containing a repeating Si-O backbone and the organic groups attached to the silicon atom via silicon-carbon bonds define the class of silicone. The most common example is poly(dimethylsiloxane) or PDMS. This synthetic polymer has a repeating $[(CH_3)_2SiO]$ unit. This is the basic building block of silicones. Depending upon the number of repeat units in the polymer chain and the degree of crosslinking (tying the polymer chains together) at least six classes of commercially important products can be produced. They are fluids, emulsions, compounds, lubricants, resins, and elastomers or rubbers.

The Production of Silicones

The first step in the production of a commercial silicone is the preparation of elemental silicon (see Fig. 1). Since silicon itself does not exist free in nature it must be separated from its naturally occurring oxide. This sand, quartz, or silica is reduced to elemental silicon by heating in the presence of a carbon source, typically wood or other forest products, in a carbon furnace.

$$SiO_2 + 2C \xrightarrow{\text{about } 1400\,^{\circ}C} Si + 2CO$$

Fig. 1. Carbothermic Reduction of Silica to Silicon

After the preparation of silicon the next step toward the formation of silicone is that of converting the element to a compound containing chlorine, specifically, dimethyldichlorosilane. This is efficiently achieved via the direct reaction or direct process. In this reaction silicon is reacted directly with methyl chloride in the presence of copper and other transition metal catalysts. A typical distribution of materials from this reaction would include about 70-90% dimethyldichlorosilane, 3-15% methyltrichlorosilane, 3% trimethylchlorosilane, 0.5% dimethylchlorosilane, 0.1% tetramethysilane, and 1-6% polysilanes.

The next step in the process is the hydrolysis of dimethyldichlorosilane to yield a mixture of silicones, both cyclics and linears. The linear siloxane can be reacted further through a condensation reaction to yield molecules of greater molecular weight, they may be endblocked to give fluids, or cracked with base to give cyclics siloxanes. The cyclics can be polymerized via either anionic or cation routes to give fluids, gums or compounds. These polymerizations may occur in bulk, emulsion, solution or via phase transfer routes.

Silicone Fluids

Fluids are usually straight chains of poly(dimethylsiloxane), PDMS, which are chain terminated with a trimethylsilyl groups. The smallest PDMS is hexamethyldisiloxane [Me_3Si-O-$SiMe_3$] while longer siloxanes can have many thousands of repeating Me_2SiO units in their chains. PDMS fluids come in all viscosities from water-like liquids to non-pourable fluids and all of them are essentially water insoluble.

Liquid PDMS has a very low surface energy, 20-23 dynes/cm^2, and a glass transition temperature of -123 °C! These unusual properties are due in part to the unique flexibility of the siloxane backbone, the high bond energy of the siloxane bond, the low intermolecular forces between the methyl groups on silicon, and the partially ionic nature of the siloxane bond. The Si-O-Si bond angle varies between 140-180 degrees with only a 0.3 kcal/mol barrier to linearization. The activation energy for backbone relaxation is 2.75 kcal/mol above the glass transition temperature and 75 kcal/mol at temperatures below its glass transition temperature. This compared to polystyrene whose glass transition temperature is 110 °C and has a surface energy of about 40 dynes/cm^2.

Gels

Silicone gels are relatively lightly crosslinked PDMS matrixes. This chemical tying of siloxane chains produces a three-dimensional network which can be swollen with PDMS fluids to give a sticky, cohesive mass without form. Its physical appearance is dictated by the amount of crosslinking and how much fluid is added to the network.

Elastomers

Silicone elastomers are crosslinked polymers whose three-dimensional structure is much more intricate than a gel. In addition, there is very little free, non-crosslinked, polymer in the matrix. Amorphous silica is frequently added to the matrix to give greater reinforcement of the network and thereby increase the strength of the article.

Silicone Gel-filled Breast Implants

Basic Components

The basic components of silicone gel-filled breast implants manufactured by Dow Corning Corporation and Dow Corning Wright are shown in Fig. 2.

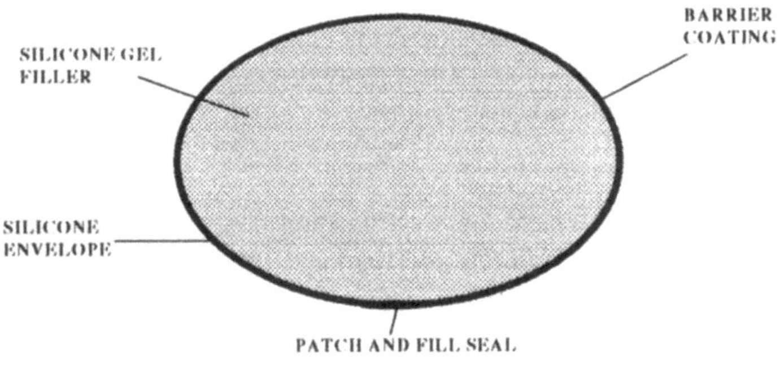

Fig. 2. Silicone-gel breast implant components

The implants are composed of the following: a silicone elastomer outer shell or envelope; a silicone gel filler; a patch made of a silicone elastomer, and; a fill seal composed of a silicone adhesive. During approximately the last ten years of sales, the envelope contained a fluorosilicone elastomeric barrier coating.

Historically, there were three types of gel used as filler materials: the original firm gel (sold from 1964 to approximately 1977), a slightly modified firm and, a responsive gel (both sold from approximately 1975 to 1992).

Three elastomers were used in the manufacture of the envelope. The first was a peroxide cured silicone. Later the elastomer was converted to a standard platinum-cured system. The most recent envelope was a two-layer system consisting of a high performance silicone elastomer outer shell and a fluorosilicone elastomer barrier layer, designed to minimize the diffusion of gel components through the silicone envelope. This high performance silicone elastomer has excellent physical properties and tear resistance. Dow Corning markets its silicone elastomers into the health care industry using the registered trademark, Silastic®.

Manufacturing Steps

The general manufacturing process for silicone breast implants can be described in three basic steps. The first, envelope preparation, consists of dipping stainless steel mandrels into a solvent dispersion of the uncured silicone elastomer base. Several mandrels were each attached by metal arms to a rack that was automated to provide for controlled submersion of the envelope forms into the dip coating tank. Upon removal from the tank and air drying, the coated mandrels were heated in a dry heat oven where the silicone base polymer is converted to a cured elastomer. The process of curing converts the silicone base to a crosslinked network, resulting in an elastomeric material. After curing, the silicone elastomer was removed from the mandrels. The empty envelope had a circular opening on the posterior, this being the former point of attachment of the mandrel to the metal arm. A patch of uncured silicone elastomer was placed over this hole using controlled pressure and cured. If the product was barrier coated, the patch-placed envelope was then injected with a fluorosilicone elastomer dispersion. The patched envelope was placed onto fixtures that rotated to allow the dispersion to coat the interior surface of the envelope. Following coating and air drying, the fluorosilicone barrier coating was cured. The unfilled patched envelope was then filled with a liquid silicone gel formulation by inserting a needle through the patch and injecting the uncured fluid material. The fill hole was then sealed with a silicone adhesive. The implants were cleaned and heated to accelerate the cure of the fluid components to form a cohesive gel. Each gel-filled mammary implant was submitted for primary packaging, sterilization and final packaging.

Platinum Curing of Silicones

Curing or crosslinking of silicones can be thought of as the process of chemically linking polymers together to form a three-dimensional network. This can be accomplished using a variety of bimolecular reactions. A review of crosslinking of silicones was recently published [10]. One of the more common is the platinum catalyzed addition reaction. In a very simplified way platinum catalyzed curing can be described as linking polymer chains together with a short chain oligomer (often referred to as the crosslinker), forming new covalent bonds. The polymer chains generally contain one type of reactive functional group and the crosslinker, another. In the application of this curing system, both the polymer and crosslinker can have multiple functional groups (located terminal or pendant on the siloxane chain) and mixtures of polymers may be used to control crosslink density and degree of polymerization between crosslinks.

The chemistry of platinum catalyzed crosslinking of silicones is shown in Fig. 3. This shows the linking of one polymer chain with the crosslinker. Here, the polymer is PDMS which contains some methylvinylsiloxane units in the backbone. The crosslinker is a short chain silicon hydride functional oligomer. In the presence of a platinum catalyst, the silicon hydride effectively adds across the double bond of the vinyl group, forming an ethylene linkage. This reaction, called hydrosilylation, was discovered by Speier [11]. The extensive field of hydrosilylation has been recently reviewed by Ojima [12]. Advantages of hydrosilylation crosslinking include: no cure by-products, controllable cure rates and no post cure requirements. The reaction occurs at room temperature and often inhibitors must be formulated into the system to allow for proper working time of the elastomer prior to cure. The inhibitors are either volatilzed from or reacted into the matrix during cure.

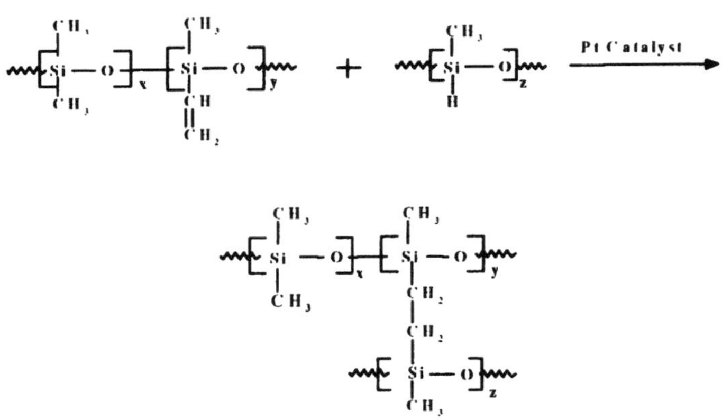

Fig. 3. Chemistry of platinum catalyzed crosslinking.

Silicone Elastomer Matrix

The elastomer formulation used in the envelope manufacture consists of a high molecular weight PDMS polymer that contains vinyl functionality. The vinyl groups can either be in the terminal or pendant positions along the polymer chain. Fumed, amorphous silica is mixed into these polymer gums with the aid of a silica treating agent or process aid. These are either short-chain, silanol-terminated oligomers or hexamethyldisilazane (which silylates the silica surface). The process aids serve to render silica surface hydrophobic and allows for dispersion into the high molecular weight polymers. This polymer base is then mixed with the catalyst system.

The platinum catalyst system is composed of a platinum complex with vinyl siloxanes, a short-chain silicon-hydride functional fluid (crosslinker) and an inhibitor. The catalyst system and the polymer base were dispersed in 1,1,1-trichloroethane for use in the dipping process.

The silicone elastomer network that forms the envelope is figuratively shown in Fig. 4. It is composed of a crosslinked network of very high molecular weight polydimethylsiloxane. Dispersed in this network is fumed amorphous silica which has been treated or silylated. This silica serves to improve the physical properties and tear resistance of the elastomer.

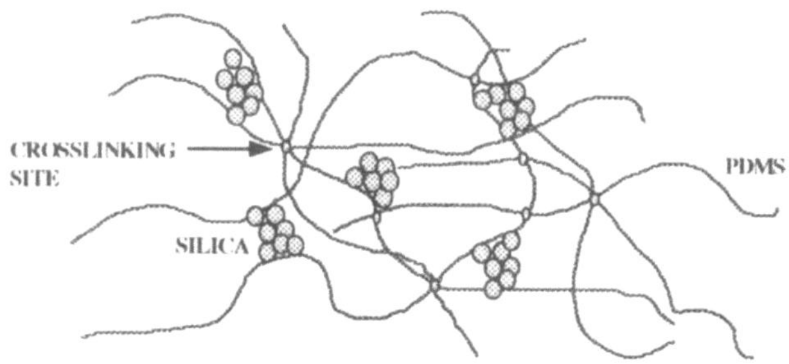

Fig. 4. Silicone Elastomer Matrix.

To illustrate this, an amorphous silica-filled high performance silicone elastomer has very good physical properties, as shown in Table VI. When the silica is removed from the system, these properties decrease significantly, particularly the tear strength.

Table VI. Physical properties of silica filled and unfilled elastomer

Property	Silicone Elastomer With Silica	Silicon Elastomer Without Silica
Tensile, psi	1650	375
Elongation, %	1100	485
Tear strength, ppi	220	23

Silicone Gel Matrix

The silicone gel matrix differs from elastomer matrix in several ways (see Fig. 5). First, the network is composed of shorter chain vinyl-functional fluids (~300 repeat units) as compared to the very high molecular weight vinyl-functional polymers (~5,000 repeat units) used in the elastomer matrix. These fluids contain pendant vinyl functionality and are crosslinked using a similar platinum system as described above. Crosslinks are formed using a silicon hydride terminated short chain crosslinker. The gel network is crosslinked in the presence of a non-functional PDMS fluid. Effectively, this fluid serves to swell the gel and give it a soft consistency and its gel-like properties. Because the reactive functionalities are diluted in the non-functional fluid, inhibitors are not used in the manufacture of the gels as cure at room temperature is relatively slow, allowing for adequate working time. There is no amorphous fumed silica in the gel.

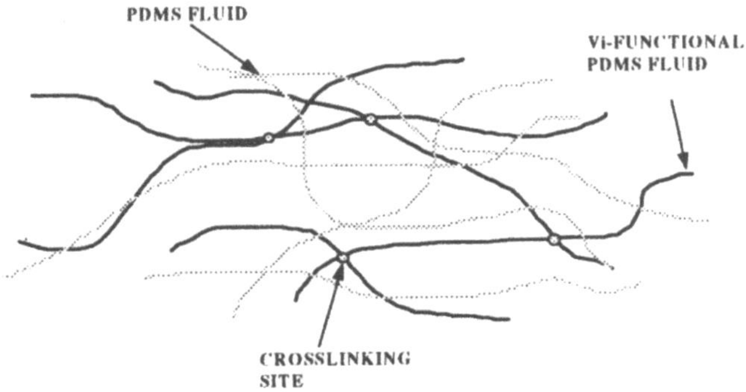

Fig. 5. Silicone Gel Matrix.

Silicone chemistry, its application to medical devices and interactions with biological systems is not simple. However, silicones remain one of the most studied and best tested biomaterials in the history of the science.

References

1. Davy H (1808) XXIII. Electro-Chemical Researches, on the Decomposition of the Earths; with Observations on the Metals Obtained From the Alkaline Earths, and on the Amalgam Procured from Ammonia, Phil. Trans. R. Soc. London 98:333
2. Partington JR (1964) A History of Chemistry, Vol. 4, MacMillian: London, pp 150.
3. Weeks ME (1956) Other Elements Isolated With the Aid of Potassium and Sodium; Beryllium, Boron, Silicon, Aluminum, published in Discovery of The Elements, J. Chem. Ed., Easton, PA, pp 586
4. Berzelius JJ (1820) Versuch uber die Theorie der Chemischen Proportionen, Dresden
5. Berzelius JJ (1824) Unterfuchungen Uber die Flufsfpathfaure und deren Merkwurdigften Verbindungen, Ann. Phys. Chem. 1:169 and 204
6. Friedel C, Crafts JM (1863) Some New Organic Compounds of Silicon and The Atomic Weight of this Element, Ann. 127:28
7. Kipping FS (1904) Organic Derivatives of Silicon. Preparation of Alkylsilicon Chlorides, Proc. Chem. Soc. 20:15
8. Rochow EG (1945) The Direct Synthesis of Organosilicon Compounds, J. Am. Chem. Soc., 67:963
9. Bondi A (1964) van der Waals Volumes and Radii, J. Phys. Chem. 68 (5):441
10. Calrson SJ, Semlyen JA (ed.) (1993) Siloxane Polymers, Prentice Hall, New Jersey
11. Speier JL, Webster JA, Barnes G (1957) Addition of Silicon Hydrides to Olefinic Double Bonds. Part II. Use of Group VIII Metal Catalysts, J. Amer. Chem. Soc. 79:974
12. Ojima I (1989) The Chemistry of Organic Silicon Compounds, Wiley, New York, pp 1479

Silicone Degradation Reactions

By Chris Batich*, Don DePalma, James Marotta, Guy Latorre
Materials Science and Engineering Department, University of Florida
and N.S. Hardt
Department of Pathology, University of Florida

INTRODUCTION

Silicone (polydimethylsiloxane, PDMS) is generally a very stable polymer. Because of this, it is used in a wide variety of adverse environments such as those with high temperature or as electrical insulation. However, a great deal of this stability derives from the fact that hydrolysis reactions which occur are reversible and the polymer essentially heals itself. It is likely that such reversibility would not occur in the surface region where high concentrations of other components, such as water, can exist. Because of the significant concern about the fate of silicone released from breast implants in particular, it is important to understand the types of chemical changes which may occur in silicone upon exposure to physiological environments so that the data on various silicon-containing species can be correlated with other physiological studies on known compounds. Accordingly, this chapter will focus on the known silicone degradation reactions which occur within normal physiological ranges (37° and mixed aqueous environment). Various other studies will be drawn upon to evaluate the possible changes since the literature on silicone modification under physiological situations is sparse at this time. Three main reactions discussed are hydrolysis, oxidation, and addition.

The physical form of the silicone is also an important parameter in this evaluation since one expects changes and tissue interaction to occur on the surface. Hence, the greater the dispersion, the greater the amount of surface area and consequently, the greater possibility for reaction. As shown in Table I, a drop of silicon oil with a radius of one centimeter can be divided into smaller droplets and this will sharply increase the total surface area. Hence, such a drop, if divided to smaller drops with a radius of approximately one micron (as is seen in normal tissue slides of phagocytized silicone) would generate 10^{12} spheres with a total surface area of about 10 square meters. If the particles were smaller, for instance 0.1 micron radius, there would be 10^{15} particles with about a 100 square meter surface area. With particles this small, the surface chemistry becomes a major determinant of the properties of the material and needs to be determined as carefully as the bulk properties.

Table I: Changes in radius, volume and area of spheres as their size is reduced from dividing a 1 cm. radius drop of liquid (adapted from Hiemenz, 1986).

Radius (cm)	Number of Spheres	Volume per Sphere (cm^3)	Area per Sphere (cm^2)	Total Area (cm^2)
1	1	4.2	12.6	12.6
0.5	8	0.5	3.1	25.1
1.25×10^{-1}	512	.008	.19	101
10^{-4} (1μ)	10^{12}	4×10^{-12}	1×10^{-7}	1×10^{5} (10m^2)
10^{-5} (0.1μ)	10^{15}	4×10^{-15}	1×10^{-9}	1×10^{6} (100m^2)

Assuming that no changes take place in silicone, four basic questions can be asked about an implant: How much silicone is released from it? What is the composition of the material which is released? Where does the material go within the body? What effects does it have when it gets there? We will address only the first two questions and will also discuss the changes which might occur in the silicone during the course of its dispersion through the body which may influence some of the behavior seen.

The phenomenon of gel bleed has been known for two decades and has been described as "inevitable" (Brody, 1977). An early *in vitro* bleed study of silicone gel-filled breast implants (Bergman and van der Ende, 1979) consisted of placing an implant on a pre-weighed piece of filter paper in a desiccator for 2 and 12 weeks. At each time period the paper was weighed and the weight gain calculated. Bergman, et al. concluded that there was a "progressive oozing" of silicone gel through the implant shell in all five implant manufacturers. One method used to measure silicone release rate in simulated body fluid at 37°C gave a value of about 1 mg./day for most implants (Yu, et al.).

There is little data in the literature on the composition of gel bleed. The most comprehensive study (Varaprath, 1991) showed very little vinyl siloxane contained in gel bleed (about 100 ppm). Most oil from gel bleed was somewhat reduced in molecular weight as described below. A significant amount of very low molecular weight material was found in the gel bleed from several implants which may represent octamethycyclotetrasiloxane (D_4), the cyclic tetramer (mol. wt = 297). The unreactive internal fluid used to make the bulk of the gel was shown by Varaprath to have a weight average molecular weight (Mw) of about 37,000 and a number average molecular weight (Mn) of about 14,000. There was no low molecular weight material reported. In contrast, the gel bleed from an implant was found to have mostly material with a slightly lower molecular weight (Mn = 5,000-13,000 and Mw = 9,000-24,000), but also included about 4% of very low molecular weight components (approximately Mn = 530 and Mw = 540) and 3-15% very high molecular weight components (about 300,000 molecular weight).

An analysis of extraction liquids from gel sheeting used as a topical, semi-occlusive dressing found that the most abundant siloxane oligomers were cyclic components, octamethycyclo-tetrasiloxane (D_4), decamethycyclopentasiloxane (D_5), dodecamethycyclohexasiloxane (D_6), and other larger cyclic siloxanes (Haggard, et al., 1993). The identification of these low molecular weight components is of interest because they can diffuse faster and enter a cell more readily than higher molecular weight components, and thus may show changes in degradation.

In Figure 1 is a schematic diagram showing the interface between an implant and the fibrous capsule and surrounding tissue. The "gel" filling material consists of a true cross-linked section called a gel making up roughly 10-20% of the material and a lower molecular weight soluble fraction (sol) which can be extracted and can also largely pass through the elastomer shell. This sol can be picked up by the synovium-like cells and transported to the tissue much as in a synovial capsule. The fibrous capsule appears to reach a certain saturatable concentration of silicon which is transported through this structure. However, very high levels of silicone can build up between the fibrous capsule and the implant, depending on the relative rate of release from the implant and the rate of transport through the capsule. Trapped silicone will continuously be released from an essentially zero order release device into the surrounding tissue. There is indication that macrophages and other cells pick up this silicone which is then transported to lymph nodes and other locations, including the liver. It is uncertain how much other silicone is emulsified at this point and carried with interstitial fluid to distant locations, although it is likely that this occurs to some extent because of the large number of natural surfactants present in interstitial fluid and blood (e.g., membrane components, oligopeptides). The main point of interest here is that these mechanisms produce a large surface area of particulate material which will have a significant surface chemistry. This ignores rupture and migration along tissue planes by large pieces of PDMS, although there is indication that subsequent to rupture, the material is also incorporated into cells by phagocytosis and distributed to distant locations. Because of the present poorly characterized distribution of this variable material, establishing dose response relationships is difficult. A number of studies suggest that the capsule, as well as the blood, is a saturatable transport system for the distribution of this finely divided silicone. This is inferred from demonstration of increased levels of silicone in blood and capsules of women with implants, and its detection in distant organs. In a similar manner, low levels of PDMS may be degraded actively when phagocytized, but higher levels may swamp cellular degradation mechanisms.

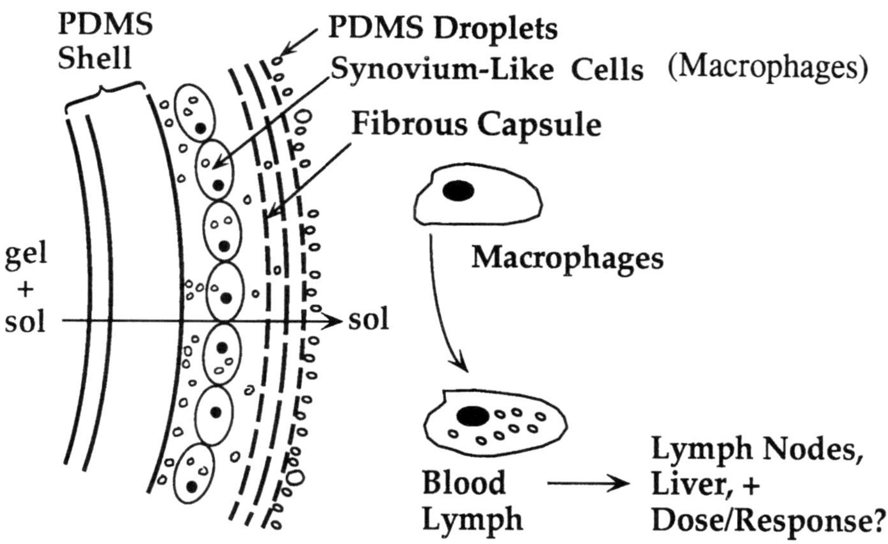

Figure 1: **Schematic generation of PDMS droplets formed from an unruptured gel-filled implant by "gel bleed" ie. permeation of oil.**

HYDROLYSIS

As shown in Figure 2, the siloxane bond can be hydrolyzed by exposure to water, creating two silanol groups. As mentioned, this reaction is highly reversible, tending to form the siloxane bond when high enough concentrations of silanol groups are present. This explains, for instance, the equilibrium aqueous solution concentration value of about 50 parts per million for silicic acid $Si(OH)_4$, in glass containers. Above 50 parts per million, silanol groups condense and reform silica. The same reaction occurs with silicone polymers and is accelerated greatly in both directions by the presence of acid or base catalysts. This can happen even in cross-linked networks in air at room temperature if the air is moist, as seen in stress relaxation studies (Vondracek, 1982). Some of the catalysts for the condensation reaction have been strong acids and bases and also amines (Saam, 1990).

$$R_3Si\text{-}O\text{-}SiR_3 + H_2O \underset{\text{Condensation}}{\overset{\text{Hydrolysis}}{\rightleftharpoons}} 2\,R_3\,Si\text{-}OH$$

Figure 2: Hydrolysis and condensation reactions between a siloxane band and two silanol groups.

We conducted a hydrolysis study as part of a master's thesis (DePalma, 1992). The surface chemistry of silicone is somewhat difficult to follow because of the extreme mobility of the polymer which allows low molecular weight materials to routinely rise to the surface and create a fresh silicone layer whenever the material was exposed to air. In addition, many of these changes happened rapidly due to the low glass transition temperature of the silicone. Eventually we settled on working with a piece of elastomer which had been extracted extensively with toluene to remove the approximately 5% extractable, low molecular weight material present. The elastomer was a peroxide-cured silicone film which would have the same general properties as the platinum-cured elastomer used in most breast implants. Studies were conducted at elevated temperatures to speed the reaction and the results were extrapolated to 37°C. The extrapolations were not strictly linear and showed a lag period before the reaction seemed to follow a linear period. This lag, we feel, was due to the influence of silanol groups on subsequent reaction, i.e., it acted as a catalyst itself and hence, speeded up the reaction once it formed. Despite these variations, there was generation of a more hydrophilic surface in each case after extended exposure of a PDMS solid to a saline solution. Other groups reported similar behavior [M. Morra, et al., "on the aging of oxygen plasma-treated PDMS surfaces" J. Col. & Interface Science 137, 11-24 (1990)], in that control samples which had been stored in water at room temperature eventually became hydrophilic. Most of our study was directed towards understanding the kinetics of this reaction and extracting an activation energy for it. The activation energies determined and those reported in the literature for similar systems are indicated in Table III (DePalma, 1992).

Table II: Activation energy summary for hydrolysis reactions of PDMS.

A.C. Martellock	Q (Kcal/mol)	viscosity average molecular weight change
uncatalyzed	23	
catalyzed	6	
R.C. Osthoff, et al.		thermal stress-relaxation
uncatalyzed	22.8	
catalyzed	5.1	
DePalma (1992)		contact angle goniometry
	4.5	3 pts (333°, 343°, and 353° K)
	6.8	4 pts (333°, 343°, 353° and 373° K)
		XPS derivatization
	4.1	3 pts (333°, 343°, 353° K)
	3.3	4 pts (333°, 343°, 353° and 373° K)

Surface changes were monitored by two methods. The first method used contact angle goniometry for air measured under water. The other method involved a surface derivatization method combined with x-ray photoelectron spectroscopy and, we believe, showed reaction with surface silanol groups. The two methods yielded essentially the same general numbers, which give us the activation energy reported and allowed us to produce the following extrapolation for the surface hydrolysis reaction at 37°C. As seen in Addendum, a fairly rapid initial reaction would take place which would slowly increase with time, leading to a significant fraction (about 25-30% change) in somewhere between two and ten years. The exact numerical agreement between this saline, elevated temperature study and the in vivo environment may vary, however, it is very likely that the hydrolysis reaction occurs on the surface relatively slowly over a period of, roughly, five years in both saline and tissue.

The change in the surface from a siloxane bond to a silanol containing structure would lead to profound changes in behavior. Silanols are acidic and have a pK_a similar to that of phenol. Hence, they would likely be ionized to some extent. Because of the presence of "reactive silanol groups" on fumed amorphous silica, the particles are treated with silicone polymer to reduce their surface density (Levier, 1993). The presence of the silanol group has been linked to the activity of silica in various biological evaluations such as fibrosis and cell lysis (Razzaboni, 1990). There are numerous reports indicating that crystalline silica is more damaging than amorphous silica. However, if the materials are adjusted for similar surface silanol concentration, they both appear to be about as physiologically damaging to nearby cells. The crystalline/amorphous difference appears to result from the difference in the method of preparation of the materials. Crystalline silica or quartz is ground in water, which leads to hydrolysis of the fractured siloxane bonds. In fact, the crack propagation velocity in silica is much higher in the presence of water than it is in the absence of water because of the enhanced effect on breaking this bond (Ritter, 1991). Amorphous silica, on the other hand, is formed in a high temperature fuming process and generates siloxane bonds on the surface (Kingery, et al., 1976). These siloxane bonds have been detected by a variety of methods and are shown to slowly hydrolyze on storage in a moist environment to produce surface silanol groups. When the amorphous silica has been so allowed to hydrolyze on the surface, it also has activity similar to that of the crystalline material. Relating this to the PDMS behavior, it appears that the hydrolyzed particles would likely be more physiologically active than the unhydrolyzed PDMS.

The binding of PDMS to proteins is an interesting area where the presence of silanols would likely lead to different behavior (Shi, et al., 1989). In electrophoresis, for instance, it is considered important to block surface silanol groups to prevent binding of proteins (Towns, 1990). However, proteins also have hydrophobic regions which would bind strongly to the siloxane area. Many questions remain in this area and it is uncertain at this point whether the binding of the hydrophobic interior of the proteins would cause a different kind of response than binding of the hydrophilic exterior of many proteins, exposing a more hydrophobic interior. It is likely that the binding will be different in quantity as well as quality and lead to different types of denaturization as well as amounts bound, depending on the state of the PDMS.

Silanol groups can also interact with carbohydrates to form structural polymers in animals (Mathews, 1990).

The hydrolysis reaction occurs also in the bulk to some extent, possibly due to the transport of acids and bases into the gel by complexation with cyclic siloxane species (Saam, 1990). This degradation was demonstrated in a study (McCoy, 1987) of factors influencing the stability of mammary gel. It was shown that residual catalyst concentrations above about two parts per million led to depolymerization when the gel was stored at 36°C. The degradation in this case was measured by a penetrometer and essentially measured the extent of cross-linking of the gel.

Concentrations above this level occasionally occurred during production and the recommendation of the report was that extraction be carried out with testing afterwards to keep the levels low.

OXIDATION

As shown in Figure 3, oxidation basically involves the removal of a methyl group from the PDMS side chain, replacing it with a silanol group. It would be expected that such a reaction would occur through free radical attack on the methyl hydrogens, leading to substitution. It has been demonstrated that having a silicon adjacent to an alkyl carbon hydrogen bond increases the propensity for free radical extraction by a factor of about five (Barton, 1990). As shown in Figure 3, the oxidation leading to production of silanols on side chains would lead to gelation if the main backbone chain was intact. In other words, the formation of a gel from a liquid would occur if oxidation were occurring and the silanol groups were, in turn, reacting with each other. This kind of reaction might be expected from superoxide or hydroxyl radical generation, such as has been postulated to occur in an oxidative burst during an inflammatory response. If this reaction were occurring, one would expect the liquid "gel bleed," which had been through the elastomer shell, to slowly turn into a gel (cross-linked) material. This point would be significant because it has shown (Naim, 1993) that the gel form of PDMS is a strong adjuvant while the liquid form is not. The NMR methods developed by Garrido in this volume demonstrate that oxidation occurs since silicon is observed with more than two oxygens attached to it. Additionally, one can look at the physical state of silicone in preserved tissue slides. During normal processing of histological samples, the tissue is extracted with various solvents of decreasing polarity, eventually being extracted with xylene before being infiltrated with paraffin wax. Such a processing would remove liquid which is soluble in xylene, but would not remove gel, which could only swell. We attempted to determine whether the small amounts of silicone remaining in tissue slides were soluble in xylene and the results are shown in Figure 4. We concluded that some cross-linking had taken place in this tissue sample which is from a woman with a non-ruptured implant. This shows that liquid released by gel-bleed has gelled at the point where a tissue analysis has taken place. These results are consistent with oxidation during residence in the tissue or during tissue processing. The specific mechanism shown in Figure 3 (first step) is for high temperature oxidation of PDMS. Other physiological oxidants such as superoxide, hypochlorous acid or hydroxyl radical may not proceed through a hydroperoxide intermediate, but would also lead to a cross-linked structure as a final product.

Oxidation leads to silanols.

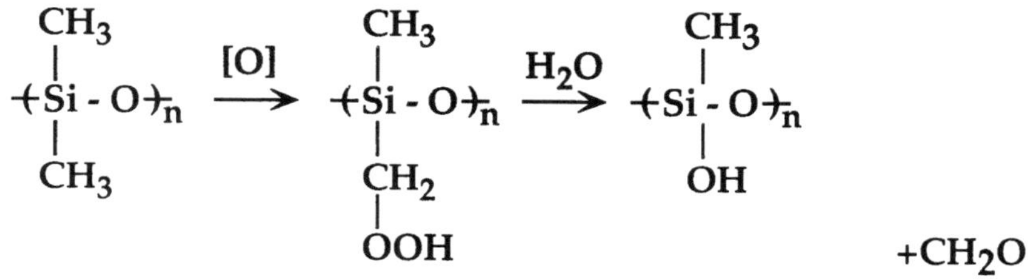

Which leads to cross-linking (gelation).

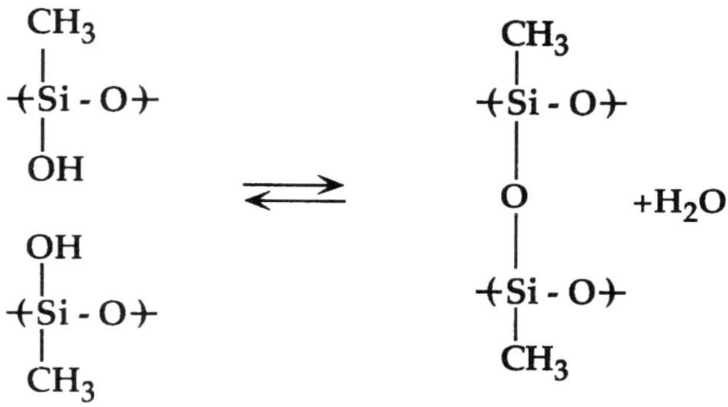

Figure 3: Removal of methyl groups from PDMS by oxidation with subsequent cross-linking.

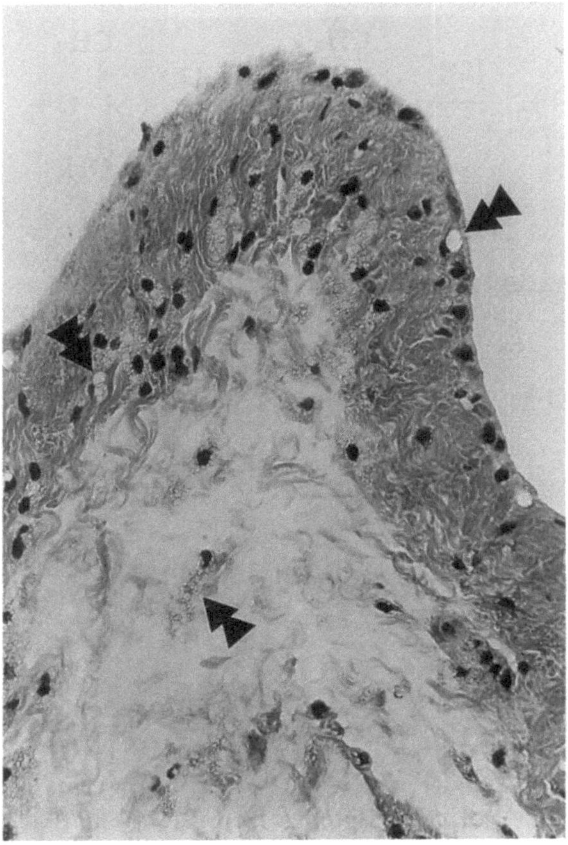

Figure 4: This patient underwent bilateral subcutaneous mastectomies for fibrocystic disease with subsequent placement of silicone gel filled implants. Three years after surgery she developed signs and symptoms of autoimmune disease, and was eventually diagnosed with scleroderma. She did not improve after medical therapy, and the implants were removed. At surgery, the elastomer shells were intact. The capsular tissue was routinely processed with xylene as a dehydrating agent. During hematoxylin and eosin staining, xylene was again used as a clearing agent. Microscopic examination of the capsules revealed numerous intracellular vacuoles of refractile, water clear, foreign material (arrows). The identity of this material was confirmed to be silicone using microscopically guided Fourier transform infrared spectroscopy. Since the elastomer shell was intact, the origin of the silicone is presumed to be gel bleed. Hematoxylin and eosin at 200X.

ADDITION TO VINYL GROUPS

As shown in Figure 5, the small amount of vinyl groups which are present in gel bleed can react with other components having them add to the vinyl groups. This reaction is the basis for the platinum cross-linking reaction, leading to the gel originally. However, other functional groups are known to add to vinyl substituants in various organic molecules and such behavior would also be expected here. Almost no information on this reaction has been found in the literature.

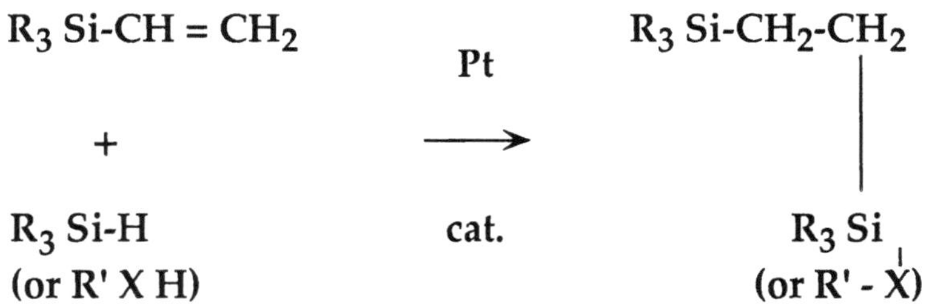

Figure 5: Addition: forms conjugates/crosslinks.

CONCLUSION

These various results suggest that at the surface of PDMS droplets, hydrolysis and oxidative changes take place, leading to a surface which is a cross-linked silanol containing composition. This composition would not be unlike that of silica which had been hydrolyzed to a form which would have a significant biological effect. The interior of such droplets may be largely normal PDMS at this point, depending on their size. If this mechanism is true, then methods which would address silicosis may also function, to some extent, to ameliorate other silicone induced diseases. One method proven to be successful with silicosis is treatment with polyvinylpyridine-N-oxide. The N-oxide group is believed to complex selectively with the silanol groups and block them from interacting in an adverse way with cell membranes (Shi, et al., 1989).

ACKNOWLEDGEMENT

We acknowledge the Society of Plastic Surgeons Educational Foundation for partial support of this project.

* Chris Batich has worked with attorneys representing women in suits against some manufacturers.

REFERENCES

Barton, T. and P. Boudjouk, "Organosilicon Chemistry," Ch. 1 in Silicone-Based Polymer Science, Amer. Chem. Soc. (1990), ed. J. Zeigler and F. Fearon.

Bergman, R., A. van der Ende, "Exudation of Silicone Through the Envelope of Gel-Filled Prostheses: An In Vitro Study," Brit J. Plast. Surg., 32:31-34, 1979.

Brody, G., "Fact and Fiction About Breast Implant 'Bleed,'" (Editorial), Plast. Reconstr. Surg. 30:615-616, 1977.

Haggard, W., J. Lemons, J. Mays, C. Prince, "Investigation of Cellular Responses to the Components of Silicone Gel Sheeting," Abstract Society For Biomaterials Proceedings, 280, 1993.

Hiemenz, P., "Principles of Colloid and Surface Chemistry," 2nd ed. (1986), Marcel Dekker, New York, NY, p. 7.

Kingery, W., H. Bowen, D. Uhlmann, Introduction to Ceramics, 2nd ed., John Wiley & Sons, 1976.

LeVier, R., et al., "What is Silicone?" Plast. Recon. Surg. 92, 163-167 (1993).

Martellock, A., "The Hydrolytic Degradation of Silicone Polymers," Elastoplastics Technology Conf., March 24, 1966.

Mathews, C. and K. van Holde, Biochemistry, Benjamin/Cummings Pub., Redwood City, CA (1990), p. 287.

McCoy, S., "Factors Affecting the Integrity and Stability of Q7-2159A Mammary Gel and Intermediates," Dow-Corning Quality Assurance Report, April 1, 1987.

Naim, J., et al., "The Adjuvant Effect of Silicone-Gel on Antibody Formation in Rats," Immun. Invest., 22, 151-161 (1993).

Osthoff, R., et al., "Chemical Stress Relaxation of PDMS Elastomers," J. Amer. Chem. Soc., 76, 4659 (1954).

Razzaboni, B. and P. Bolsaitis, "Evidence of an Oxidative Mechanism for the Hemolytic Activity of Silica Particles," Environ. Health Persp. 87, 337-341 (1990).

Ritter, J., Crack Propagation in Ceramics in Engineered Materials Handbook, Vol. 4, Ceramics and Glasses, ASM International, 1991.

Saam, J., "Formation of Linear Siloxane Polymers," Chapter 3 in Silicone-Based Polymer Science, Amer. Chem. Soc. (1990), ed. J. Zeigler and F. Fearon.

Shi, X., et al., "The Chemical Properties of Silica Particle Surface in Relation to Silica-Cell Interactions," J. Tox. Env. Health, 27, 435-454 (1989).

Towns, J. and F. Regnier, J. Chromotog. 516, 69-78 (1990).

Varaprath, S., memo to R. LeVier, "Composition Analysis of Mammary Gel Bleed," Internal Dow-Corning Wright Study, June 19, 1991.

Vondracek, P. and A. Gent, "Slow Decomposition of Silicone Rubber," J. Appl. Polym. Sci., 27, 4517-4523 (1982).

Yu, L., G. LaTorre, J. Marotta, C. Batich, N. Hardt, "In Vitro Measurement of Silicone Bleed from Breast Implants," Submitted for Publication, Plastic and Reconstructive Surgery.

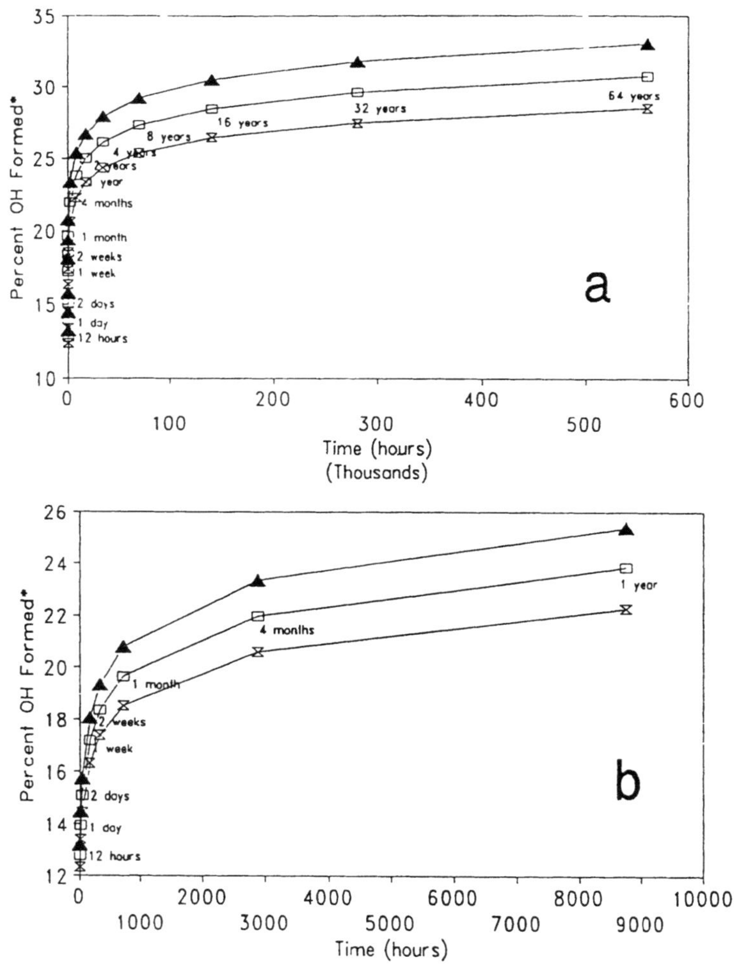

Addendum: Figure from DePalma (1992) showing general increase in hydrophilicity with time at 37°C extrapolated from calculated measurements at higher temperatures.

Chemical, Physical and Mechanical Analysis of Explanted Breast Implants

C. J. Wolf, H. J. Brandon, V. L. Young, K. L. Jerina, and A. P. Srivastava
Washington University, St. Louis, MO 63130

Introduction

The slow degradation or deterioration of a material due to the long-term effects of the environment are usually referred to as aging. Aging is an extremely complex process which may represent a myriad of physical and/or chemical processes. In polymeric materials the physical processes accompanying aging range from loss of additives, such as plasticizers or anti-oxidants to swelling by liquids. Chemical aging includes diverse phenomenon such as cross-linking, depolymerization, or reaction with environmental species, such as oxygen, to produce new or different compounds. The aging of silicones is of great interest, particularly with respect to changes which may occur in body implants during long-term implantation.

We report preliminary results on the chemical and mechanical analysis of explanted silicone gel filled implants which had been implanted for time periods ranging from zero to 21 years. All the mechanical measurements were conducted using standard ASTM approved procedures where possible and the primary physical chemical analysis method utilized matrix assisted laser desorption ionization (MALDI) mass spectrometry to analyze both extracted gels and the silicone rubber casing or shell. MALDI is a recent mass spectrometric development, specifically designed to analyze high molecular weight materials such as polymers.

The implant is a two part system, composed of a gel and a casing or shell. The shell is a cross-linked silicone rubber containing amorphous (fused) silica. The silica is added to enhance the mechanical properties, primarily tensile strength and tear resistance, of the rubber. The silica is usually treated with a surface active agent to promote coupling between the silica and the silicone polymer.

Long-term environmental aging of a silicone rubber may lead to any one of several deleterious effects:

1) degradation of the base polymer to a lower average molecular weight material,

2) degradation leading to the production of cyclic compounds, such as octamethylcyclotetrasiloxane (also known as D_4),

3) additional cross-linking to embrittle the rubber,

* This study was partially funded by a grant from the Plastic Surgery Educational Foundation.

4) degradation or weakening of the overall bonding between the silicone polymer and the silica reinforcing agent, and/or

5) swelling of the silicone shell by the low molecular weight components of the gel it encapsulates.

In several instances the shell surrounding the gel was not found during explantation. This suggests a strong interaction between the liquid gel and the shell which may lead to destruction of the cross-linking of the silicone rubber. The uncross-linked shell is then readily assimilated into the gel.

Experimental Procedures

Chemistry (Shell): Approximately 300 mg sections of a shell were cut into small pieces, of the order of 1 x 1 mm, and extracted with chloroform (Chromatographic grade) for 72 hours at 40°C in a Soxhlet extractor. The extract was concentrated by gentle evaporation of the solvent to a total volume of approximately 3 ml. A small aliquot of the extract was placed directly on the MALDI matrix (2,5 dinitrobenzoic acid) and analyzed after the solvent was removed.

Chemistry (Gel): Approximately 300 mg of gel were dissolved in 10 ml chloroform and analyzed by MALDI mass spectrometry.

MALDI: MALDI is a recent development specifically designed to utilize the tremendous analytical capability of mass spectrometry for the analysis of high molecular weight compounds [1,2,3]. The MALDI mass spectrometer used in these studies was a Per Septive Biosystems Voyager RP with a nominal resolving power of approximately 300. A few picograms of a polymer extract is placed on an inert matrix, 2,5 dinitrobenzoic acid, dried, and ionized with a N_2-laser (338 nm). The radiation is absorbed by the matrix and "transferred" to the polymer and little or no fragmentation of the molecular ions occurs. However, the ionized species normally observed in MALDI is the sodium adducts of the parent molecule. In dimethyl silicones, the de-methylated ion is quite stable and an ion corresponding to the replacement of a methyl group by sodium is usually observed. In many instances another ion is observed, corresponding to the replacement of a hydrogen by sodium. The resulting spectrum is relatively simple and a molecular ion peak corresponding to each molecule of the polymer distribution is observed [3]. The peaks of a given series are separated by 74 mass units, corresponding to the repeat unit of the polydimethyl siloxane polymer, $-(CH_3)_2SiO-$ and the remainder method is used to determine molecular structure. The "Remainder" procedure is described in the Appendix.

One of the primary objectives of the chemical analyses discussed in this paper is to compliment a series of biomechanical analyses. These analyses are being conducted on breast implants of various types and manufacturers explanted following durations of implantation ranging from one month to more than 20 years. The analyses consist of mechanical tests, microscopic examinations, and physical measurements for explanted clinically used breast implants. Experimental data are being correlated with implantation time to ascertain the degree of structural change due to exposure of breast implants to the physiological environment of the human body. All the mechanical property data presented in this particular paper were obtained from the same type of silicone gel implants with smooth shells produced by the same manufacturer.

ASTM testing procedures are utilized wherever possible. Extreme care is taken to remove the gel from the implant shell. Each shell is cleaned of gel by light rubbing with isopropyl alcohol. Test samples were prepared from the cleaned shells. All specimen preparation and test procedures have been standardized so that data from all implants are obtained under identical conditions. Shell thickness distributions were measured prior to mechanical testing.

Results and Discussion

The detailed design and the specific construction for each of the silicone implants depends on the manufacturer as well as the time period for which they were made. In general they all consist of a cross-linked silicone rubber shell containing a lightly cross-linked silicone gel. The overall consistency of the gels vary considerably. We have arbitraryly classified the many gels we have at our disposal into five major categories, based on their rheology: they are summarized in Table 1. The distribution of gels is approximately 30, 30, 30, 7, 3% for Types I, II, III, IV, and V, respectively.

The chemical composition of the gels is quite different. The composition of Type I is far more complex than that of Type V. The MALDI spectra of gel Types I and V are shown in Fig. 1a and 1b, respectively. An expanded view of the mass range 1000 to 2000 for these two gels is shown in Fig. 2a and 2b. Note the simplicity of gel Type V indicating only the presence of dimethyl siloxane.

A summary of the "Remainder" analysis is given in Table 2. The general conclusions are as follows:

Type I: the spectra is complex and indicates the presence of at least five different series of silicone polymers. The primary polymers are methyl terminated, vinyl terminated, and high molecular weight cyclic (or a hydrogen terminated linear polydimethyl siloxanes).

Type III: at least four different series of polymers were observed, the primary polymer is a 60-mass terminated material. The identity of this series is not known at the current time. Two other minor series, a methyl terminated and a vinyl PDMS series are also present.

Type V: the spectrum from the Type V gel is quite simple: only a single polymer series consisting of dimethyl PDMS was observed. This is consistent with the observation that the material is a relatively non-viscous liquid.

Analysis of Shell: The MALDI remainder analysis from a typical shell, which had been implanted for 21 years, yielded a vinyl terminated polymer series, and two smaller series, one dimethyl terminated and the other methyl/hydrogen (silane) terminated. Another shell, prepared by the same manufacturer at a different time which had been implanted 15 years exhibited similar silicone polymers, but the primary series was composed of the high molecular weight cyclic compounds (or hydrogen terminated silanes), accompanied by a large amount of dimethyl silicone and a much smaller amount of vinyl terminated material.

Transport of Fluids in Silicone Shells: The transport of the low molecular weight cyclic silicone, octamethylcyclotetrasiloxane (also known as D_4), through a typical silicone rubber implant shell was determined from a weight gain curve. A thin rectangular strip, approximately 1 x 4 cm cut from an unfilled silicone shell, was immersed in D_4 at 22°C and the weight gain measured as a function of time. The data for two implants plotted in standard Fickian form, i.e., weight gain versus square-root time, is shown in Fig. 3. Solubility (S) corresponds to the equilibrium weight gain, i.e., 213 wt%, and the diffusion coefficient (D) was determined from the slope of the initial portion of the sorption curve, and is given by [4]:

$$D = \pi(slope)^2 \ell^2 / 16S^2$$

where ℓ is the thickness of the sample. The diffusion coefficient determined from this plot corresponds to 1.2 x 10^{-11} m^2/s. These two quantities, D and S can be used to estimate the transport of D_4 through a silicone membrane of known thickness provided that the concentration of the D_4 in the gel in contact with the membrane is known.

The cross-link density, i.e., the effective number of cross-links per unit volume, can be estimated from the swelling coefficient of a known penetrant. An unfilled piece of silicone shell, approximately 2 x 3 x 0.05 cm, was swollen in hexane at 22°C. The weight gain was 152 wt%; this corresponds to a volume fraction of 0.746 (the polymer volume fraction in the swollen polymer (υ_2) was 0.254).

According to the Flory-Rehner theory for polymer swelling [5], the cross-link density (υ_c) is given by:

$$\upsilon_c = \left[-\ln(1-\upsilon_p) + \upsilon_p + \chi\upsilon_p^2\right] / \left[V\left(\upsilon_p^{1/3} - \frac{1}{2}\upsilon_p\right)\right]$$

where χ is the solvent interaction parameter (χ = 0.48 for the hexane-polydimethyl siloxane system) and V is the molar volume for the swelling agent (for hexane V = 130 cm^3/mol). The average molecular weight between cross-links (M_c) is given by the reciprocal of υ_c,

$$M_c = \frac{\rho}{\upsilon_c}$$

where ρ is the density of the polymer. The tensile modulus (Young's)E, for the membrane can also be estimated by the relation:

$$E = 3RT\upsilon_c$$

where R is the universal gas constant and T is the temperature (K):

The values from the swelling measurements are:

$$\upsilon_c = 1.25x10^{-4} mol/cm^3$$

$$M_c = 1x10^4 Da$$

$$E = 0.93MPa(136\,psi)$$

Mechanical Studies (Shell): Typical thickness ranges are presented in Fig. 4 for five explanted implants and two control implants. Control implants are plotted at "0" years. We estimate that the controls were manufactured after 1979. The explanted implants had implantation times ranging from eight to twenty-one years. The year that each explanted implant was placed in the body is listed above the thickness range. The two controls had different volumes (500 cc and 340 cc) and shell thicknesses. The considerable variation in shell thickness for a given implant is indicated by the range bars associated with each implant.

The tensile strength, maximum elongation at break, breaking energy, and the tear resistance were also determined. Data for these parameters were measured using an Instron testing machine. The tensile strength data are shown in Fig. 5 for six implants as a function of the implantation time. Each data point in this figure represents the average of at least five tensile specimens. Some of the implants appear to exhibit little change in tensile strength, while others show an appreciable decrease. More data are needed before a definitive statement regarding the effect of implantation time on tensile strength can be formulated. The ultimate elongation of the samples appears to decrease with implantation time (see Fig. 6). It is important to note that the elongation at the time of implantation is not known because a limited number of controls have been tested. However, the observation that there is a decrease with time is consistent with the hypothesis that the rubber degrades with time. It is expected that extensive data will result in a better understanding of the effect of implantation time on elongation.

The breaking energy is the total area under the stress-strain curve up to the point of rupture. It represents the work required for rupture (see Fig. 7). Again, the breaking energy exhibits a decrease when plotted as a function of implantation time, but the breaking energy at the time of implantation is not known. The tear resistance, measured in a separate experiment, also decreased as a function of implantation time for all implants, as shown in Fig. 8. Unfortunately, tear strength was not measured for the shell implanted for 21 years.

Summary

The chemical and biomechanical properties of explanted implants whose time of implantation ranged from zero to 21 years were measured. The properties appear to decrease with time. However it is important to note that proper controls have yet to be tested. The consistency of the gel varied considerably with manufacturer and date of manufacture. The data will be correlated with control samples when they become available. The data are consistent with the hypothesis that in some instances, the gel does affect the cross-linking, i.e., strength, of the silicone rubber shell. At the present time only a limited number of samples have been tested in this on-going program. One of our major objectives, to determine the influence of the physiological environment of the human body on the durability of the silicone implant, has yet to be quantified.

Appendix

"Remainder" Analysis of Polymer Functionality

The spectrum is composed of several series of peaks (m/z), each component separated by the mass of the base polymer. For dimethylsiloxanes this corresponds to 74 mass units. However, the isotopic distribution of the elements must be considered; this is particularly important for silicon which has three stable isotopes a) (Si^{28} (92.2%), b) (Si^{29} (4.7%), c) (Si^{30} (3.1%). Since the resolving power of the MALDI time-of-flight mass spectrometer is approximately 300, the observed peak is actually a composite peak whose centroid can be estimated from the atomic masses. The measured peak mass is corrected for the isotope effect and the mass comprising the polymer molecule is determined. The remainder is indicative of the functionality, or terminal groups, on the polymer chain. In order to obtain a more accurate value, the "remainder" of a series of 8-10 mass peaks in the mass range 1000 to 2000 is averaged. A sample calculation is given below: a series of peaks shown in Fig. 1 are separated by 74 mass units, a typical peak has a measured mass of 1283.28 Da, the isotope correction yields a nominal mass peak of 1280.7 Da, which corresponds to a polymer chain containing 17 siloxane units and a "remainder mass" of 22.7 Da. The average "remainder mass" in the mass region 1200 to 2400 is 23.3 ± 0.5 Da: this ion is due to de-methylated siloxane sodium ion and corresponds to the 17th-mer of a polydimethyl siloxane polymer.

References

1. F Hillenkamp, M Karas, RC Beavis, and BT Chail, Matrix-assisted laser desorption/ionization mass spectrometry of biopolymers, Anal. Chem. 63 1193 (A) 1991.
2. M Karas, U Bahr, and U Giessmann, Matrix-assisted laser desorption ionization mass spectrometry, Mass Spectrum Reviews, 10, 335 (1992).
3. PO Davis and DE Kars, A Facile Sample Preparation for the Analysis of Synthetic Organic Polymers by Matrix-assisted Laser Desorption/Ionization, Org. Mass Spectrum (Lett), 28, 923 (1993).
4. J Crank in The Mathematics of Diffusion, 2nd Edition Clarendon Press, Oxford, England, 1979.
5. PJ Flory and J Rehner, Statistical Mechanics of Cross-Linked Polymer II Swelling, J. Chem Phys., 11, 521 (1943).

Table 1. Gel Classification

Type I	Extremely viscous, does not flow under the influence of gravity, but retains its shape
Type II	Very viscous, exhibits some flow under the action of gravity, but retains general shape even after months at ambient
Type III	Viscous liquid like, but does not completely conform to the shape of the containing vessel
Type IV	Milkish white, grease-like looking substance, exhibits little flow
Type V	Clear viscous liquid, conforms to the shape of the retaining vessel, has the appearance of a heavy oil

Table 2. Summary of MALDI Mass Spectrometry Analysis of Explanted Silicone Gels

Type	Mfg	Years Implanted	Peaks*	Comment
I	B	19	L 37.2 ± 0.3, L 23.3 ± 0. S 53.0 ± 0.6	ruptured
III	B	21	L 40.6 ± 0.6, L 26.4 ± 0.6, M 11.9 ± 0.7	intact
III	B	14	L 59.7 ± 1,4, S 27.0 ± 0.6	ruptured
IV	?	13	L 36.8 ± 0.3, S 22.6 ± 0.3	ruptured**
V	A	5	L 22.5 ± 0.7, S 36.6 ± 0.5	ruptured**

*Prefix letter: L, M, S indicate a large, medium, or small peak
Number corresponds to average of 6-8 separate peaks with the associated standard deviation (10-)
**No apparent shell

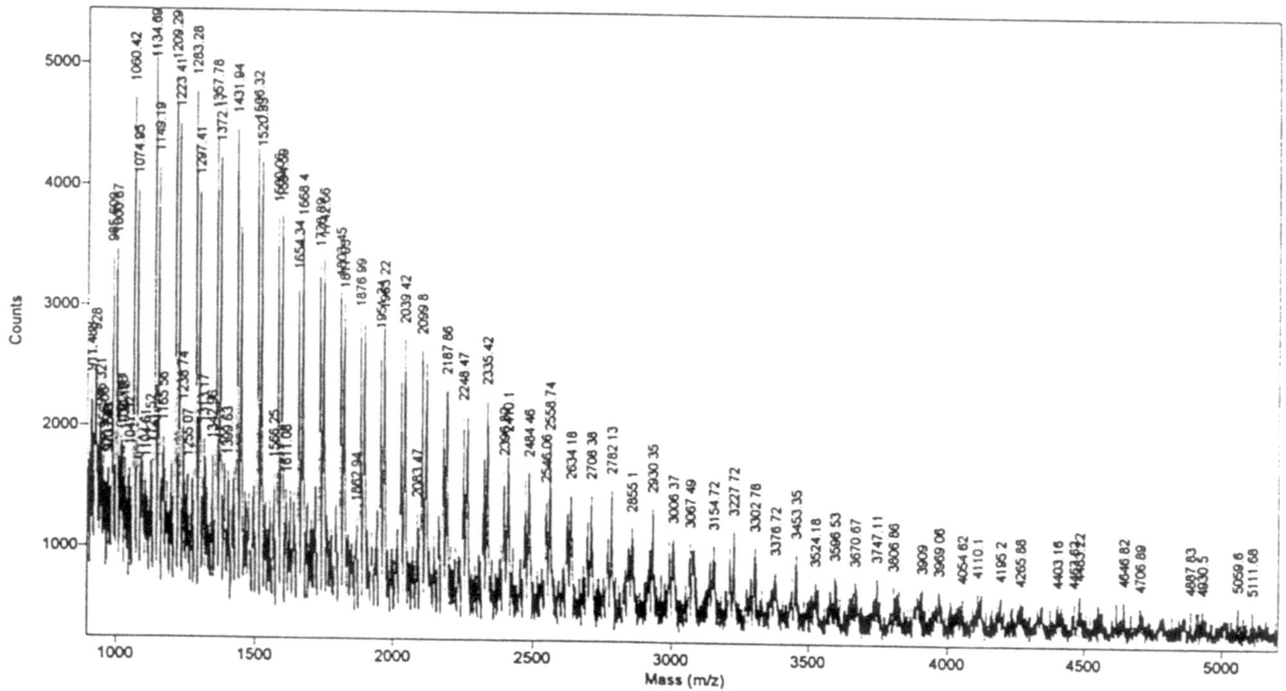

(a)

Fig. 1 MALDI mass spectrum of extracts of explanted silicone gels. The numbers above the peaks correspond to the mass of that particular polymer molecule. a) Type I gel implanted for 19 years.

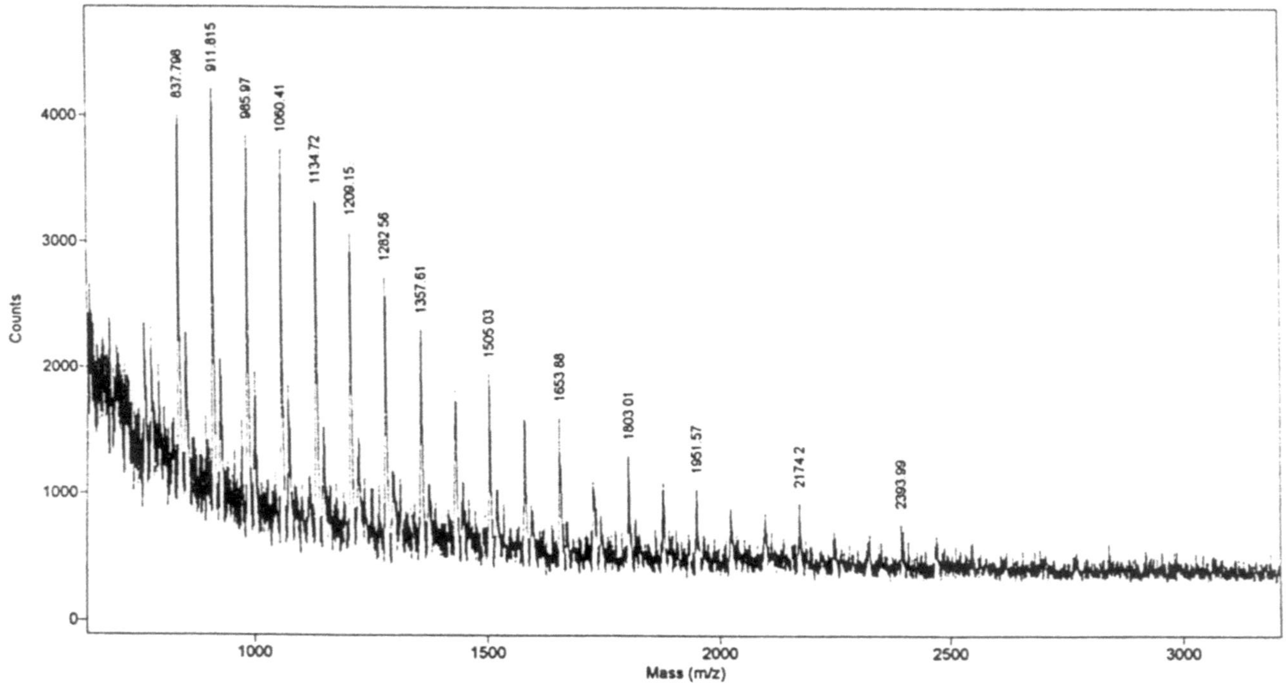

(b)

b) Type V gel implanted for 17 years.

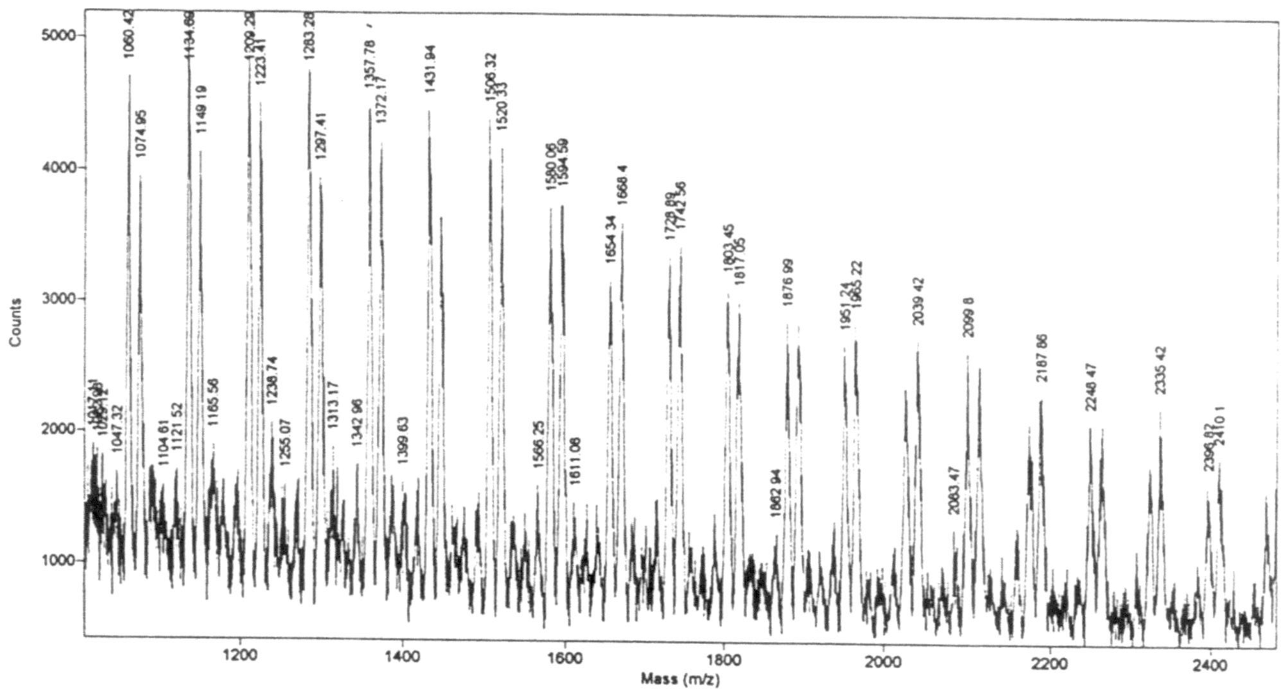

(a)

Figure 2 Expanded MALDI mass spectrum of samples shown in Figure 1. a) Type I gel.

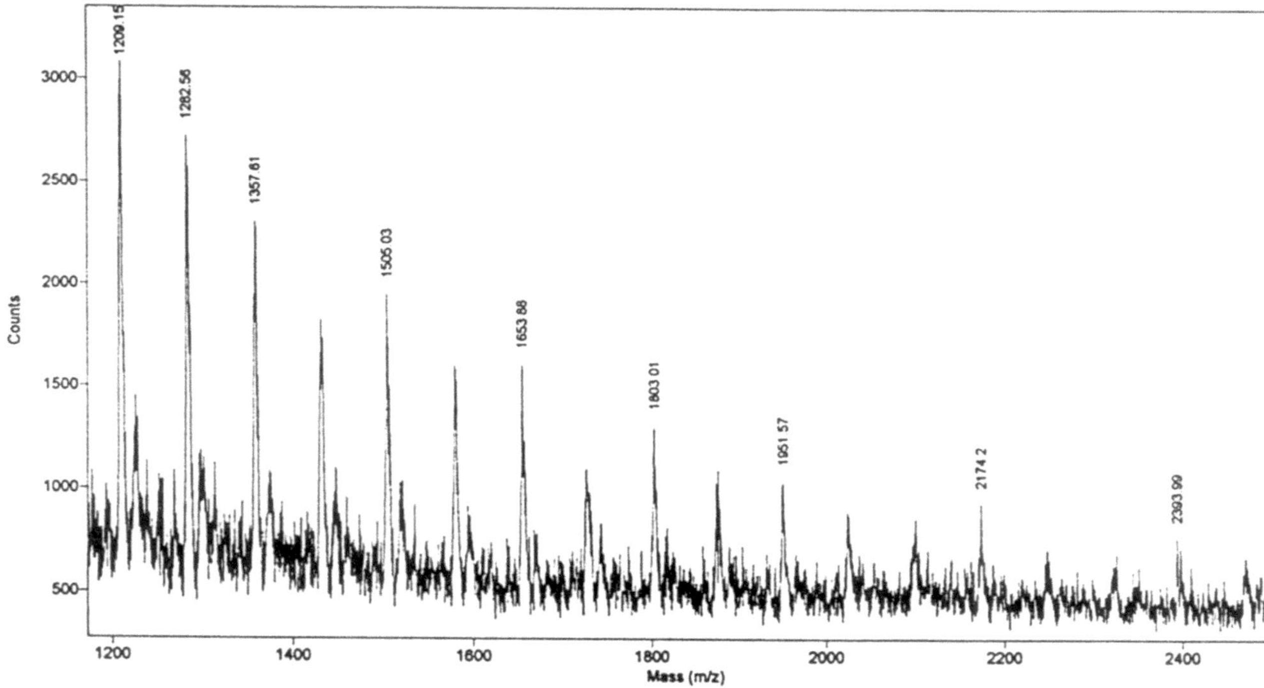
1209.15
1282.56
1357.61
1505.03
1653.88
1803.01
1951.57
2174.2
2393.99
Counts
3000
2500
2000
1500
1000
500
1200
1400
1600
1800
2000
2200
2400
Mass (m/z)

(b)

b) Type V gel.

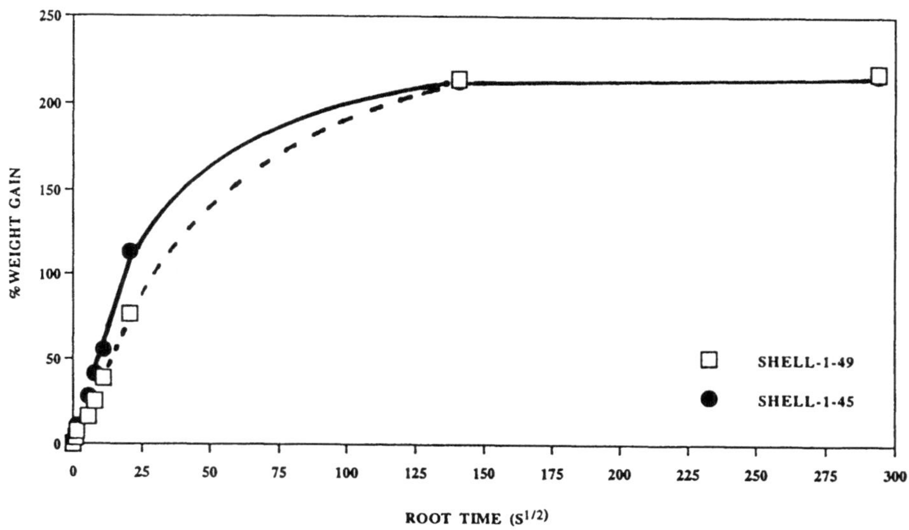

Figure 3 Typical Fickian diffusion plot showing the weight gain in a silicone rubber implant (control) as a function of square root time (seconds).

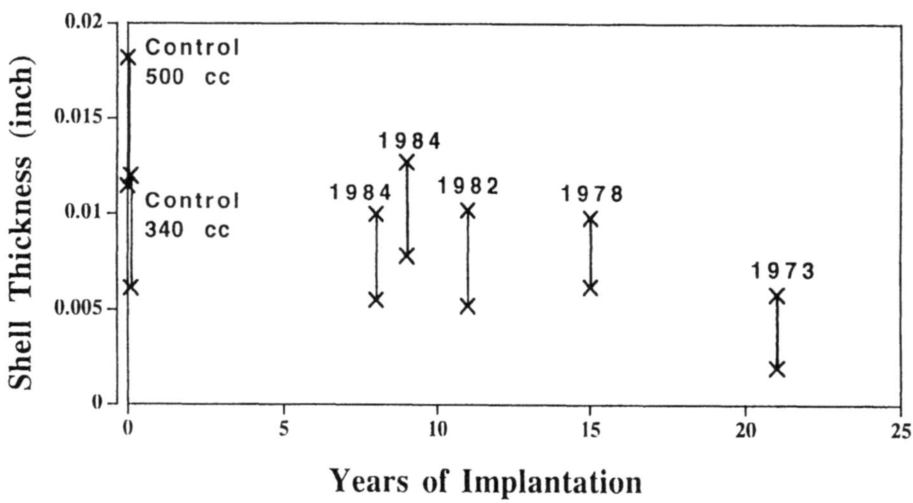

Fig. 4 Thickness (inch) of silicone shell breast implant.

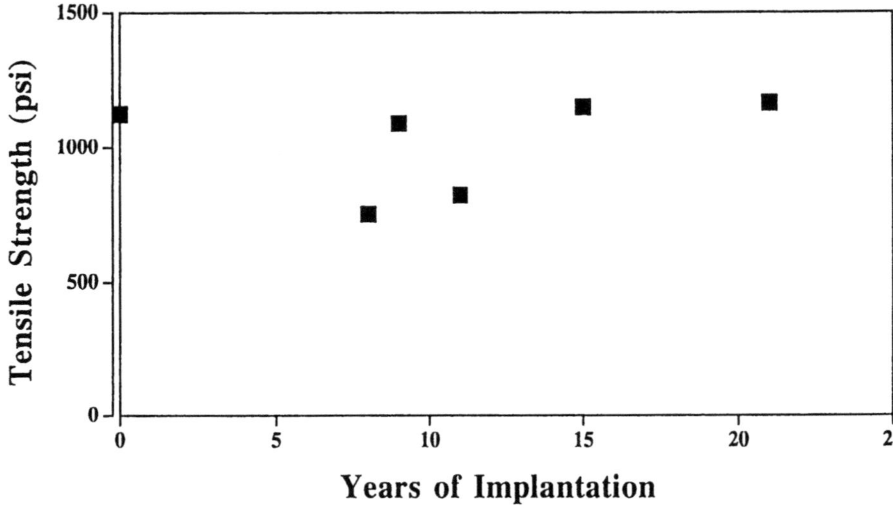

Fig. 5 Tensile strength (psi) of silicone shell breast implant.

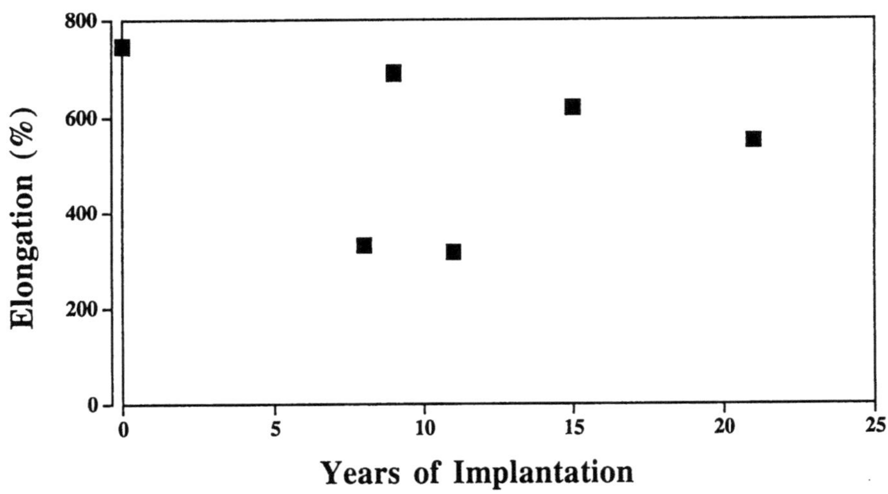

Fig. 6 Elongation ($\Delta l/l_o$) of silicone shell breast implant.

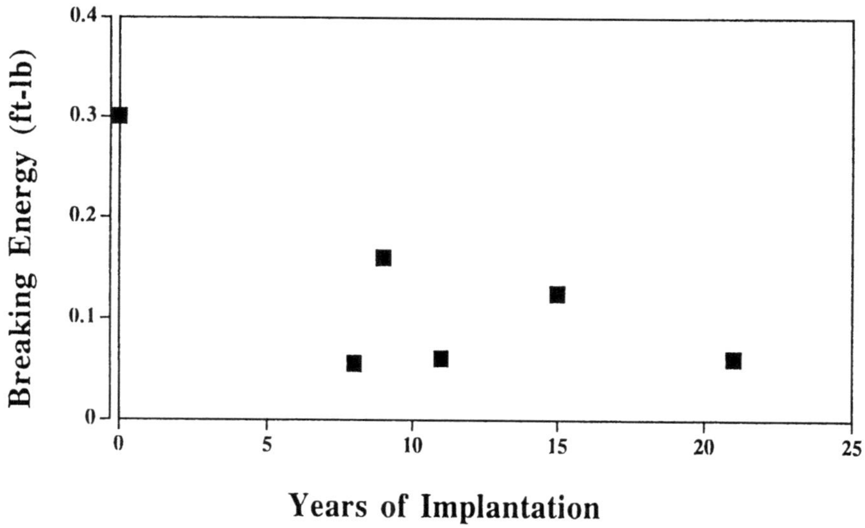

Fig. 7 Breaking energy (ft-lb) of silicone shell breast implant.

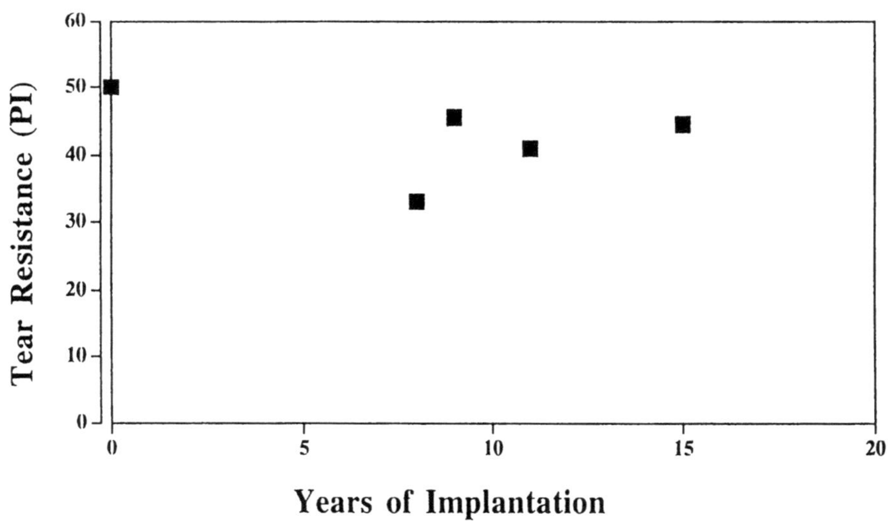

Fig. 8 Tear resistance (pounds/inch) of silicone shell breast implant.

Silicon and Silicone Levels in Patients with Silicone Implants

W. Peters, PhD, MD, FRCSC [1], D. Smith, PhD, DSc, FRCS [2], S. Lugowski, MSc [2], A. McHugh, BSc [2], P. MacDonald, MSc [2] and C. Baines, MD [3]

[1] From the Division of Plastic Surgery, Wellesley Hospital, [2] the Centre for Biomaterials, and [3] the Division of Preventive Medicine and Biostatistics, the University of Toronto, Toronto, Ontario, Canada

Address correspondence to Dr. Peters, Suite 418, Jones Bldg., Wellesley Hospital, 160 Wellesley St. East, Toronto, Ontario M4Y1J3, Canada
This research was funded by a Medical Research Council of Canada University Industry Grant and by Dow Corning

Summary

Although a potential link between silicone gel breast implants and autoimmune connective tissue disease has been suggested, none has been proven. The potential role of silicone as an immune adjuvant remains very controversial. Currently available techniques do not easily allow precise measurements of silicone in tissues. However, all compounds containing silicon (which would include silicone) can be measured accurately. The present study was designed to measure silicon levels in the fibrous capsules of patients with silicone-gel breast implants, saline breast implants and silicone inflatable penile prostheses. Baseline control silicon levels were obtained from the breast tissue of patients undergoing breast reduction, who had no exposure to breast implants. All silicon measurements were carried out using atomic absorption spectrometry with a graphite furnace.

The mean silicon levels in 16 breast tissue control samples from 8 patients undergoing breast reduction varied from 0.046 to 0.742 µg/g dry weight, with the median mean being 0.0927. The median silicon level in capsules from 6 patients with saline implants was 7.7 µg/g (range 36.6). The median silicon level in capsules from 5 patients with silicone inflatable penile prostheses was 19.5 µg/g (range 34.8). Although the levels of silicon in capsules of patients with saline breast prostheses and penile implants were higher than in control samples, they were much lower than those from the capsules of the 58 gel implants (median 9979 µg/g).

Of the 58 silicone gel breast implants (from 20 patients with bilateral implant removal and 18 patients with unilateral removal) which had been inserted from 1974 to 1990, 28 were intact, 8 had pinhole leaks, and 22 were ruptured. Median capsule silicon levels and ranges for all 58 implants, for intact only, for leaking, and for ruptured were: 9979 (152,000), 10,477 (88,703), 6592 (65,396), and 9922 (152,387) µg/g respectively. There were no significant differences in silicon levels associated with implant status, duration *in situ*, or year of implantation. Capsule contracture was not associated with higher levels of capsule silicon. Capsule silicon levels were about 10^6 times higher than previously assayed blood silicon levels. This may be because silicone released from implants remains localized in capsular tissue, or because blood-borne silicone is quickly excreted. Using ^{29}Si nuclear magnetic resonance spectroscopy, no detectable silicone was found in the blood of 7 control women and 7 women with silicone-gel implants (5 with known implant rupture).

Introduction

A silicone-gel breast implant consists of a rubber-like silicone (siloxane) elastomer envelope enclosing a volume of silicone-gel. The exact composition of the gel has been changed over the years, and it remains confidential proprietary information. However, based on testimony presented at the FDA hearing in 1992, the gel consists of a mixture of 76% low molecular weight (6,000-19,000) and 24% high molecular weight (300,000-400,000) components [1,2]. The envelope consists of a polydimethyl-siloxane elastomer, extensively cross-linked to form a network of extremely high molecular weight and contains amorphous silica as a reinforcing agent [1]. Solvent extraction of the envelope and the gel has revealed 30 different linear and cyclic components, some of which have adjuvant activity in animals [3].

Since 1978, it has been recognized that silicone can be expected to "bleed", by diffusion, from all clinically intact gel implants [4]. Laboratory studies have demonstrated that this phenomenon increases under load, and that primarily low molecular weight (6,000-10,000) components are involved [2]. These compounds would be expected to be capable of diffusing into surrounding tissues. Low molecular weight silicone compounds have been shown to be more soluble in body fluids, and to have greater biological activity than higher molecular weight compounds [1,2].

In 1986, "low-bleed" implants were introduced by Dow Corning [1]. The outer elastomer envelope of these implants was made thicker and more uniform than previously. The envelope was also coated on the inner surface with a fluorosilicone polymer [5], in which liquid silicone is only poorly soluble. These structural changes were reported to reduce the diffusion ("bleed") rate to about 10% of that formerly encountered [5]. Dow Corning has recently reported "bleed" rates of 60 to 100 mg per year for implants made before 1986, and 5-10 mg per year for implants made from 1986 onwards [6]. From 1986 onwards, other implant manufacturers also made changes to the structure of the elastomers of their implants, to increase their strength and to reduce their "bleed" properties [1].

In addition to the "bleed" phenomenon, silicone-gel implants can leak or rupture [7,8]. Studies by Peters and colleagues [7,8] and de Camara and co-workers [9] demonstrated a positive co-relation between the time since implantation and the number of leaking or ruptured implants, in prostheses inserted from 1975 to 1991. In the study by Peters and colleagues, only 23.2% of the implants which had been in place from 1971 to 1984 remained intact [7,8]. In the study by de Camara's group, all 22 implants inserted between 1975 and 1982 were leaking or ruptured [6].

Currently available techniques do not easily permit accurate measurements of silicone in tissues. However, all compounds containing the element silicon - which would include silicone - can be measured accurately. Modern techniques, such as atomic absorption spectrometry with a graphite furnace [10], direct current plasma emission spectrometry [11], and inductively coupled plasma emission spectroscopy [12] have allowed precise measurements of silicon in body fluids and tissues. Using these techniques, recent studies have shown normal plasma silicon levels of 140 ± 10 and normal serum levels of 170 ± 100, and 10-250 ng/ml [10, 11, 12]. In addition, Peters and colleagues (using atomic absorption spectrometry with a graphite furnace) [13] have recently shown that whole blood silicon levels in 30 patients with silicone-gel implants were significantly higher than those of age-matched control patients without implants (median 33.45 vs. 17.05 ng/ml P=0.005). In 1994, Evans and co-workers (using direct current plasma atomic emission spectroscopy) demonstrated measurable baseline silicon levels (varying from 0.2 to 45 μg/g tissue - wet weight) - in fat, nipple, breast tissue, liver, spleen, and axillary lymph nodes - in 9 of 10 cadaveric patients who had not received breast implants [14]. In contrast, 4 cadaveric patients who had received silicone breast implants had silicon levels in capsule and breast tissue, varying from 200 to 1600 μg/g tissue [14].

Materials and Methods

The objective of the present study was to assess the silicon levels, originating from silicone, in fibrous capsule specimens removed from a series of patients who had received silicone-gel breast implants. These values were then compared to capsule samples from other patients, who had received either saline breast implants or inflatable penile prostheses. Baseline control silicon tissue levels were determined in 16 breast tissue samples from 8 patients (with no exposure to breast implants) who had undergone breast reduction surgery.

From January 1990 to August 1994 over 600 patients with silicone-gel implants were clinically evaluated. These patients were either self-referred or physician-referred to a clinical plastic surgery practice. All patients sought further consultations regarding their implant status. During the study interval, 82 patients requested removal of their implants (150 implants). The most common reason for removal was capsular contracture with pain; other reasons included suspected rupture, "silicone phobia", and asymmetry [7].

All breast implants were removed by one surgeon (WP) usually through an inframammary approach. If gel implants appeared to be clinically intact, capsular specimens were excised and placed in silicone-free vials. If gel implants were leaking (with a sticky film of material on their surface) or ruptured, they were removed, and the capsular specimens were wiped repeatedly with dry gauze, until no further visible material was seen on their surface. Capsule specimens were then placed in silicone-free vials and frozen and stored at -70 °C until subsequent assay. Capsule specimens from patients with saline breast implants and penile prostheses were also placed in silicone-free vials and stored under identical conditions.

All reagents, plastic ware, equipment, and methods for preparations of plastic ware, blood collection, silicon analyses, and instrumentation have been described in previous communications from our laboratory [13, 15].

Analysis of Data

Because the data for capsule silicon levels were not normally distributed, they were analyzed with non-parametric tests using Kruskal-Wallis One-Way ANOVA on ranks (Sigmastat statistical software, Copyright © 1992-94, Jandel Scientific).

^{29}Si Nuclear Magnetic Resonance Studies

Duplicate blood samples from 7 control patients and 7 patients with silicone-gel implants (5 patients with known implant rupture) were assayed for silicone using ^{29}Si nuclear magnetic resonance (NMR) spectroscopy [29]. Blood samples were stored at 4 °C until use (within 5 days of collection). Volumes of 250 μL of blood were loaded into a standard Varian 7 mm internal diameter zirconium magic angle spinning (MAS) rotor and the ^{29}Si NMR spectrum was acquired under previously described conditions [29]. The acquisition parameters included slow spinning of the MAS rotor (~1000 Hz), a sweep width of 33,000 Hz digitized into 2048 data points at the ^{29}Si NMR frequency of 79.459 Mhz (i.e. a magnetic field strength of 9.40 Tesla = 400 Mhz for protons), a 3.5 μs radio-frequency pulse, a recycle delay of 10 s, and averaging together 8000 such scans to yield the so-called free induction decay.

Results

Capsule Silicon Studies

A total of 58 silicone gel breast implants, which had been inserted from 1974 to 1990, were removed from 38 women, during the period 1990 to 1994. All patients had received their implants for cosmetic breast enlargement reasons. None had any history of breast cancer. Implants from Heyer Schulte, Dow Corning, Surgitek, McGhan, and Cox Uphoff were represented in these 58 implants. Of the 58 gel implants, 28 were intact, 8 were leaking (pinhole), and 22 were ruptured (Table 1). Duplicate measurements of silicon levels were made from single samples of each capsule. The median silicon level for all 58 capsules was 9,979 μg/g (range 152,000). Table 1 shows the capsule silicon level according to implant status. The medians for these groups of implants were not significantly different (P=0.69). Thus, there was no significant difference between the silicon levels in the capsules from intact, leaking, and ruptured implants.

Table 1. Silicon levels (μg/g dry weight) in 58 capsules from silicone gel breast implants, as a function of implant integrity.

Implant Status	Number of Capsules	Mean	(SE)	Range	Median
Intact	28	19,079	(4399)	88,703	10,477
Leaking	8	15,051	(7847)	65,396	6,592
Ruptured	22	27,173	(8412)	152,387	9,922

Figure 1 shows the frequency distribution of capsular silicon levels according to implant status. The histogram supports the observation that silicon levels were not significantly influenced by implant status. Approximately 50% of capsules had silicon levels less than 10,000 μg/g. In this category, there were proportionately more ruptured (54%) and leaking (75%) implants than intact (43%) implants. In capsules with silicon levels in excess of 10,000 μg/g, there is no pattern associating implant status with silicon level. There was no significant relationship between capsule silicon levels and years of duration *in situ*.

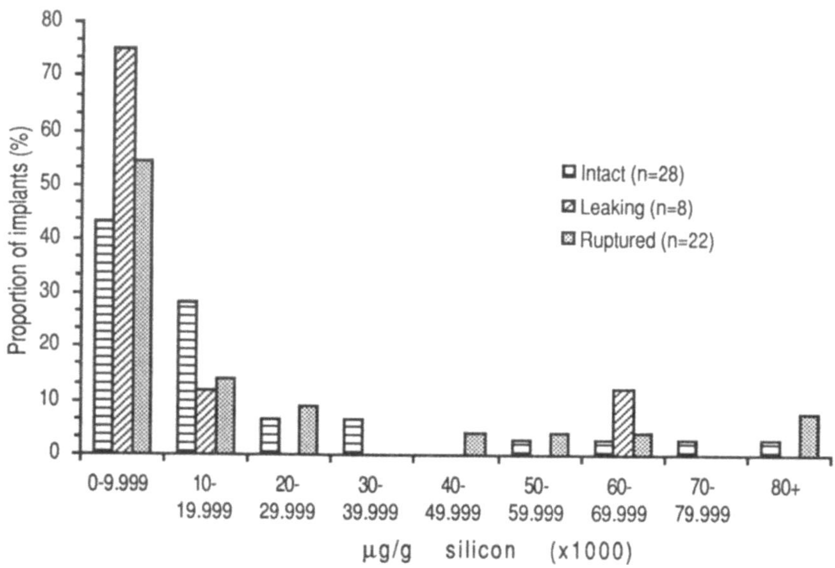

Fig. 1. Frequency distribution of silicon levels by implant status

Of the 38 patients in this study, 20 had bilateral implants removed and 18 had unilateral removal. After calculating the within-patient differences among women who had two implants removed, the median difference was 3900 μg/g and the range was 60,462. This range was strongly influenced by a single outlier of 60,642 which, if disregarded left a range of about 33,000.

In the patients with the 58 silicone-gel implants, there was no association between higher levels of silicon and capsule contracture. In 13 of these capsules, silicon levels were over 26,000 μg/g. However, in this group, 9 breasts demonstrated a Baker class I-II contracture, whereas 4 demonstrated a class III-IV contracture.

Table 2 shows the median silicon levels in capsules from 5 patients with inflatable penile prostheses (inserted for 1-14 years), and 6 patients with saline implants (inserted for 4-18 years). Breast tissue samples were removed bilaterally from 8 patients with no exposure to breast implants, who were undergoing reduction mammoplasty. Mean silicon levels in these patients ranged from 0.046 to 0.742 μg/g dry weight, with the median mean being 0.0927.

Table 2. Median silicon levels (µg/g dry weight) from capsules of saline implants and inflatable penile prostheses.

Source	Number	Median	Range
Capsules from inflatable penile prostheses	5	19.5	34.8
Capsules from saline breast implants	6	7.7	36.6

Blood ^{29}Si NMR Studies

Using ^{29}Si NMR spectroscopy, no detectable levels of silicone were found in 7 women with silicone-gel breast implants and 7 age-matched control patients without implant exposure. The implants had been inserted for a median of 13 years (range 13 years). Five of the 7 implant patients subsequently demonstrated implant rupture at explantation.

Discussion

Earlier chemical methods to determine silicon levels were frequently complicated by contamination from silica in environmental dust and silicone on glassware [16]. Phosphate in biological fluids also interfered with many early forms of analysis. More recently, several developments have facilitated much more accurate silicon analyses. The use of a dedicated, class 100, dust-free, meticulously clean facility minimized environmental contamination. The advent of laboratory plastic ware minimized silicone contamination. Special methods have been developed to decontaminate other laboratory ware. In addition, the development of modern methods of silicon analysis, such as atomic absorption spectroscopy and inductively coupled plasma atomic emission spectroscopy have provided very sensitive and accurate methods of measuring silicon levels [10-12].

Silicon is a naturally-occurring essential trace element which, in the last decade, has been recognized to participate in the normal metabolism of higher animals and to perform an important function in connective tissue, especially in bone and cartilage [16,17]. Silicon is found in the brain, liver, lung, kidney, bone, blood and urine and the sweat of humans [18]. Analysis of such tissues would therefore be expected to yield measurable silicon levels even in the absence of silicone implants. Data are lacking, however, to demonstrate the "normal" range of values that would be expected in such tissues and the effects of factors such as environment and diet. In the present experiments, dried tissue samples were extracted with n-heptane and centrifuged. The data thus represent extractable silicon probably in the form of silicone and colloidal material and not total silicon in the original sample.

This study provides several surprising findings. First, there was no significant difference among the median values of silicon levels in capsules from intact, leaking, and ruptured implants. This finding may reflect the fact that silicone-gel is now known to consist typically of a mixture of 76% low molecular weight (6,000 - 9,000), and 24% high molecular weight (300,000 - 400,000) components [1,2]. The high levels of silicon in capsules of all implants may reflect the high proportion of low molecular weight components which could have diffused from these implants. In their study of 8 capsules from patients with gel implants, Evans and colleagues also found higher levels of silicon in the capsules of intact implants than ruptured implants [14].

Another surprising finding was that the distribution of capsule silicon levels was not related to the years of duration of the gel implants *in situ*. In intact implants, this may again be explained by the high proportion of low molecular weight gel components, which may have diffused across the elastomeric shell, soon after implantation. In the ruptured and leaking implants, the time of implant failure after implantation is usually not ascertainable. Also unknown is the rate of silicone clearance from the body. From 1986 to 1990, many gel implants were constructed with a "barrier" layer to reduce silicone "bleed" through the elastomeric shell of gel implants [1]. In this study all implants inserted from 1986 onwards were inserted by the same surgeon (WP) and were Surgitek SCL "low bleed" implants. In the present study, capsule silicon levels were unrelated to calendar year of implantation, suggesting either that the layer was not effective or that, if it was, other variables were responsible for overcoming the protective effect.

Within-patient differences in the 20 patients who had bilateral implant removal demonstrated a large range (median difference 3900 µg/g, range 60,462). Many factors could contribute to these differences. Original pairs of implants may have been heterogeneous. One implant may have been traumatized more than the other during insertion. One implant may have been traumatized more than another during its *in situ* lifespan from: closed capsulotomy, activities of daily living, athletic activities, or accidents. In addition, single measurements of capsule silicon may have been unrepresentative of levels elsewhere in the capsule.

The silicon levels in the capsules reported in the present study were higher than those of the study of Evans and co-workers [14]: median silicon levels of 9,979 µg/g (range 152,000) vs. about 500 µg/g (range 1600). These differences may be explained by the different method of silicon assay (atomic absorption spectrometry with a graphite furnace vs. direct current plasma atomic emission spectroscopy), different tissue status (dry weight vs. wet weight), and differences in sample size.

Although saline breast implants have been shown to shed silicone particles from the elastomeric envelope [19] and others have suggested that silica could be released from the elastomer [20], our results clearly demonstrate that silicon levels in capsules around saline implants were elevated to a much lesser degree than those of gel implants. The mean silicon levels in the 16 control breasts without implant exposure varied from 0.046 to 0.742 µg/g, with a median mean being 0.0927. The median silicon levels in capsules from saline breast implants and penile prostheses were 7.7 µg/g (range 36.6) and 19.5 µg/g range 34.8 respectively. The median capsule silicon level for all 58 gel implants was 9979 µg/g (range 152,000). Genito-urinary silicone prostheses have also been found [21] to shed particles into the local tissue. These observations together with possible diffusion of leachable material may account for the significant silicon levels observed for the penile prostheses and the saline-filled breast implants in contrast to the low levels found for the normal breast tissue samples.

In their studies of the immunological activity of the components of silicone gel breast implants, Naim and co-workers [3,22] showed that the gel was a very potent humoral adjuvant, capable of inducing the production of autoantibodies in rats. The solid silicone elastomer had only minimal adjuvant properties. The fact that the gel promotes immunological activity in rats, however, does not necessarily mean that it would have similar activity in humans [23].

Peters and colleagues [13] have previously shown that the whole blood silicon levels in 30 patients with silicone gel breast implants were significantly higher than those of controls (median 33.45 vs. 17.05 ng/ml, P=0.005). There were no significant differences between patients who received their implants between 1973-1985 ("high bleed") and those who received implants between 1986-1991 ("low bleed"). In the present study, the median capsule silicon levels with gel implants was 9979 μg/g. Capsule silicon levels were about 10^6 times higher than blood silicon levels. This may be because silicone released from implants remains localized in capsular tissue, or because blood-borne silicone is quickly excreted.

Little is known about the metabolism or excretion of silicon or silicone from the body. Certain foods and beverages (notably vegetables, grain, rice, and beer) have been shown to contain significant levels of silicon [16,24]. There is geographical variation in the silicon content of tap water. Studies from Great Britain have shown that the concentration of soluble silicon was higher in the hard water of nongranite areas than in soft-water areas where granite rocks were widespread [16,25]. In certain areas of Yugoslavia, Bulgaria, and Romania, the high silicon content of local drinking water has been linked to a form of chronic interstitial nephritis known as Balkan nephropathy [26]. This disorder progresses slowly but inevitably to renal failure.

Urine silicon levels exceed serum levels by 20 to 100 fold and have ranged from 1.8 to 51.6 mg/l [11, 27]. These differences appear to reflect different dietary (particularly vegetable) intakes of silicon. Urine silicon assays are, therefore, thought to be useful only in metabolic studies in which the diet is well controlled.

Silicates, which are constituents of certain analgesics, antacids, and prepared foods, appear to be excreted in the urine within 24 hours of injection [16]. Adults who were given a 5 g dose of magnesium trisilicate (a silicate antacid) demonstrated a three-fold increase in serum and urine silicon levels 1-2 hours after injection. Serum and urine levels in these patients subsequently returned to normal within 24 hours. Similarly, silicon from beer ingestion is rapidly excreted in urine [28]. Beer is rich in silicon and contains about 300 μmoles per pint. It is derived from hot mashing techniques, which extract orthosilic acid from the phytolythic silica in barley. When 6 male volunteers were given 2 pints of beer each, plasma silicon was markedly increased one hour later, and the profile of urinary silicon concentration showed a marked rise in the subsequent 8-hour collection (from a mean of 190 μmol to a mean of 485 μmol per 8 hr urine fraction). Within 8 hours of ingestion, a mean value of 56% of the injested silicon had been excreted in the urine. Silicone released from gel implants may also be rapidly excreted in the urine.

The 1994 study by Garrido and co-workers [29] used ^{29}Si NMR spectroscopy to assess the level of silicon compounds in six patients with breast implants versus three control patients without implants. There were no measurable levels of silicon compounds in the control patients. However, all six implants patients had measurable amounts of serum silicon compounds, which were identified as unchanged silicone, hydrolyzed silicone, silica gel, and highly coordinated silicon. These results suggested that silicone may be altered *in vivo* and may appear in multiple forms. The levels of silicon compounds were much higher than those of previous studies and those of the current study.

In the present ^{29}Si NMR spectroscopy study, no detectable levels of silicone (or any other chemical form of silicon) were found in the blood of 7 control patients and 7 patients with silicone-gel implants (5 of whom subsequently demonstrated implant rupture at explantation). This is consistent with the low levels of total silicon compounds (which would include silicone) which we have previously demonstrated in the blood of 30 patients with silicone-gel implants. Subsequent investigations in our laboratory have demonstrated a sensitivity limit for the ^{29}Si NMR detection of silicon compared to be 10^4 higher than that of atomic absorption spectroscopy with a graphite furnace.

Conclusion

The median level of silicon in 58 capsules from patients with silicone-gel breast implants was approximately 10,000 times greater than that of control breast tissue. The immunological significance of this elevated silicon level is not known. The potential role of silicone as an immune adjuvant remains very controversial. Although a potential link between silicone-gel breast implants and autoimmune connective tissue diseases has been suggested, none has been proven. This study demonstrates that levels of capsular silicon in women with silicone-gel breast implants are not associated with implant status. Further, it demonstrates that, although capsular silicon from saline breast and inflatable penile silicone implants is higher than that of control tissue, it is negligible compared to gel implants.

References

1. FDA Hearing: General and Plastic Surgery Devices Panel Meeting (1992) Transcript Vol I: 1-459, Vol II: 1-560, Vol III: 1-362.
2. Callahan T(1992) Tensile strength and liquid silicone bleed in FDA General Plastic Surgery Devices Panel Meeting. Transcript Vol I: 73-84.
3. Naim JO, Lanzafame RJ, van Oss CJ (1993) The adjuvant effect of silicone-gel on antibody formation in rats. Immunol Invest 22:151-161.
4. Barker DE, Retsky MI, Schultz S (1978) "Bleeding" of silicone from bag-gel breast implants and its clinical relation to fibrous capsule reaction. Plast Reconstr Surg 61:836-841.
5. LeVier RR. (1992) Dow Corning presentation in FDA General Plastic Surgery Devices Panel Meeting Transcript Vol II: 31-49, 142, 219.
6. Baines CJ, Arseneau J, Smith DC. (1992) Summary of the report on silicone gel-filled breast implants Can Med Assoc J 147:1141-1146.
7. Peters WJ, Keystone E, Smith DC (1994) Factors affecting the rupture of silicone gel breast implants. Ann Plast Surg 32:449-451.
8. Peters WJ (1994) The rupture of silicone gel breast implants. Ann Plast Surg 33:462-463.
9. de Camara DL, Sheridan JM, Kammer BA (1993) Rupture and aging of silicone gel breast implants. Plast Reconstr Surg 91:829-834.
10. Gitelman HJ, Alderman FR (1990) Determination of silicon in biological samples using electrothermal atomic absorption spectrometry. J Anal At Spectrosc 5:587-589.
11. Roberts NB, Williams P (1990) Silicon measurement in serum and urine by direct current plasma emission spectrometry. Clin Chem 36:1460-1465.

12. Marco-Franco JE, Torres VE, Nixon DE, Wilson DM, James EM, Bergstralh EJ, McCarthy JT (1991) Oxalate, silicon and vanadium in acquired cystic kidney disease. Clin Nephrol 35:52-58.
13. Peters WJ, Smith DC, Lugowski S, McHugh A (1995) Do patients with silicone gel breast implants have elevated levels of serum silicon compared to control patients? Ann Plast Surg 34:343-347.
14. Evans GRD, Slezak S, Rieters M, Bercowy GM (1994) Silicon tissue assays in non-augmented cadaveric patients: is there a baseline level? Plast Reconstr Surg 93:1117-1122.
15. Peters WJ, Smith D, Lugowski S, McHugh A, Keresteci A, Baines C (1995) An analysis of silicon levels in capsules of gel and saline breast implants and of penile prostheses. Ann Plast Surg , in press.
16. Dobbie JW, Smith MJB. Urinary and serum silicon in normal and uremic individuals. In: Evered D, O'Connor M (1986) Silicon Biochemistry: Ciba Foundation Symposium 121. New York: Wiley 194-213.
17. Carlisle EM (1986) Silicon as an essential trace element in animal nutrition. In: Silicon Biochemistry. Ciba Foundation Symposium 121. Evered D, O'Connor M (ed). New York: John Wiley and Sons 123-129.
18. Hosokawa S, Yoshida O (1990) Trace elements and complications in patients undergoing chronic hemodialysis. Nephron 55: 375-379.
19. Vargas A (1979) A shedding of silicone particles from inflated breast implants. Plast Reconstr Surg 64: 252-253.
20. Heggers JP, Kossovsksy N, Parsons RW (1983) Biocompatibility of silicone implants. Ann Plast Surg 11:38-41.
21. Barrett DM, O'Sullivan D, Malizia AA (1991) Particle shedding and migration from silicone genito-urinary prosthetic devices. J Urolog 146: 319-322.
22. Naim JO, van Oss CJ, Lanzafame RJ (1993) The induction of autoantibodies to thyroglobulin in rats with silicone gel as adjuvant. Surg Forum 44: 676-678.
23. Rose NR. Invited comment (1992) Ann Plast Surg 28: 499-501.
24. LeVier RR, Harrison MC, Cook RR, Lane TH (1993) What is silicone? Plast Reconstr Surg 92:163-167.
25. Dobbie JW, Smith MJB (1982) The silicon content of body fluids. Scott Med J 27:17-19.
26. Marcovic BL, Abrambasic MD (1971) Experimental chronic interstitial nephritis compared with endemic human neuropathy. J Pathol 103:35-40.
27. Belliveau JF, Griffiths WC, Wright GC, Tucci JR (1991) A direct current plasma emission spectrometric procedure for the assay of silicon in urine. Ann Clin Lab Sci 21:328-334.
28. Bellia JP, Birchall JD, Roberts NB (1994) Beer: a dietary source of silicon. Lancet 343:235.
29. Garrido L, Pfleiderer B, Jenkins BG (1994) Migration and chemical modification of silicone in women with breast prostheses. Magn Reson Med 31:328-330.

Detection of Silicone Migration and Biodegradation with NMR[1]

L. Garrido, A. Bogdanova, L.L. Cheng, B. Pfleiderer,† E. Tokareva, J.L. Ackerman and T.J. Brady.
NMR Center, Department of Radiology, Massachusetts General Hospital and Harvard Medical School, Charlestown, MA, USA. †Present address: Institute of Clinical Radiology, Westfalian Wilhelms-University, Münster, FRG.

Introduction

Silicones, generic name of synthetic polymers with a backbone of SiO bonds and organic side groups (aliphatic and/or aromatic), are among the most widely used materials for biomedical purposes [1]. In particular, it is estimated that about 1.5 million silicone gel-filled breast prosthesis are presently implanted in the U.S. for the purpose of reconstruction and augmentation mammaplasty. Although silicones have been assumed to be stable, their benign nature has been questioned recently, and in April 1992 the Food and Drug Administration (FDA) severely restricted the use of silicone gel-filled prostheses for breast augmentation arguing that the risks have not been adequately defined [2].

The exposure of women with silicone gel-filled breast implants to silicone can occur in two ways: "bleed" through or rupture of an implant. Silicone gel-filled breast implants consist of an outer shell (200 to 300 μm thick) made of silicone rubber surrounding a silicone gel, a copolymer of dimethylsiloxane and vinylmethylsiloxane slightly crosslinked to form a three-dimensional structure. The crosslinking is achieved by the reaction of vinyl groups present in the copolymer chains [3,4] and the resulting gel is swollen with polydimethylsiloxane (PDMS) fluid to yield a sticky, cohesive mass without form [4]. Light-microscopy has demonstrated microscopic droplets beyond the implant capsule and the energy-dispersive X-ray analysis of the tissue samples showed a silicon peak [5]. Thus, implants bleed silicone with passage of free silicone or PDMS (removable fraction) through an intact envelope, presumably due to the permeability of the rubber to the components of the gel [4,6].

In addition, the silicone rubber shell of the implant may rupture exposing body tissues to the silicone gel. It is estimated that implants are ruptured in 4-6% of asymptomatic women [7]. A recent study of 51 implants found that the number of intact implants declines over time and all implants older than 10 years were leaking or ruptured [8]. The chemical composition of the extract may include not only linear polymer chains (PDMS), but also cyclic chains with different molecular weights and functionality present as impurities in PDMS and as a consequence of an incomplete crosslinking reaction [3].

The health consequences of exposure to the gel, or to silicone that passes through the envelope are unclear. Results of various studies have associated silicone implants with the development of connective tissue disease [9-14] while

[1]This work was supported by the MGH-NMR Center. No benefit of any kind is received either directly or indirectly by the authors.

others suggested that there is little or no relationship [15-17]. The most common complication of breast augmentation is periprosthetic capsular contraction. The periprosthetic breast capsule has been described by most investigators as a foreign body response involving macrophages and other types of cells [18,19].

Silicon of undetermined chemical form has been found in periprosthetic capsule and macrophages, as well as in the lymph nodes of patients with silicone gel-filled implants [5,20]. Because of the ubiquitous presence of silicone products in the environment and the lack of appropriate analytic techniques, researchers have been unable to accurately determine the presence of silicone. Analytical methods such as histopathology, energy dispersive X-ray elemental analysis and transmission electron microscopy, which have been used to study the side effects of silicone in living subjects, are not chemically specific. These techniques are unable to distinguish between silica, silicone, and silicone's various degrees of chemical functionality. Therefore, they can neither provide a direct measurement of the metabolic activity involving silicone, nor reveal alterations in the chemical nature of this complex polymeric material.

Nuclear magnetic resonance (NMR) is able to provide detailed information about a substance's chemical composition and molecular architecture, both reflected in the chemical shift spectrum, as well as about the molecular and polymer chain dynamics related to NMR parameters, such as the spin-lattice (T_1) and spin-spin (T_2) relaxation times. NMR is a standard characterization technique in polymer science for the study of the kinetics of polymerization, crosslinking, hydrolysis, degradation, etc.[21,22]. Thus, we have used a combination of *in vivo* ^{1}H NMR localized spectroscopy and *in vitro* ^{29}Si NMR spectroscopy to investigate the migration and chemical modification of silicones in animal models and humans. The results have shown that silicone migrates from the implant to local and distant sites [23-25], and degrades *in vivo* [26].

As mentioned above, macrophages are involved in the body's response to implanted silicone breast prostheses and, in particular, are involved in the transport of silicone to various tissues and organs. Thus, it is likely that biotransformation occurs in mononuclear cells (monocytes, macrophages, etc.) local to the implant or at distant sites (e.g. lymph nodes and liver). In this study we present the ^{29}Si NMR results of our investigations about the distribution of silicone metabolites in various compartments of blood samples from women with silicone gel-filled breast implants. The biodegradation of PDMS in the presence of macrophage-like cells is analyzed.

Experimental Details

Blood Samples

As part of a research protocol, informed consent was obtained and blood samples were collected from five volunteers without implants and 23 patients with silicone gel-filled breast implants. All blood samples were collected in heparinized tubes following exactly the same protocol. Blood components (e.g., lymphocytes/monocytes, plasma proteins, etc.) were separated using standard procedures. For example, the blood samples (~8 ml) were centrifuged at 2000 rpm for 15 min at 4 °C. The plasma then was collected by aspiration and fractionated according to molecular size by ultrafiltration. In particular, four fractions Cn were obtained by using membranes (Amicon) with molecular weight cutoffs at: C1>300,000 daltons; 300,000>C2>50,000; 50,000>C3>10,000; 10,000>C4. Each fraction was lyophilized and stored at 4 °C prior to analysis.

The cell fraction was washed three times with isotonic saline solution. The lymphocyte/monocyte cell fraction was separated from the other cells present in blood using Ficoll-Hypaque gradients [27]. The fraction was washed three times, then lyophilized and stored at 4 °C prior to analysis. The other cell fraction was washed and stored following the same procedures.

For the NMR measurements, plasma and cell fractions were resuspended in isotonic saline solution.

Cell Cultures

A macrophage-like J-774 cell line, kindly provided by Dr. Joel Swanson (Harvard Medical School, Boston, MA) was used to study the biodegradation of PDMS (the main extractable compound from silicone gel-filled implants) in an *in vitro* model system. To ensure homogeneous distribution of PDMS in the culture medium, water soluble complexes of PDMS with cyclodextrins were prepared by mixing 7.5 mg of PDMS, molecular weight of 16,000 g mol^{-1}, (Polysciences) with 1 ml of an aqueous solution of γ-cyclodextrin (Sigma) (10% w/v). The mixture was sonicated for 8 min. and placed in a shaker bath at moderate speed for 60 h at room temperature. J-774 cells (0.8 to 1 x 10^6) in DMEM culture medium with 10% FBS (Gibco), supplemented with sodium bicarbonate and antibiotics (mixture of penicillin/streptomycin) were plated in a T75 plastic cell culture flask, in duplicate, and incubated at 37 °C in a humidified atmosphere at 6% CO_2. After 24 hours, the culture medium was removed, and new culture medium containing 3.3 mg of PDMS was added to the flasks to a total volume of 4 ml. After three more days, 2.5 ml of fresh medium was added and the culture was stopped at the end of the eighth day. The cells were trypsinized and the whole sample (cells and medium) were lyophilized and prepared for NMR analysis. These experiments were repeated three times.

NMR Measurements

The measurements were performed at 9.4 T (^1H and ^{29}Si resonance frequencies of 400.13 and 79.48 MHz, respectively). The spectra were acquired at ambient temperature using a broad band magic angle spinning probe (Bruker Instruments, Inc., Billerica, MA) with a sample size of ~200 mg. The pulse sequence employed was a single read pulse (tip angle 45° or 80°) followed by acquisition at a recycle delay of 10 s. All free induction decays were subjected to Fourier transformation, 400 Hz exponential line broadening, and phasing. All chemical shifts were referenced externally to tetramethylsilane at 0 ppm. The areas of the individual peaks in the ^{29}Si spectra were determined using a Gaussian addition program (GLINFIT, Bruker Instruments). The areas were normalized to the number of averages and the weight of the samples. Quantitation was performed by comparison of spectral areas with a standard having a concentration of silicon of 44 mM.

Results and Discussion

Fig. 1 shows the ^{29}Si spectra corresponding to samples of whole blood from (A) a volunteer with no implant and (B) a patient with silicone implants for 17 years.

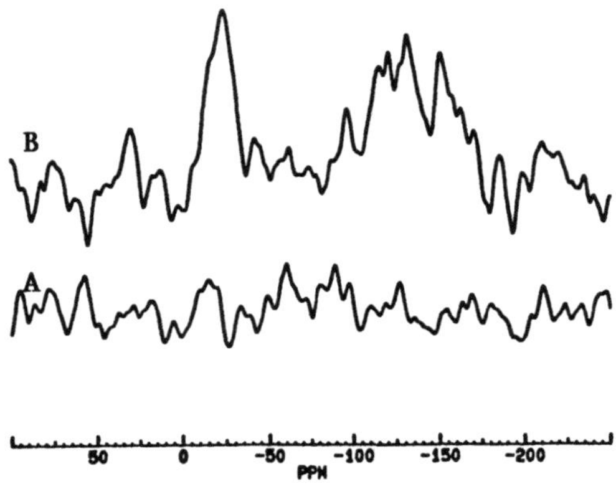

Fig. 1. ^{29}Si NMR spectra corresponding to blood samples from (A) a woman with no implants and (B) a woman with silicone gel-filled breast implants (17 years). These results are similar to those obtained in rodents [23,26], and are an indication of the chemical modification of silicones *in vivo*.

After 6,000 averages no ^{29}Si resonances (peaks) are observed in control spectrum A indicating that under our experimental conditions silicon compounds are not present in detectable amounts in non-implanted volunteers. Samples from five other controls gave similar negative results. Spectrum B (6,000 averages) shows several resonances from 0 to -160 ppm that can be attributed to various Si functional groups [23,26] present as a consequence of the biotransformation of silicone. The resonance at approximately -22 ppm in Fig. 1B corresponds to the resonance frequency of silicon bound to two oxygens and two methyl groups which is the structure of the repeat unit of PDMS (chemically unchanged silicone). The ^{29}Si NMR results further indicate that other silicon compounds, in addition to silicone, are also present. Possible reactions which could lead to the formation of other compounds are polymer chain scission with formation of terminal hydroxyl groups and the substitution of methyl groups by hydroxyl groups (see Fig. 2), which are consistent with the appearance of peaks at 0 to -20 ppm and -25 to -65 ppm, respectively. The initial oxidation will be followed by the formation of silicates and silica gel as indicated by the appearance of peaks at -70 to -115 ppm. The appearance of ^{29}Si resonances between -120 and -160 ppm can be explained by the presence of high coordinated oxygen-silicon complexes [23,26,28].

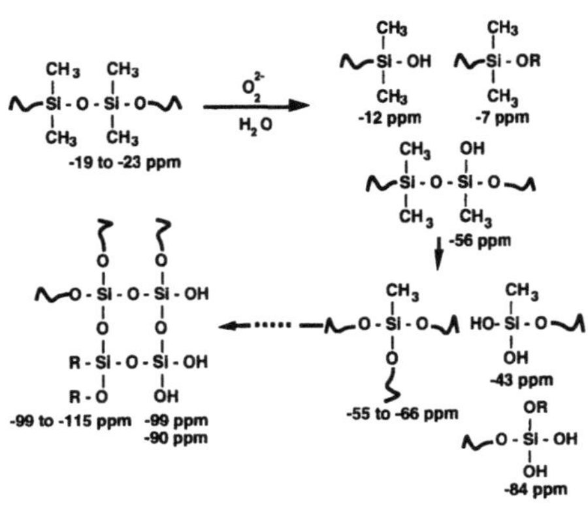

Fig. 2. Diagram showing a possible reaction path for the degradation of silicone to silica or silicate *in vivo*.

Table 1. ^{29}Si NMR chemical shifts of various Si functional groups.[a]

Functional Group	δ (ppm)
$- O_{0.5}Si(CH_3)_2(OR)$	-5
$- O_{0.5}Si(CH_3)_2(OH)$	-11
$- (O_{0.5})_2Si(CH_3)_2$	-22
$- O_{0.5}Si(CH_3)(OH)_2$	-42
$- (O_{0.5})_2Si(CH_3)(OH)$	-54
$- (O_{0.5})_3Si(CH_3)$	-60
$- (O_{0.5})_4Si^{2-}$(monosilicate)	-70 to -73.5
$- (O_{0.5})_2Si(OH)_2$	-91
$- (O_{0.5})_3Si(OH)$	-99
$- (O_{0.5})_4Si$	-99 to -115
$[- (O_{0.5})_4Si(CH_3)]^+$	-129[b]
$[- (O_{0.5})_4Si(CH = CH_2)]^+$	-141[b]

[a] ^{29}Si NMR chemical shifts from reference 28 and references cited therein.
[b] Pentacoordinated silicon

In addition, proteins and other biomolecules may form covalent bonds with silicone and its byproducts, generating unidentified peaks in the observed silicon spectrum. A summary of silicon functional groups with their corresponding chemical shifts is shown in Table 1. The physical association of silicone and silica with proteins and other macromolecules could cause broadening and small shifts (~0 to 5 ppm) of the NMR peaks observed. Similar results were obtained for all blood samples from 23 patients with implants as shown in Table 2 and Fig. 3.

Table 2. Total concentration of Si containing compounds in the blood of women with silicone breast implants measured by ^{29}Si NMR spectroscopy.

Implantation Time (years)	Implant status (Diagnosis by MRI)	Total [Si] (mM)
23	rupture	66
21	rupture	143
20	rupture	111
20	rupture	54
20	rupture	58
19	rupture	109
18	rupture	86
17	no rupture	112
17	no rupture	93
16	no rupture	67
14	rupture	43
14	rupture	53
14	rupture	104
14	no rupture	49
12	rupture	83
11	rupture	42
11	rupture	96
10	rupture	46
9	rupture	57
9	rupture	55
7	rupture	31
6	no rupture	70
5	not conclusive	48

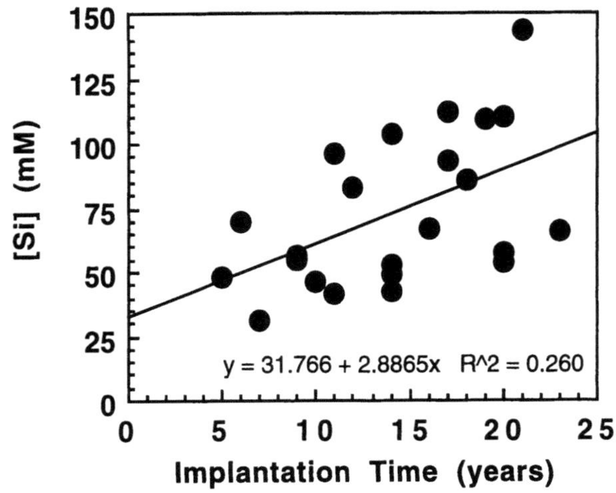

Fig. 3. Plot of the dependence of the total concentration of silicon containing compounds in whole blood on the implantation time. Essentially no correlation between [Si] and implantation time is found.

These NMR results confirm our preliminary findings which provided the first experimental evidence to support the hypothesis that silicone can degrade in humans [18,29]. PDMS has been shown to degrade under mild conditions of temperature and humidity in the laboratory [30] and in soil [31].

In this study, the concentrations of the silicon species detected in the blood of women with implants were found to vary substantially (a slight trend is observed in total [Si] in the blood which increases with increasing implantation time, see Fig. 3) and there was no correlation with the status of the implant. To interpret the data correctly, we must take into consideration the error associated with the NMR measurements (i.e., saturation of nuclei response due to their long T_1 and short recycle delay used) which will alter the NMR signal intensity, and other factors that can affect significantly the concentration of silicone in the blood. These factors include, the characteristics of the implant (i.e., manufacturer, type, size), the time of rupture, the presence of a fibrous tissue capsule around the implant, and individual metabolic activity. The chemical composition and physical properties of breast implants have changed significantly since they were first available for cosmetic and reconstructive surgery of the breast modulating the migration of silicone to the surrounding tissue and blood. Some examples of these changes in the gel are: the relative amount of crosslinked and free polymer, types of crosslinking agent and catalyst, degree of crosslinking, viscosity of the free polymer. Similarly, changes in the shell include: thickness, chemical treatment of silica filler to improve polymer-filler interaction and reduce migration of silica particles, presence of external and/or internal coatings to improve tissue adherence, reduce capsule formation, reduce permeability to free polymer.

In a recent study [32], using electrothermal atomic absorption spectrophotometry, the concentration of silicon in the blood of women with silicone gel-filled breast implants was found to be double that of women with no implants, and significantly lower than the silicon concentration measured in the present study. The difference between the values obtained using AA and ^{29}Si NMR techniques could be due to the fact that part or all the silicone and partially hydrolyzed silicone present in the blood, a consequence of the migration of silicone from the implants, may be lost during the preparation steps (i.e., drying and oxidation) and prior to detection by AA. The total concentration of silicon in blood measured in ref. 32 is 10 times lower than that of silicon present as soluble silicic acid in serum measured by direct current plasma emission spectrometry [33]. Teuber et al. [34] measured silicon levels in serum of women with silicone implants using inductively coupled plasma atomic emission spectroscopy and found concentrations on the order of 10 μM. The analysis of blood by NMR does not require any sample preparation and all silicon compounds present in blood are measured at the same time.

After determining the presence of silicon containing compounds in whole blood of women with silicone gel-filled implants, we investigated the distribution of silicone and its metabolites in several components of blood. The ^{29}Si NMR spectra of various blood compartments show significant differences as illustrated in Fig. 4.

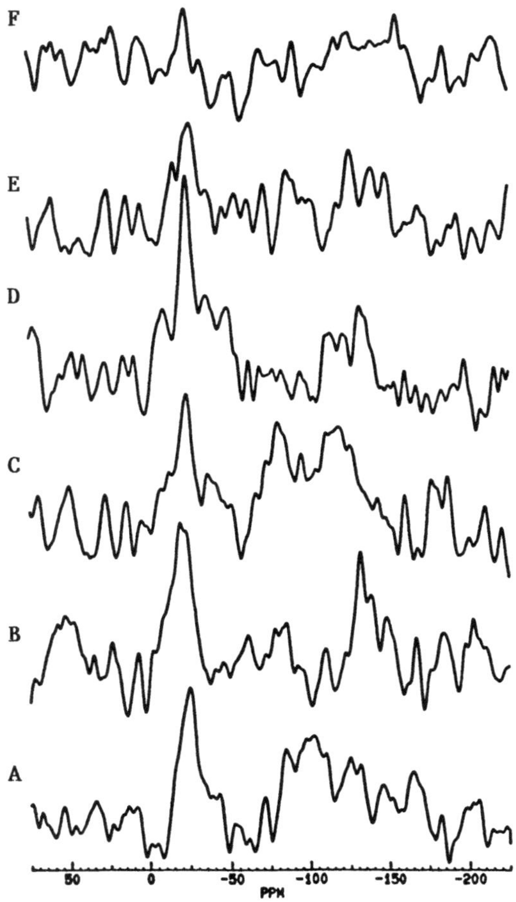

Fig. 4. ^{29}Si NMR spectra of plasma and cell fractions from a blood sample previously analyzed (Fig. 1B). The spectra 3A, 3B, 3C and 3D correspond to plasma fractions C1>300,000 daltons, 300,000>C2>50,000, 50,000>C3>10,000 and 10,000>C4, respectively. Fig. 3E and 3F illustrate the ^{29}Si spectra associated with the lymphocyte/monocyte cells and the rest of the cells in the same blood sample, respectively. The presence of silicon resonances in the spectra is significant in all of them except in Fig. 4F (blood cells not included in the lymphocyte/monocyte fraction).

All fractions have a peak at ~ -20 ppm that corresponds to the silicons in the structural unit of PDMS (chemically unchanged silicone). The broadening of this peak with increasing molecular size of the plasma fraction could be due, in part, to the restriction in molecular mobility of the polysiloxanes (silicone) associated with other macromolecules present in the plasma. The presence of terminal hydroxyl groups, peaks at about -10 ppm, and disilanols, resonances at ~ -40 ppm, are more apparent in the plasma fraction with the lowest molecular weight (Fig. 4D). The region of the ^{29}Si spectrum between -70 and -160 varies greatly for the plasma fractions studied, suggesting that some of the peaks observed are a consequence of the association and/or bonding of silicone metabolites with specific plasma proteins. These metabolites, partially hydrolyzed silicone, silicates and silica, have hydroxyl groups that are likely to interact with amino, phosphate and other functional groups present in proteins, phospholipids, etc., giving rise to new silicon functionalities with resonances not yet assigned. The biotransformation (oxidation) of silicone most probably requires the action of macrophages and other phagocytic cells (i.e., monocytes) at the implant site, in distant tissues and organs, and in blood. This hypothesis is supported by the results shown in Fig. 3E which shows the ^{29}Si NMR spectra corresponding to the lymphocyte/monocyte cells from the blood sample studied previously (Fig. 1B). The spectrum shows peaks at -22 ppm (silicone), -80 and -120 ppm (silicates and silica). The ^{29}Si NMR spectrum of the remaining cells did not show any resonances.

Furthermore, we investigated the biodegradation of PDMS incubated with a macrophage-like J-774 cell line. Fig. 5 shows the ^{29}Si NMR spectra corresponding to (bottom) an aqueous solution of the PDMS-cyclodextrin complex and (top) a PDMS-cyclodextrin solution after incubation with macrophage-like J-774 cells. The spectrum at the bottom shows only one peak at -22 ppm associated with silicon in the structural unit of chemically unchanged PDMS. The spectrum at the top shows, in addition to the resonance at -22 ppm, other resonances at -5 to -15, -70 to -80 and -110 ppm consistent with hydrolyzed PDMS (end groups), mono- and di-silicates, polysilicates and silica, respectively. The resonance at 90 ppm has not yet been identified.

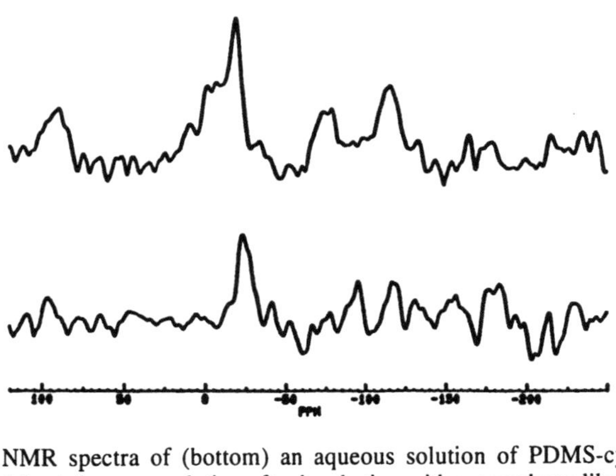

Fig. 5. ^{29}Si NMR spectra of (bottom) an aqueous solution of PDMS-cyclodextrin complexes and (top) the same solution after incubation with macrophage-like J-774 cells for 8 days. The spectrum at the bottom shows one peak at -22 ppm consistent with chemically unchanged PDMS, while the top spectrum shows multiple resonances indicating the presence of chemically unchanged PDMS (-22 ppm), hydrolyzed PDMS end groups (-5 to -15 ppm), mono- , polysilicates and silica with peaks at -70 to -80, and -110 ppm. These results indicate the degradation of PDMS by macrophage-like J-774 cells *in vitro* .

These results clearly indicate that PDMS is degraded by macrophage-like cells *in vitro* and support the hypothesis that macrophages are integrally involved in the biodegradation of silicones in living systems as well as previous findings in animal models and humans that silicones are not stable in living systems.

4 Conclusions

This work clearly shows that women with silicone gel-filled breast implants have measurable amounts by ^{29}Si NMR of silicon containing compounds in their blood, most likely due to the migration of PDMS and other polysiloxanes present in these prostheses. The total amount of silicon seems to be independent of the apparent status of the implant. The NMR results show that silicon containing compounds are present in various plasma fractions and in the lymphocyte/monocyte cell fraction. It is found that polysiloxanes are not biostable but undergo oxidation by the activity of macrophage-like cells *in vitro* and monocytes/macrophages *in vivo*.

5 References

1. Van Noort R, Black MM (1981) Silicone rubbers for medical applications. In Williams DF (ed) Biocompatibility of clinical implant materials. CRC Press, Boca Raton, pp 79-98.
2. Kessler DA (1992) The basis for the FDA's decision on breast implants. N Eng J Med 326:1713-1715.
3. Picha GJ, Goldstein JA (1991) Analysis of the soft-tissue response to components used in the manufacture of breast implants: rat animal model. Plas Reconstr Surg 87:490-500.
4. LeVier RR, Harrison MC, Cook RR, Lane TH (1993) What is silicone? Plas Reconstr Surg163-167
5. Truong LD, Cartwright J, Goodman MD, Woznicki D (1988) Silicone lymphadenopathy associated with augmentation mammaplasty. Am J Surg Pathol 12:484-491.
6. McGrath MH, Burkhardt BR (1984) The safety and efficacy of breast implants for augmentation mammaplasty. Plast Reconstr Surg 74:550-560.
7. Angell M (1992) Breast implants -protection of paternalism? N Eng J Med 326:1695-1696.
8. de Camara DL, Sheridan JM, Kammer BA (1993) Rupture and aging of silicone gel breast implants. Plast Reconstr Surg 91:828-834.
9. Weiner SR, Paulus HE (1986) Chronic arthropapthy occuring after augmentation mammoplasty. Plast Reconstr Surg 77:185-192.
10. Endo LP, Edwards NL, Longley S, Corman LC, Panush RS (1987) Silicone and rheumatic diseases. Semin Arthritis Rheum 17:112-118.
11. Brozena SJ, Fenske NA, Cruse CW, Espinoza CG, Vasey FB, Germain BF, et al (1988) Human adjuvant disease following augmentation mammoplasty. Arch Dermatol 124:1383-1386.
12. Varga J, Shumacher HR, Jimenez SA (1989) Systemic sclerosis after augmentation mammoplasty with silicone implants. Ann Intern Med 111:377-383.
13. Sahn EE, Garen PD, Silver RM, Maize JC (1990) Scleroderma following augmentation mammoplasty. Arch Dermatol 126:1198-1202.
14. Bridges AJ, Conley C, Wang G, Burns DE, Vasey FB (1993) A clinical and immunologic evaluation of women with silicone breast implants and symptoms of rheumatic disease. Ann Inter Med 118:929-936.
15. Fiala TGS, Lee WPA, May JW Jr (1993) Augmentation mammoplasty: results of a patient survey. Ann Plast Surg 30:503-509.
16. Sanchéz-Guerrero J, Schur PH, Sergent JS, Liang MH (1993) Silicone breast implants and rheumatic disease. J Arthritis Rheum 37:158-168.

17. Gabriel SE, O'Fallon WM, Kurland LT, Beard CM, Woods JE, Melton LJ (1994) Risk of connective-tissue diseases and other disorders after breast implantation. New Engl J Med 330:1697-1702.
18. Heggers JP, Kossovsky N, Parsons RW, Robson MC, Pelley RP, Raine TJ (1983) Biocompatibility of silicone implants. Ann Plast Surg 11:38-45.
19. Thomsen JL, Christensen L, Nielsen M, Brandt B, Breiting VB, Felby S, Nielsen E (1990) Histologic changes and silicone concentrations in human breast tissue surrounding silicone breast prostheses. Plast Reconstr Surg 85:38-41.
20. Gutierrez FJ, Espinoza LR (1990) Progressive systemic sclerosis complicated by severe hypertension: reversal after silicone implant removal. Am J Med 89:390-392.
21. Komoroski RA (ed) (1986) High resolution nmr spectroscopy of synthetic polymers in bulk, Deerfield, FL.
22. Koenig JL (ed) (1991) Spectroscopy of polymers, ACS Publications, Washington, D.C.
23. Garrido L, Pfleiderer B, Ackerman JL (1993) Migration and biodegradation of free silicone from silicone gel-filled implants after long-term implantation. Mag Reson Med 30:534-543.
24. Garrido L, Pfleiderer B, Jenkins BJ, Hulka CA, Kopans DB (1994) Migration and chemical modification of silicone in women with breast prostheses. Mag Reson Med 31:328-330.
25. Pfleiderer B, Garrido L (1995) Migration and accumulation of silicone in the liver of women with silicone gel-filled breast implants. Mag Reson Med 33:8-17.
26. Garrido L, Pfleiderer B, Papisov M, Ackerman JL (1993) In vivo degradation of silicones. Mag Reson Med 29:839-843.
27. Djeu JL (1992) Monocyte/macrophage functions. In: Rose NR, de Macario EC, Fahey JL, Friedman H, Penn GM (eds) Manual of clinical laboratory immunology. 4th Ed. American Society for Microbiology, Washington, D.C. pp 231-235.
28. Marsmann H (1981) ^{29}Si NMR spectroscopic results. In: Diehl P, Fluck E, Kosfeld R (eds) Oxygen-17 and Silicon-29. NMR, basic principles and progress. Springer-Verlag, New York, v 17, pp 65-235.
29. Touchette N (1992) Silicone implants and autoimmune disease: studies fail to gel. J NIH Research 4(5):49-52.
30. Vondrácek P, Gent AN (1982) Slow decomposition of silicone rubber. J Appl Polym Sci 27:4517-4523.
31. Lehmann RG, Varaprath S, Frye CL (1994) Degradation of silicone polymers in soil. Environ Toxicol Chem 13:1061-1064.
32. Peters W, Smith D, Lugowski S, McHugh A, Baines C (1995) Do patients with silicone-gel breast implants have elevated leves of blood silicon compared with control patients? Annals Plast Surg 34:343-347.
33. Roberts NB, Williams DP (1990) Silicon measurement in serum and urine by direct current plasma emission spectrometry. Clin Chem 36:1460-1465.
34. Teuber SS, Saunders RL, Halpern GM, Brucker RF, Conte V, Goldman BD, Winger EE, Wood WG (1995) Serum silicon levels in women with silicone gel breast implants. Biol Trace Elem Res 48:000-000.

Serum Silicon Levels are Elevated in Women with Silicone Gel Implants

S.S. Teuber[1,2], R.L. Saunders[1], G.M. Halpern[1], R.F. Brucker[3], V. Conte[3], B.D. Goldman[3], E.E. Winger[3], W.G. Wood[3], and M.E. Gershwin[1*].
[1]Department of Internal Medicne, Division of Rheumatology, Allergy and Clinical Immunology, University of California, Davis, School of Medicine, Davis, California, 95616, USA.
[2]Department of Veterans Affairs Northern California System of Clinics, Pleasant Hill, California, 94523 USA.
[3]Bay Area Laboratory Co-operative (BALCO), 1520 Gilbreth Road, Burlingame, California, 94010, USA.

Abstract

The metabolic fate of silicone gel leaked into the body from an implant is unknown. In this study, serum from 72 women with silicone gel breast implants and 55 control women was blindly assayed by inductively coupled plasma atomic emission spectroscopy (ICP-AES) for elemental silicon. Samples were processed using materials free of silicon. The mean silicon level in controls was 0.13 ± 0.07 mg/l (range 0.06 - 0.35 mg/l), while in implant patients, the mean was significantly higher at 0.28 ± 0.22 mg/l (range 0.06 - 0.87 mg/l) ($P< 0.01$, Student's *t*-test with correction for unequal variances). Using the mean of the control group + 2 SD as a cutoff for normal range (0.27 mg/l), 25/72 (34.7%) implant patients exceeded this value, compared with 2/55 (3.6%) controls. There was no significant correlation between past rupture of one or both implants, current rupture at the time of the blood draw or the number of years with implants and silicon levels. The results suggest that elevations of serum silicon are seen in many women with silicone gel breast implants. The kinetics of this elevation and the actual chemical species of the measured silicon remain to be determined.

Introduction

There are current concerns that long-term exposure to polydimethylsiloxane (PDMS) or other components of gel-filled breast implants, such as amorphous silica in the implant shell [1], may be associated with autoimmune or inflammatory diseases in some individuals [2]. It is well-known that the gel will bleed through the implant shell over time [3]. In addition, there is potential for mechanical breakdown and degradation of the implant shell due to hydrolysis, mechanical forces, and perhaps effects of oxidative attack from the body's

*Disclosures: M.E. Gershwin has served as an expert witness for plaintiff's attorneys. BALCO is a reference lab for trace mineral analysis. This presentation was based on a paper currently in press in Biological Trace Element Research (1995) [9].

inflammatory cells [4]. Elemental silicon, which accounts for 35 - 40% of the implant by weight [5], can be quantitated by methods which include ICP-AES, while direct, accurate, quantitative measurements of organosilicon compounds such as PDMS are not technically feasible at this time. If implant components are degraded with time and gain access to the circulation after leakage or rupture, circulating silicon might be elevated in the blood or serum of such women in the form of soluble silicic acid, or an elevation may be noted due to measurement of the silicon contained in circulating PDMS fragments or PDMS degradation products. In the current study, we hypothesized that silicone gel implants would serve as an endogenous source of ongoing elevation of serum silicon levels, especially in those women who had ruptures at the time of the blood draw or a history of past rupture.

Methods

Subjects. A local press release aided in recruitment of women with silicone gel breast implants and age-matched controls. Some women were referred for the study after evaluation of their implants by ultrasonography. Informed consent was obtained from all volunteers. Since the implant-related factors affecting serum silicon levels are unknown, we excluded women if they had only one implant, dual lumen or saline implants, or polyurethane coating. Women were also excluded if their implants had been removed prior to the blood draw. Women with a history of renal disease were ineligible because of the known relationship between renal insufficiency and elevated blood silicon levels [6,7]. The subjects were instructed to fast, discontinue any medication (prescription or over-the-counter), and drink only bottled or municipal water (not well water which has been reported to contain higher levels of silicon [8]) for 12 hours before the serum samples were collected.

The samples were collected using silicon-free polypropylene syringes (10 ml Neutral Luer-Monovette, Sarstedt, Inc., Newton, NC) and 21G x 1" Precision Glide needles (Becton Dickinson, Franklin Lakes, NJ). After clotting and centrifugation, the serum was removed with disposable polyethylene pipettes and stored in polypropylene tubes (Sarstedt, Inc.) at 4 °C. An additional aliquot was removed for creatinine determination if a sufficient volume of sera had been obtained. Samples for silicon analysis were labeled with an accession number and sent by overnight express mail on ice to the laboratory for blinded assay.

Equipment. Serum samples were analyzed using an inductively coupled plasma atomic emission spectrometer (Applied Research Laboratories, Dearborn, MI; Model 34000 simultaneous ICP) equipped with a C-3 type concentric nebulizer (Precision Glassblowing, Englewood, CO). A peristaltic pump (Gilson Medical Electronics, Inc., Middleton, WI; Model Minipuls 2) and autosampler (Gilson Model SC-15B) were used to introduce samples into the argon plasma. The serum samples and calibration standards were weighed in 12 ml polypropylene centrifuge tubes (Sarstedt, Inc.).

Reagents. Doubly deionized water was used for the preparation of all solutions and was prepared by passing reverse osmosis purified water (Premier, Phoenix, AZ; Model ROTFC 4SV) successivly through combination organic mixed bed and ultrapure mixed bed exchange cartridges (Barnstead/Thermolyne, Dubuque, IA).

A commercial 1000 mg/L certified standard silicon solution (Lot 982DB, SPEX Industries, Inc., Edison, NJ) was diluted with 10 mL/L HNO_3 (Redistilled Nitric Acid, GFS Chemicals, Inc., Columbus, OH) to prepare the silicon stock standard solution (1.0 mg/L).

Sample Preparation and Analysis. A target weight of 2.5 grams of serum was brought up to 10 grams with the 10mL/L HNO_3 diluent. The samples were vortex mixed for 20 seconds and then transferred into 5 ml polypropylene autosampler tubes (Sarstedt, Inc.).

ICP-AES measurements were performed under the operating conditions previously described [9]. A 10mL/L HNO_3 solution was used as a blank. The instrument was calibrated with 5 standards that were gravimetrically prepared by diluting the primary 1.0 mg/L silicon solution in 10 mL/L HNO3 to give final concentrations of 0, 0.1, 0.25, 0.5 and 1.0 mg/L. The standards were freshly prepared and vortexed before each analytical run. No spectral or matrix interference was observed. Solutions of silicon added to serum gave the same signal response as aqueous standards; thus, aqueous calibration appears suitable for measurements of silicon in serum [6].

The samples were nebulized into the argon plasma and integrated intensities at 251.61 nm (Si) were compared to the analytical calibration curves. The samples were analyzed by making 3 consecutive 10 second integration measurements per determination. The average value was reported. Under the conditions of this quantitative assay of silicon, the detection limit (defined as 3 SD above the mean determined with a zero concentration of silicon) was 0.006 mg/L. The method was linear up to 1.0 mg/L.

Accuracy and Precision. Using pooled serum from healthy subjects obtained from Peninsula Blood Bank, Burlingame, CA, the method was tested for accuracy and precision by performing spike/recovery tests. 2.5 grams of pooled serum, mean Si level 0.109 mg/L (n = 60 measurements), was added to 2.5 grams of 0.1 mg/L or 0.5 mg/L silicon solution and 5 grams of 10ml/L HNO_3 diluent to give spiked serum silicon levels of 0.1 and 0.5 mg/L . The percent recovered was 103% of the 0.1mg/L added (recovered mean 0.103 mg/L, n = 60) and 101% of the 0.5 mg/L added (recovered mean 0.508, n = 60). Intra- and interassay precision measurements were also tabulated (Table 1).

Creatinine Measurement. Numbered specimens were submitted blindly for serum creatinine determination using a Boehringer Mannheim/Hitachi 747 Analyzer (Boehringer Mannheirm, Indianapolis, IN).

Statistics. Student' *t*-test was used for comparison of paired groups. Students' *t*-test with Cochran's corrections for unequal variances was used to compare groups of values with unequal variances. Pearson's simple correlations were performed. The results are presented as mean $\pm$ SD. $P < 0.05$ was considered significant.

Table 1. Precision of silicon measurements by ICP-AES using blood bank sera.

	Silicon Added (mg/L)	Number	Measured Mean (mg/L)	SD	%CV
Intra-assay	0.0	10	0.107	0.005	4.7
	0.1	10	0.211	0.005	2.3
	0.5	10	0.617	0.15	2.4
Inter-assay	0.0	60	0.109	0.005	4.9
	0.1	60	0.212	0.008	3.8
	0.5	60	0.617	0.021	3.5

Results

110 women volunteered for the study, but 38 were excluded from analysis for the following reasons: 5 had polyurethane implants, 12 had dual lumen implants, 12 had only one implant, and 9 had undergone explantation prior to the blood draw. Of the remaining 72 women, the average age was 48.1 $\pm$ 9.6 years. Implants had been in place for a mean of 13.8 $\pm$ 5.8 years with a range of 1 - 27 years. The 55 control women had a mean age of 47.7 $\pm$ 10.7 years (P = NS). The mean silicon level in women with implants was 0.28 $\pm$ 0.22mg/L with a range of 0.06 to 0.87 mg/L. The mean level in the control women was significantly less at 0.13 $\pm$ 0.07 mg/L with a range of 0.06 to 0.35 mg/L ($P < 0.01$, t-test with correction for unequal variances). Figure 1 shows the distribution of silicon values for the two groups. The mean silicon level of the control group + 2 SD, 0.27 mg/L, can be used to designate a normal range for serum silicon in this population. Using this value as a cutoff, 25/72 (34.7%) of the implant patients exceeded this value, while only 2/55 (3.6%) of the controls were elevated.

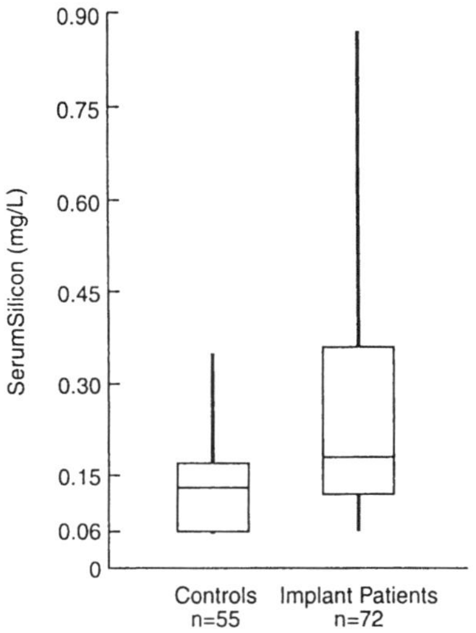

Fig. 1. Serum silicon distributions in control and implant patient populations as depicted by box and whisker plots. The box represents the population median value and upper and lower quartiles.

Eleven patients were available as a subgroup with current ruptures to test the hypothesis that women with rupture would have higher serum silicon levels than the rest of the women with implants. Additionally, 8 were found to have had past ruptures. Another woman was excluded from analysis because she had history of a past rupture as well as a current rupture. Four of the eleven patients with current rupture had surgery shortly after the blood draw which confirmed rupture, in some cases intracapsular, and in others, with extension beyond the implant connective tissue capsule. Seven patients have not had surgery yet, but are included in the group with current rupture based on MRI results in four and ultrasound in three. The mean silicon value for these women with current rupture was 0.24 $\pm$ 0.15 mg/L, with a value of 0.27 $\pm$ 0.22 mg/L in the 52 other implant patients without any known history of rupture (P = NS). The 8 patients with a history of past rupture and subsequent replacement of implants had a mean silicon level of 0.35 $\pm$ 0.25 (P = NS). Pearson simple correlations also did not show significant correlations between serum silicon levels and the status of either current or past implant ruptures. In addition, there was no significant correlation between silicon levels and the number of years silicone gel implants had been in place. Since the 52 women without any known history of rupture have not all had their implants subsequently removed, it is possible that some of these women also have ruptures, which would make comparison between groups invalid.

Creatinine levels were performed on 62 patients and 49 controls and all were within normal range. The mean creatinine in patients was 0.67 $\pm$ 0.14 while the mean value in controls was 0.66 $\pm$ 0.18 (P = NS). We did not measure creatinine clearances directly, but a previous study did not show significant elevations of serum silicon until renal insufficiency was marked with creatinine clearance less than 40 mL/min [7] and another study showed good correlations between elevation of blood creatinine and silicon level [6].

Discussion

ICP-AES appears to be a sensitive and precise means of measuring serum silicon levels, which should also reflect the presence of non-volatile organosilicon compounds since these contain silicon. The mean level of silicon in healthy individuals reported here, 0.13 mg/L, is similar to the mean values found in other studies: 0.11 mg/L by ICP-AES on whole blood [6], 0.14 mg/L by direct current plasma - atomic emission spectrometry (DCP-AES) on serum [7] and 0.15 mg/L and 0.17 mg/L on plasma by furnace atomic absorption spectrometry [8,10]. This is a procedure that will enable investigators to further gather analytical data on serum silicon levels in health and disease. There are no confirmed adverse health effects caused from accumulation of silicon from silicon dioxide in the dialysis bath water or drinking water in hemodialysis patients (with serum levels up to 4.6 mg/L [8]). In fact, some have hypothesized that the high levels of silicon in blood may help protect hemodialysis patients from aluminum toxicity [11]. However, another group reported that high levels of silicon, comparable to levels found in patients with renal failure, inhibit the activity of the anti-oxidant enzyme superoxide dismutase (SOD), which they propose could result in excess oxygen free radical production and deleterious complications such as inflammatory conditions and cellular damage. The effect of silicon on SOD was studied *in vitro* and the degree of inhibition was directly proportional to silicon levels [12]. This same group also reported that SOD levels in red blood cells were significantly lower in renal failure patients known to have elevated serum silicon levels compared to controls [13]. SOD plays a major role in the destruction and elimination of the damaging oxygen-free radicals in the body and inhibition of this enzyme could could have clinical importance.

However, patients with silicone gel implant represent a completely different situation, since the presumed source of the elevations of serum silicon - as compared to hemodialysis patients - is a complex chemical polymer whose intermediate metabolic degradation products may have unknown and perhaps even deleterious effects. The fact that elevations are detected is significant, because for years it had been felt that silicones were biologically inert and would not break down in the body. However, evidence has accumulated that silicones can induce significant local inflammatory reactions [14] and migrate from the site of implantation. Garrido et al., in a series of publications [15-17], have shown both in animal models and in women with silicone gel implants that silicone can clearly migrate from the site of implantation in an enclosed silicone rubber bag to distant sites such as liver, and that the chemical species detected by nuclear magnetic resonance spectroscopy are not present in the original implant material, thus substantiating metabolic degradation in vivo.

It is interesting that women who had confirmed current ruptures of one or both implants did not necessarily have an elevated serum silicon level. Conversely, several women who underwent surgery after their blood was drawn were found to have intact implants and yet had elevated silicon levels. We presume that this is reflective of the gel bleed that can occur from all implants [3]. The chemical species present in the sera, the kinetics of the significant elevations seen, and the clinical relevance of elevated serum silicon levels in women with breast implants are worth further evaluation.

References

1. LeVier RR, Harrison MC, Cook RR, Lane TH (1993) What is silicone? Plast Reconst Surg 92: 163-167
2. Yoshida SH, Chang CC, Teuber SS, Gershwin ME (1993) Silicon and silicone: theoretical and clinical implications of breast implants. Reg Toxicol Pharmacol 17: 3-18
3. Barker DE, Retsky MI, Schultz S (1978) "Bleeding" of silicone from bag-gel breast implants, and its clinical relation to fibrous capsule reaction. Plast Reconstr Surg 61:836-841
4. Yoshida SH, Teuber SS, German JB, Gershwin ME (1994) Immunotoxicity of silicone: implications of oxidant balance toward adjuvant activity. Fd Chem Toxicology 32:1089-1100
5. Thomsen JL, Christensen L, Nielsen M, Brandt B, Breiting VB, Felby S, Nielsen E (1990) Histologic changes and silicone concentrations in human breast tissue surrounding silicone breast prostheses. Plast Reconst Surg 85: 38-41
6. Mauras Y, Riberi P, Cartier F, Allain P (1980) Increase in blood silicon concentration in patients with renal failure. Biomedicine 33:228-230
7. Roberts NB, Williams P (1990) Silicon measurement in serum and urine by direct current plasma emission spectromety. Clin Chem 36: 1460-1465
8. Gitelman HJ, Alderman FR, Perry SJ (1992) Silicon accumulation in dialysis patients. Am J Kidney Diseases 19:140-143
9. Teuber SS, Saunders RL, Halpern GM, Brucker RF, Conte V, Goldman BD, Winger EE, Wood WG, Gershwin ME (1995) Elevated serum silicon levels in women with silicone gel breast implants. Biol Trace Element Res (in press)
10. Gitelman HJ, Alderman FR (1990) Determination of silicon in biological samples using electrothermal atomic absorption spectrometry. J Analytical Atomic Spectrometry 5:687-689
11. Dobbie JW Smith MJB (1986) in Silicon Biochem: Urinary and serum silicon in normal and uremic individuals. Ciba Foundation Symposium 121, Wiley, New York, NY, pp 194-213
12. Shainkin-Kestenbaum R., Adler AJ, Berlyne GM (1990) J Trace Elem Electrolytes Health Dis 4: 97-99
13 Shainkin-Kestebaum R, Caruso C, Berlyne GM (1990) Reduced superoxide dismutase activity in erythrocytes of dialysis patients: a possible factor in the etiology of uremic anemia. Nephron 55:251
14. Picha GJ, Goldstein JA (1991) Analysis of the soft-tissue response to components used in the manufacture of breast implants: rat animal model. Plast Reconstr Surg 87:490-496
15. Garrido L, Pfleiderer B, Jenkins BC, Hulka CA, Kopans DB (1994) Mag Resonance Med 31:328-330
16. Garrido L, Pfleiderer B, Papisov M, Ackerman JL (1993) In vivo degradation of silicones. Mag Resonance Med 29:839-843
17. Pfleiderer B, Ackerman JL, Garrido L (1993) Migration and biodegradation of free silicone from silicone gel-filled implants after long-term implantation. Mag Resonance Med 30:534-543

Interaction of Silicones with Proteins and Tissues

The Development of an ELISA Method for the Detection of "Antibodies" to Silicone

by B. Rosenau ScD, A.B. Schneebaun MD*, and P. H. Schur MD
From the Department of Rheumatology and Immunology, Harvard Medical School, at Brigham and Women's Hospital, Boston Mass. and * the Lahey Clinic, Burlington Mass.

This study received support only from a grant from the USPHS, NIH AR 42630

Dr Schur was a consultant and expert witness regarding breast implant litigation from Nov.1993 to Dec. 1994--unrelated to the present investigation.

Introduction: As part of an ongoing study to determine whether there is an association between silicone implants and connective tissue diseases, symptoms and/or immune phenomena, we undertook an investigation to determine whether individuals have/make antibodies to silicone. We chose the ELISA technique as a method to demonstrate the possible presence of antibodies to silicone. In developing an ELISA we considered the following:

1. What form of silicone to use as antigen.
2. How to coat ELISA plates with antigen.
3. How to block plates to prevent nonspecific binding of serum
4. How to wash plates.
5. Choice of microtiter plate.
6. What dilution of serum to use
7. Quality Control: What to use as positive and negative controls, and an internal standard to account for day to day variation in ELISA
8. What conjugated anti-immunoglobulin to use, and at what dilution
9. How to calculate results
10. What statistics to use.

1. Antigen: (The experiments described in this section used Costar #3590, Cambridge, Mass., EIA/RIA plates.--For further discussion of plate selection see section 3 below). We wanted to use an antigen as identical as possible to the "silicone" used in breast implants. We were kindly provided medical grade polydimethylsiloxane (PDMS) (Dow Corning 360 Medical Fluid, Midland, Michigan--viscosity 100CS) and hydroxy-terminated PDMS (Dow Corning Q1-3563--contains dimethyl cyclosiloxanes and hydroxy-terminated PDMS). Hydroxy-terminated-PDMS was also used based on the rationales given by Wolf et al (1). When PDMS or hydroxy-terminated PDMS (OH-PDMS) was diluted with water or phosphate-buffered saline (PBS) the two liquids easily separated (as with oil and water). Therefore, equal volumes of organic solvents (e.g. chloroform, toluene) and PDMS were added to microtiter plate wells in a fume hood, and allowed to dry overnight at room temperature. The plates were then washed 3 times with 95% alcohol to remove the organic solvent, aspirated to remove any remaining fluid, and then washed with PBS-Tween 3 times. Plates were reacted with an antinuclear antibody (ANA) negative pool of 50 normal human serums plus a serum from a patient with systemic lupus erythematosus (SLE), who had antinuclear antibodies and silicone breast implants.

After the sera were incubated in the wells overnight at 37 C, the plates were washed 3 times with PBS-Tween, a conjugated anti-IgG(anti-human IgG-alkaline phosphatase; Sigma (St. Louis MO)--diluted in 1%BSA/PBS/Tween) was added , and the standard ELISA procedure (see Method 1 below) followed. No color was observed in any well.

Similar experiments were performed using butane as an organic solvent. Subsequently all wells, including control wells treated with just butane, showed very high OD, suggesting nonspecific reactions.

Similar experiments were performed using PDMS and OH-PDMS in 95% alcohol vs PDMS and OH-PDMS in water. There was no difference in ODs between wells coated with PDMS in alcohol vs water in either tests or controls.

Similar experiments were performed with Silicone (Silicone Lubricant--Multi Purpose--HeavyDuty--Tru-Test--True Value, Chicago, Illinois) sprayed onto microtiter plates. When the material dried, the wells were opaque,and therefore unsuitable for ELISA testing.

Undiluted PDMS or OH-PDMS was used to coat Titertek microtiter plates (see section 3 below) overnight at 37 C. Plates were then washed once with double-distilled water and then incubated with sera as above, and then a standard (see Method 1 below) ELISA followed. There was no apparent reactivity with sera.

2. Pre-coating wells: Microtiter wells were pretreated with various substances in an attempt to improve antigen binding to microtiter wells.

Similar experiments to those described in section 1 above were performed with microtiter wells first coated with petroleum jelly (Vaseline, Chesebrough Ponds Inc, Greenwich CT) and then PDMS. The ODs obtained in wells precoated with vaseline were negligible as compared to wells receiving silicone only, suggesting that the silicone did not stick to the vaseline.

Similar experiments were performed with microtiter wells treated with colorless nail polish (Revlon--New York,NY) and then PDMS. Control wells coated with nail polish showed as much reactivity as wells coated with nail polish and silicone. Similar experiments were performed with Whatman #54 filter paper dotted with PDMS and allowed to dry in a hood overnight. The dots were punched out and placed in microtiter wells. The plates were washed and the pieces of paper stayed in the wells. Subsequently the Method 1 ELISA protocol (see below) was followed and wells were reacted with serum as above. Prior to reading ODs filter paper was removed with a forceps. There was no difference between wells containing filter paper treated with PDMS vs control wells.

Similar experiments were performed with nitrocellulose membranes (Biorad (Melville, NY) #162-0115; 0.45 micron). Optical densities were higher in wells without silicone than in those containing silicone indicating that serum proteins had probably been transferred to the membrane without interacting with silicone.

Wells in Costar plates were pretreated with 0.1% BSA (Miles Scientific, Naperville, Illinois) as per Wolf et al (1) and Voller et al (2) to enhance silicone binding. Plates were then treated as per the Method 1 ELISA (see below). The ODs for wells containing 0.1% BSA were comparable to those in uncoated wells, suggesting that this low concentration of BSA did not provide for ample binding of the silicone. Similar experiments were performed using 1%BSA and sera diluted 1/200 and weak reactivity was observed, so similar experiments were performed using sera diluted 1/25 and 1/50. Sera diluted at 1/25 yielded a great deal of nonspecific reactivity; at a dilution of 1/50 there was little nonspecific reactivity.

Tests were also performed to determine whether either human serum albumin (HSA) (Sigma, St. Louis, MO) or gelatin (Fisher,

Fairlawn, NJ) would be a better precoat than BSA. However, there was more nonspecific reactivity with 0.1% HSA or 0.1% gelatin than with 1% BSA.

3.Plates: Three plates were compared:

(1):Titertek (Flow Labs--McLean VA) (Linbro) polystyrene, 96 well flat bottom treated to reduce charge to neutral to prevent "skipping" of droplets--Flow #76-331-05

(2): Costar (Cambridge MASS) polystyrene, 96 well, flat bottom, high binding, gamma irradiated; Costar #3590

(3): Costar-polystyrene, 96 well, tissue culture clusters, gamma irradiated, treated chemically to give a negative charge; Costar #3594

Plates were precoated with 1% BSA followed by a silicone coat, and subsequently the Method 1 ELISA protocol (see below)was followed. Wells were reacted with sera as above. Titertek plates had the lowest background OD, and were selected for further studies.

4. Washing wells: Silicone was observed not to dissolve in either PBS with Tween, PBS, or Tween. Therefore the PBS Tween wash buffer used in other assays (3) was used.

5. Blocking nonspecific binding: Various substances were studied to prevent nonspecific binding of serum proteins to coated wells. Experiments were performed using 0.1% and 1% BSA in demineralized distilled water (DDW), 0.1% HSA in DDW, and 0.1% gelatin in DDW following coating plates with PDMS and OH-PDMS. Subsequently sera were added as per Method 1 (see below). 1%BSA was found to be even better in blocking nonspecific binding based on ODs--results similar to other assays in this laboratory (4).

Because the majority of test sera (see results below) showed reactivity with BSA, attempts were made to lessen that reactivity by diluting test sera with 5%BSA (5) and the conjugate with 1% BSA. The rest of the ELISA was performed as per Method 1 (see below). However, at the completion of this assay there was no color, suggesting that all anti-BSA and other antibodies had been removed.

In further attempts to get rid of anti-BSA reactivity, we compared the Method 1 ELISA (see below) to the following: sera were diluted instead in 10% bovine serum in WS (4). Results showed that more anti-BSA reactivity was removed when test sera and conjugate were diluted in 10% bovine serum in WS then when test serum was diluted in WS and conjugate diluted in 1% BSA/WS. We therefore incorporated these changes into Method 2 and 3.

6. Quality control: Each serum was tested in duplicate vs wells precoated with BSA and then coated with silicone, vs control wells (precoated with BSA in Methods 1-3). For each run (using Methods 1-3) a diluent blank and a pool of normal serum (NSP) were run as controls.

7-10. Subsequent steps were performed as per standard ELISA protocols utilized in the BWH Clinical Immunology Lab for testing for antibodies to dsDNA and cardiolipin (3,4).

The final methods selected based on the above considerations are delineated below as Method 1 and 2 (and 3).

Calculations: The average OD of each duplicate was determined. This average was corrected as follows to correct for day to day variation in reactivity:

$$\text{Corrected OD} = \text{average OD each test sample} \times \frac{\text{mean all NSP}}{\text{mean NSP that run}}$$

"Difference": the difference in the reactivity between silicone and BSA was calculated as follows: the corrected OD of wells precoated with BSA and then coated with silicone minus the corrected OD of wells precoated with BSA alone.

Statistics : mean +/- 2SD; t test

Absorption-Inhibition: In order to determine whether reactivity could be attributed to anti-silicone antibody, sera were selected that gave high ODs in Method 3 tests vs silicone. These sera were reacted with either an equal volume of PDMS, OH-PDMS, polypropylene glycol (as suggested by Wolf et al (1))(Aldrich Comp, Milw. WI), or PBS, and incubated on a rocker to facilitate mixing for one hour at room temperature and overnight at 4C. They were then tested in the Method 3 ELISA at a dilution of 1/50.

Test Sera: 227 (discarded)sera from BWH Blood bank donors.

: 81 sera from the Lahey Clinic (courtesy of Dr Andrea Schneebaum) from women with breast implants.

: 10 sera from women with breast implants seen at the BWH

: 3 sera from Dr Goldblum (University of Texas), 2 of which are said to have antibodies to Silastic tubing (6).

: The normal serum pool (NSP) was made up of 50 sera from individuals with negative ANA tests.

Method 1:1. Precoat Titertek plates with 200 ul 1.0% BSA in DDW; cover plates and incubate for 2 hours at 4 C.
2. Decant. Wash twice with DDW. Air dry.
3. Add 100ul hydroxy-silicone (10% in DDW) to half of the plate. Wrap in plastic and incubate for 16 hours at 37C.
4. Aspirate the excess silicone. Wash once with wash solution (WS) (0.05% TWEEN in PBS).
5. Add 100 ul serum diluted in WS to make a 1/50 dilution. Incubate for 16 hours at 37C in a moist atmosphere.
6. Wash three times with WS. --soak for 2 minutes the 3rd time.
7. Add 100 ul conjugate (Sigma anti-human IgG alkaline phosphatase--A3150) (3,4) diluted in 1% BSA in WS. Incubate for 60 minutes at room temperature (RT) on a wet towel.
8. Repeat step 6.
9. Add 100 ul substrate (p-nitrophenyl phosphate disodium; Sigma 104-0) 20mg in 10 ml glycine buffer, pH 9.8 . Incubate for 15 minutes at RT on a dry paper towel.
10. Stop with 100 ul 1N NaOH/well.
11. Read the ODs at 405nm on a plate reader (Titertek, Multiscan

Method 2: 1. Precoat Titertek plates with 100 ul 1% BSA in DDW; incubate for 2 hours at 4 C, covered
2. Wash 2 times with DDW
3. Add 100 ul 10% OH-PDMS in DDW to half of the plate; incubate overnight at 37 C.--wrap in plastic to exclude air
4. Wash once with DDW
5. Add 200 ul 1% BSA in DDW to all wells; incubate 2 hours at 4 C, covered
6. Wash three times with WS (soak for 2 minutes the 3rd time)
7. Add 100ul test (and control) sera diluted 1:50 in 10% bovine serum in WS; incubate overnight at 37C in a moist chamber
8. Wash three times with WS
9. Add 100ul conjugated anti-IgG(see Method 1) in 10% bovine serum (in WS); incubate for 60 minutes at room temperature on a wet paper towel.
10. Proceed as per Method 1.

Method 3: The same as method 2, except that PDMS is used instead of hydroxy-terminated PDMS.

Results: The results for the analyses of blood bank sera, sera from women with implants, and the "Texas" controls is given in Tables 1-3. In Method 1 (Table 1) Blood Bank sera gave higher ODs (that is had more reactivity) to wells precoated with BSA and then coated with silicone, and to wells coated with BSA, than did sera from women with implants or from "Texas." Sera from Blood Bank donors, but not sera from implants or "Texas", had higher reactivity to "silicone" wells than BSA. However, there was no significant difference between the ODs for Blood Bank sera and sera from women with implants in reactivity silicone and BSA.

In Method 2, (Table 2), "Texas" sera had higher ODs than Blood Bank sera or sera from women with implants both to "silicone" coated wells and BSA coated wells. There was no significant difference in the reactivity between wells coated with silicone and BSA; there was no significant difference in reactivity between sera from Blood Bank donors and women with implants.

In Method 3, (Table 3), sera from Blood Bank donors and from "Texas" had little more reactivity in reactions to wells coated with silicone than to BSA. However, sera from women with implants had greater reactivity to silicone coated wells than to wells coated with BSA. Furthermore, the reactivity to silicone coated wells was significantly greater for sera from women with implants than for sera from Blood Bank donors.

All three methods suggested that virtually all sera had reactivity to BSA--and that the samples gave virtually the same mean degree of reactivity to BSA in Methods 2 and 3.

The differences in OD between sera diluted with PDMS, OH-PDMS or polypropylene glycol were comparable to sera diluted with PBS, suggesting that there was no specific immune reactivity.

Selected positive sera were titrated in serial dilutions from 1:25 to 1:1600. As samples were diluted their reactivity decreased proportionally down to baseline at an approximate dilution of 1:800.

Discussion: The present observations confirm the work of others (1,6) that it is extremely difficult to set up an ELISA for the demonstration of "antibodies" to silicone. After considerable trial and effort we settled on three methods which were selected because they gave positive ODs. The results from one method (Method 3) suggested that there was more reactivity to PDMS than to BSA in the sera of women with implants than in Blood Bank donors; however, the other 2 methods failed to demonstrate that. Inhibition studies failed to demonstrate immune specificity of the reactivity. All methods demonstrated that virtually all sera had reactivity to BSA.

These observations differ from those of Wolf et al (1.). When we used their method, we in fact failed to detect any significant ODs with any sera. These observations are also somewhat different from those of Goldblum et al, in that their sera failed to give positive reactivity in our hands--although the antigen they used was somewhat different.

These observations suggest that normal individuals and women with breast implants do not have/make antibodies to silicone, confirming the work in animals where direct immunization failed to demonstrate the development of antibodies to silicone.

References

1. Wolf LE, Lappe M, Peterson RD, Ezrailson EG. (1993) Human immune response to polydimethylsiloxane (silicone): screening studies in a breast implant population. FASEB J. 7: 1265-1268

2. Voller A, Bidwell D. (1986) Enzyme linked immunosorbent assay. Manual of Clinical Laboratory Immunology. Third Edition. ED by NR Rose et al. Am Soc Microbiol. Wash DC pp. 99-109

3. Eaton RB, Schneider G, Schur PH. (1983) Enzyme immunoassay for antibodies to native DNA. Arth. & Rheum 26: 52-62

4.Ginsburg KS, Liang MH, Newcomer L, Goldhaber SZ, Schur PH, Hennekens CH, Stampfer MJ (1992) Anticardiolipin antibodies and the risk for ischemic stroke and venous thrombosis. Ann Int Med 117: 997-1002

5. Carpenter AB (1992) Enzyme linked immunoassay. In Manual of Clinical Laboratory Immunology. Fourth Edition. Edited by NR Rose et al.. Amer. Soc. Microbiol. Wash DC pp 2-9
6. Goldblum RM, Pelley RP, O'Donell AA, Pyron D, Heggers JP (1992) Antibodies to silicone elastomers and reactions to ventriculoperitoneal shunts. Lancet 340: 510-513

Table 1

Method 1

Hydroxy-terminated PDMS

	BSA+Silicone	BSA	Difference
1. Blood Bank	0.249+0.716	0.175+0.462	0.074+0.376
2. Implants	0.113+0.170	0.120+0.198	-0.007+0.128
3. Texas	0.057+0.056	0.092+0.024	-0.035+0.064
t test 1 vs 2	-0.631	-1.578	1.854
p=	0.533	0.125	0.074

Table 2

Method 2

Hydroxy-Terminated DPMS

	BSA +Silicone	BSA	Difference
1. Blood Bank	0.488+.408	0.437+.414	0.052+.26
2. Implants	0.552+.582	0.478+.47	0.072+.35
3. Texas	1.041+1.262	1.031+.258	0.010+.998
t test 1 vs 2	-1.242	-.166	-1.694
p=	.218	.869	.094

Table 3

Method 3

DPMS

	Silicone +BSA	BSA	Difference
1. Blood Bank	0.499+.42	0.436+.374	0.063+.27
2. Implants	0.634+.736	0.479+.512	0.153+.488
3. Texas	0.949+.1.206	0.921+1.264	0.028+.086
t test 1 vs 2	-3.742	-1.377	-3.887
p=	0.000	0.172	0.000

The Adsorption of Proteins on a Polydimethyl-siloxane Elastomer (PEP) and Their Antigenic Behavior

J. E. Butler, E. P. Lü, P. Navarro and B. Christiansen
The University of Iowa, Department of Microbiology[1]

Introduction

One focus of our research during the last two decades has been the immunochemistry of solid-phase immunoassay (Butler, 1991a). Contemporary solid-phase immunoassay involves the interaction of bio-molecules with, on or near, the surface of synthetic polymers composed of polystyrene, polyvinyl, nylon, methylmethacrylate, nitrocellulose, PVDF and their numerous "functionalized" variants. The native form of these polymers is intrinsically hydrophobic and readily adsorbs proteins, viruses, many peptides and nucleic acids. The practical application of biomolecular adsorption to immunoassay dates to Catt and Tregear (1967) who pioneered passive immobilization of receptors[2] as a mean of simplifying the separation of bound and free ligand; this application revolutionized immunoassay. However, modern users of the technology were slow to recognize that proteins adsorbed to hydrophobic polymers do not remain in a totally native configuration although this had been shown >30 years ago (Bull, 1956; Kochwa et al., 1967; Oreskes and Singer, 1961). More recently, we have shown that only circa 20% of polyclonal and <10% of monoclonal antibodies passively adsorbed to polystyrene, remain functional (Butler et al., 1993). The subject of adsorption-induced conformational change on polymer surfaces has been reviewed elsewhere (Butler, 1991b; 1992; Butler, 1995).

Silicone, in the form of polydimethylsiloxane (PDMS), is widely used in medical prostheses and is more hydrophobic than polystyrene based on its glass transition temperature of -123° compared to 100 C for polystyrene. The capacity of silicone elastomer to adsorb proteins has been studied for nearly 15 years

---

[1] The studies reported were supported by a research grant awarded to the University of Iowa by Dow-Corning Inc. of Midland, Michigan.

[2] A receptor is here defined as the immobilized biomolecule, e.g. antibody, whereas the ligand is the biomolecule captured from solution by the receptor.

(Bornzin and Miller, 1982; Young et al., 1983a, b; Murthy et al., 1987; Darst et al., 1988; Pankowsky et al., 1990; Tilton et al., 1990; Ziats et al., 1990). Because of our laboratory's experience with solid-phase immunoassay, we were interested in protein adsorption on PDMS because of its potential consequences in human medicine. We used very low protein concentrations to investigate protein-silicone interactions so that monolayer formation and its consequences could be evaluated. This approach is similar to studying solid-phase antigen-antibody reactions, but considers the polymeric surface the receptor[2] (e.g. antibody) and the protein to be adsorbed as the ligand (i.e. antigen).

Materials and Methods

We selected two pair of soluble proteins, the members of each pair sharing similar structure and homologous sequences but differing in their mean pI. The protein pairs selected were lactoferrin (pI = 7.9); transferrin (pI = 5.3) and bovine IgG2a (pI = 8.5) and bovine IgG1 (pI = 6.0). In addition to these proteins, we also used human IgG purified in our laboratory from pooled human serum (Butler et al., 1990).

All proteins used to study adsorption, as well as some antibodies or antibody fragments used to detect them (see below), were iodinated with ^{125}I-Na using methods previously described in our laboratory (Koertge and Butler, 1985; Dierks et al., 1986). Adsorption reached equilibrium after 4 hr at 37° on both Immulon 2 Removawells (Imm 2; Dynatech, Chantilley, VA, which served as a comparative standard) and on "silicone microtiter wells" fabricated from 6.5 mm tubing and from bases punched from flat sheets of the same material. The tubing and flat sheets were provided by Dow-Corning, Midland, MI and are of the same chemistry used to make the envelope of the silicone-gel filled breast implants. This PDMS elastomer is hereafter designated PEP (Platinum catalyzed elastomer of polydimethylsiloxane). Adsorption was conducted at pH 4.0, 5.5, 7.0 8.5 and 10 at physiological ionic strength (9.0 mSiemans) or at 0.9 mS or 90 mS. In some studies, a plasma-discharged version of PEP (PD-PEP) was used to determine the role played by polar hydroxyl group in adsorption to PEP. In certain adsorption studies, adsorptions were conducted at physiological pH and ionic strength but in a solution which contained 0.05% Tween-20. This configuration simulates conditions used to measure human antibodies to the silicone elastomer by ELISA.

Following incubation to permit passive adsorption, the supernatant was collected and counted and all wells were washed through several cycles, each cycle consisting of four rapid fillings and aspirations followed by a 15 min. soak period. All washings were collected, pooled and counted. Washing was considered adequate when steady-state desorption was reached. Stably adsorbed protein was determined by separating and counting the individual wells. In some experiments, the desorption of stably adsorbed proteins was studied over a 16 hr period by collecting the supernatant after the wells had been incubated with PBS or PBS containing 20 μg/ml of free ligand.

The avidity of protein adsorption was calculated from Langmuir plots and/or expressed from percent bound plots (Fig. 1). The percentage of any ligand which becomes bound to its adsorbed receptor, when the latter is in excess (linear binding region; LBR) is a relative measure of the avidity[3] of the interaction (Joshi et al 1992).

The antigenicity of adsorbed IgG was measured by both ELISA and RIA, the latter using both intact ^{125}I-anti-IgG and its ^{125}I-Fab.

The surface architecture of PEP and Imm 2 was compared by atomic force microscopy (AFM) using a Digital Instruments NanoScope operated in the Tapping Mode™ (Martin et al., 1987).

The Avidity of Proteins for PEP

The avidity of lactoferrin and transferrin for PEP, PD-PEP and Imm 2 under various conditions is expressed in Figure 1. The data show that the avidity of PEP for both proteins is optimal at physiological pH and ionic strength (9.0 mS). Raising the ionic strength promotes more avid binding of both proteins to Imm 2, especially above their pIs, which is consistent with a classic hydrophobic effect (Tanford, 1973). In contrast to Imm 2, increasing the ionic strength and pH did not increase the avidity of these proteins for PEP and at pH 10, significantly decreased their avidity. This suggested that polar silanol groups may contribute to the initial binding and might especially inhibit adsorption of both lactoferrin and transferrin at a pH above their pIs. This hypothesis was tested using PD-PEP which is rich in silanol groups, The use of PD-PEP resulted in a significantly lower avidity of both protein at neutral and alkaline pH, especially at high ionic strength. This is consistent with the hypothesis that while both proteins avidly adsorb to both polystyrene and PEP, polar groups are more important in the initial recognition events on PEP than on Imm 2. The data of Figure 1 demonstrate that under physiological conditions, the pI of the protein has little or no effect on the avidity of adsorption indicating that hydrophobic bonding was the major force in passive adsorption to both surfaces.

When the adsorption of the second protein pair (IgG2a/IgG1) was studied, we again failed to see any effect of pI but again observed that adsorption on PEP was optimal at physiological pH and ionic strength. Whereas the avidity of transferrin/lactoferrin was similar for PEP and Imm 2 (Fig. 1), the avidity of both IgGs was circa 40% lower for PEP than for Imm 2 (data not shown).

When the Langmuir equation was employed to estimate the point of saturation and the Keq, the data in Table 1 were obtained. The saturation point data for lactoferrin and IgG1 on Imm 2 provided values for the area occupied by a single molecule at saturation the size of which is consistent with monolayer formation. However, the corresponding values for lactoferrin and IgG1 on PEP

---

[3] We consider all polymer-protein interactions to involve multiple binding sites, thus avidity would appear to be the correct term for the measured equilibrium constant (Keq).

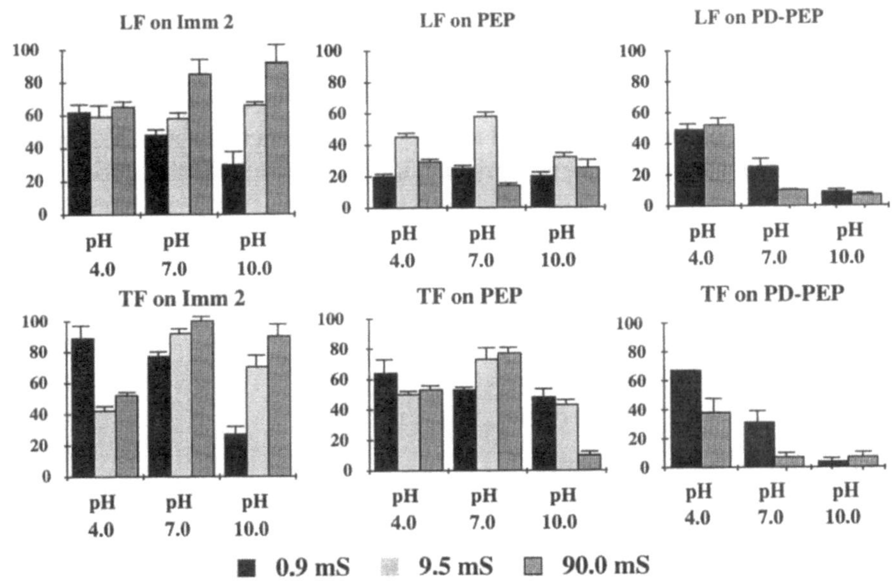

Fig. 1. The avidity of lactoferrin (LF) and transferrin (TF) for Imm 2, PEP or PD-PEP expressed as the mean percent bound in the LBR.

Table 1. Avidity Constants (Keq) and Surface Area Occupied by Single Molecules at Saturation on Imm 2 and PEP Surfaces

Protein	Surface	Keq m^{-1} e7	Area (nm^2) occupied by a single molecule at saturation
Lactoferrin	Imm 2	1.07 ± 0.12	22.66 ± 1.26
Lactoferrin	PEP	3.91 ± 0.45	60.67 ± 1.91
IgG1	Imm 2	15.84 ± 4.8	66.7 ± 4.6
IgG1	PEP	6.8 ± 0.44	108.9 ± 1.49

suggested that much less than a monolayer had formed at saturation. This prompted us to undertake studies on dissociation, to investigate multilayer formation and to comparatively examine the surface architecture of both Imm 2 and PEP using AFM.

Dissociation Analysis and Multilayer Adsorption

The percent bound data in Figure 1 suggest that passive adsorption is reversible because less than 100% of the protein added in the region of excess receptor (polymer surface) becomes stably adsorbed. This was further confirmed in monolayer desorption studies which showed a steady but slow desorption over

16 hr from both PEP and Imm 2 (Fig. 2A). The observation that free ligand promotes desorption is considered further evidence that adsorption is not irreversible as had been proposed (Bornzin & Miller, 1982) but follows the Law of Mass Action for a high avidity interaction with a very slow off rate.

Evidence from saturation analyses using Langmuir plots (Table 1) that a monolayer had not initially formed on PEP at low protein concentration, plus the fact that silicone prostheses *in vivo* would be exposed to protein concentration >1000-fold greater than in the studies reported in Figures 1 and 2A, prompted us to investigate the formation of multilayers on both PEP and Imm 2. These studies were conducted by allowing unlabelled IgG to become adsorbed as a "monolayer", washing the coated surface and then incubating the surface with the same concentration of cold or ^{125}I-labeled IgG. The last incubation was always done with labeled IgG.

These experiments showed that additional IgG became adsorbed to both surfaces after each incubation but that this was 2-fold greater on PEP than on Imm 2. When the dissociation of these "multilayers" was studied, data indicated that while each successive layer of protein adsorbed to Imm 2 had a correspondingly higher rate of dissociation, no difference in desorption rate was observed after four successive incubations with PEP (Fig. 2B).

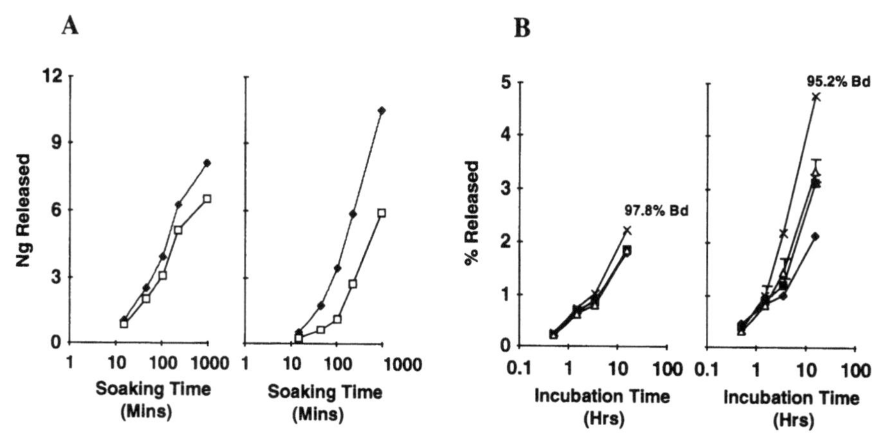

Fig. 2. A. The dissociation of the IgG monolayer from PEP or Imm 2 in the presence (•) or absence (□) of free ligand. B. Dissociation of multilayers successively adsorbed to PEP and Imm 2 expressed as the proportion of stably adsorbed protein released. The amount of the fourth layer remaining bound is given.

Atomic Force Microscopy

Figure 3 shows the surface topography of PEP and Imm 2. PEP appears to be highly textured and to have a considerably greater surface area than Imm 2. The "wind row" pattern seen for polystyrene is typical for this material (Svend-Erik Rasmussen, personal comm.).

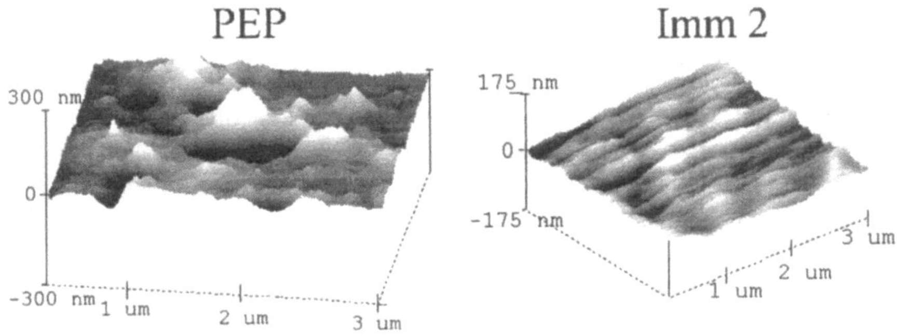

Fig. 3. The surface topography of PEP (left) and Imm 2 (right). Images are for 3μm squares obtained by AFM in the Tapping Mode. Note that the maximum surface height depicted (z axis) is 175 nm for Imm 2 but 300 nm for PEP.

The Antigenic Behavior of Adsorbed IgG

Figure 4 (top) compares the antigenicity of IgG2a and IgG1 by ELISA after adsorption on Imm 2 or PEP or after immobilization by a non-adsorptive method utilizing a streptavidin bridge (SA-PS). The amount of IgG immobilized in every case was determined from its radioactivity. IgG2a was detected using a polyclonal antibody and IgG1 using a monoclonal antibody. In all situations, protein adsorbed on Imm 2 was more antigenically detectable than when adsorbed on PEP. Non-adsorbed IgG1 (SA-PS) was most detectable.

Figure 4 (bottom) compares the antigenicity of adsorbed IgG2a using an RIA to eliminate the possible steric hindrance that might have explained the ELISA results in Figure 4 (top). Data obtained using ^{125}I-intact anti-IgG also distinguished between the antigenicity of IgG2 adsorbed on PEP and IgG2a adsorbed Imm 2. When the ^{125}I-Fab of anti-IgG was used, the detectability of IgG on Imm 2 was improved but not its detectability on PEP.

Adsorption of IgG in the Presence of a Non-ionic Detergent

The avidity of PEP for protein shown here (Fig. 1) and by others, as well as the reports of anti-silicone antibodies by Heggers (1992), Goldblum et al. (1992) and Wolf et al. (1993), in which antibody binding to PDMS was detectable in the presence of a non-ionic detergent, prompted us to investigate whether normal IgG had a relatively higher avidity for PEP than Imm 2 in the presence of detergent. Results of these tests are shown in Figure 5. Data indicate that when IgG is added at >15000 ng/well (30 μg/ml) it shows significantly greater adsorption to PEP than to Imm 2. The range from 1500-6000 ng/well of added IgG corresponds to 1:400, 1:200 and 1:100 dilutions of normal human serum, respectively.

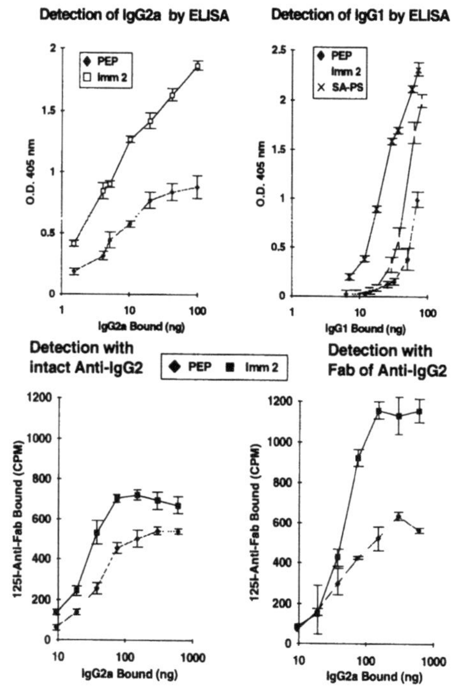

Fig. 4. The detection of IgG2a and IgG1 adsorbed as a monolayer on Imm 2 and PEP or immobilized non-adsorptively (SA-PS). TOP - Detection by ELISA. BOTTOM - Detection of IgG2a by ^{125}I-polyclonal anti-IgG or its ^{125}I-Fab.

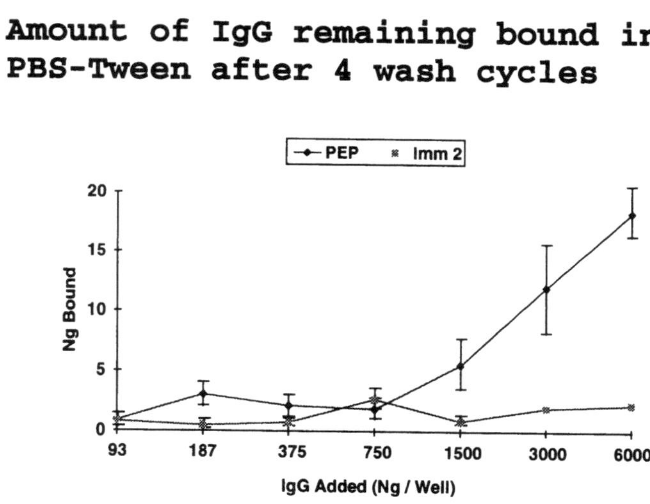

Fig. 5. Iodinated human IgG incubated over a range of concentration with PEP or Imm 2 polystyrene for 4 hr at 37°C. Wells were then washed through four cycles with PBS-Tween, counted and the bound radioactivity converted to ng of bound human IgG.

Discussion

The adsorption data presented here indicate that: (1) the avidity of globular proteins for PEP is generally similar to their avidity for a solid-phase adsorptive surface (Imm 2) that is widely used in immunoassay, (2) adsorption is optimal at physiological conditions, (3) polar interactions may be more important in initial binding to PEP than to Imm 2, (4) passive adsorption appears to be a reversible, hydrophobic interaction with a very slow off-rate, (5) the isoelectric point of proteins appears to play little or no role in the amount stably adsorbed and (6) saturation analyses of PEP suggests that the surface does not initially saturate with a protein monolayer. The data from AFM suggests that the apparent greater surface area of PEP, should have adsorbed more protein than Imm 2 at saturation. This is supported by the studies showing a similar desorption rate for each successive layer adsorbed (Fig. 2B) suggesting that protein from the first four incubations was directly adsorbing to PEP. This contrasts with the results of multilayer desorption studies on Imm 2 in which a progressive increase in dissociation was observed with each layer bound suggesting that after saturation during the first incubation (the monolayer) subsequent adsorptions involve protein-protein versus protein-polymer interactions.

The antigenic studies are both surprising and confusing. That non-adsorbed IgG is most detectable (Fig. 5, Upper Right) is consistent with all previously studies which have reported the loss of antigenicity when proteins are adsorbed on synthetic surfaces (see reviews by Butler, 1991b; Butler, 1995). Surprising is the large difference between the antigenicity of protein adsorbed on PEP versus Imm 2. While the highly textured surface of PEP might suggest that steric hindrance could be a factor on this surface when an ELISA is used for detection, the use of ^{125}I-Fab of anti-IgG failed to resolve the difference. However, it should be recalled that the protein "monolayer" on PEP tested in these studies was apparently not a true monolayer (see above). Thus, these results might be explained by the results of a previous study in our laboratory that showed when protein antigens are adsorbed at sub-monolayer concentrations, they are less detectable, probably as a result of greater conformational change due to the space available (Dierks et al., 1986). The *in vivo* significance of data in Figure 4 is in any case, questionable, because PEP *in vivo* would be exposed to much higher levels of protein such that a "true" monolayer is likely to form. Recent data from our laboratory suggest that the antigenicity of IgG on PEP following multiple incubations to yield true surface saturation, does not differ from the antigenicity of the Imm 2 monolayer (Lü et al., 1995).

The avidity of IgG for PEP is such that this protein is also able to overcome the blocking effects of non-ionic detergent when incubated at high concentration with the silicone elastomer. Thus, at serum dilutions used by others to detect anti-silicone antibodies (Heggers, 1992; Goldblum et al., 1992; Wolfe et al., 1993), normal human IgG readily adsorbs to the silicone elastomer.

In summary, silicone elastomers used in medical prosthesis, have an avidity for protein adsorption under physiological conditions which is similar to that of polystyrene widely used for solid-phase immunoassay. Adsorption to the elastomer at sub-saturating concentration results in reduced antigenicity compared to non-adsorbed protein. While the current data demonstrate the loss of antigenicity for IgGs adsorbed on both PEP and Imm 2, they do not demonstrate the expression of new, non-native epitopes; such evidence is necessary to support the hypothesis that antigenic alteration of host protein on medical prostheses results in an autoimmune phenomenon. Whether the more pronounced antigenic changes we observed at sub-saturating levels on PEP could have any *in vivo* significance because of the very high *in vivo* protein concentration., remains to be demonstrated.

The extraordinary avidity of proteins for PDMS elastomers, the vigorous washing procedures needed to study this adsorption, the adsorption of protein even in the presence of Tween-20 (Fig. 5) and the complication which may be imposed by a highly textured hydrophobic surface, create physical-chemical and technical problems which could delay a final resolution as to whether hydrophobic adsorption of host proteins by silicone medical prostheses *in vivo* has any negative medical effects.

References

Bornzin GA, Miller IF (1982) The kinetics of protein adsorption on synthetics and modified natural surfaces. J Coll Interface Sci 86:539-558

Butler JE, Spradling JE, Peterman JH, Joshi SK, Challacombe SJ (1990) Humoral immunity in root caries in an elderly population. I. Establishment of a reliable approach for measuring specific antibodies in serum and saliva, their specific activities, rate of salivary secretion and relationship to other, salivary protein. Oral Microbial Immunol 5:98-107

Butler JE (1991a) Immunochemistry of solid-phase immunoassays.(ed) CRC Press, Boca Raton, Fl 319 pp.

Butler JE (1991b) The behavior of antigens and antibodies immobilized on a solid-phase. In: Van Regenmortel MHV (ed) Structure of antigens. Vol. 1, CRC Press, Boca Raton, FL, pp 209-258

Butler JE, Ni L, Brown WR, Rosenberg B, Chang J, Voss EW Jr (1993) The immunochemistry of sandwich ELISAs VI Greater than ninety percent of monoclonal and seventy-five percent of polyclonal antifluorescyl capture antibodies (CAbs) are denatured by passive desorption. Mol Immunol 30:1165-1175

Butler JE (1995) Solid-phases in immunoassay. In: Diamandis EP, Christopoulos TK (ed) Textbook of immunological assay. Amer Assoc Clin Chem Press (In press)

Bull HB (1956) Adsorption of bovine serum albumin on glass. Biochim Biophys Acta 19:464-471

Catt K, Tregear GW (1967) Solid-phase radioimmunoassay in antibody-coated tubes. Science 158:1570-1572

Darst SA, Robertson CR, Berzofsky JA (1988) Adsorption of the protein antigen myoglobin affects the binding of conformation-specific monoclonal antibodies. J Biophysical Society 53:533-825

Dierks SE, Butler JE, Richerson HB (1986) Altered recognition of surface-adsorbed compared to antigen bound antibodies in the ELISA. Mol Immunol 23:403-411

Goldblum RM, Pelley RP, O'Donnell AA, Pyron D, Heggers JP (1992) Antibodies to silicone elastomers and reactions to ventriculoperitoneal shunts. Lancet 340:510-513

Heggers JP (1992) Immunology of Silicone. Presented at Toxicology Forum Washington DC. 16 Feb. 1992

Joshi KS, Hoffmann LG, Butler JE (1992) The immunochemistry of sandwich ELISA V The capture antibody performance of polyclonal antibody-enriched fractions prepared by various methods. Mol Immunol 20:971-981

Kochwa S, Brownell M, Rosenfield RE, Wasserman LR (1967) Adsorption of proteins by polystyrene particles I Molecular unfolding and acquired immunogenicity of IgG. J Immunol 99:981-986.

Koertge TE, Butler JE (1985) The relationship between the binding of primary antibody in solid-phase microtiter assays and its detection using ELISA technology. J Immunol Meth 83:283-299

Lü EP, Navarro P, Djavadi L, Butler JE (1995) Protein antigens adsorbed on silicone are poorly recognized compared to when adsorbed on polystyrene. FASEB J. 9:A1030 Abstr. 5968.

Martin Y, Williams CC, Wickramasinghe HK (1989) Atomic force microscope-force mapping and profiling on a 100-Å scale. J Appl Phys 61:4723-4729.

Murthy KD, Diwan AR, Simons SR, Albrecht RM, Cooper SL (1987) Utilization of immunogold to compare the adsorption behavior of fibrnogen, fibronectin and albumin on polymers. Scan Micros 2:765-773

Oreskes I, Singer JM (1961) The mechanism of particulate carrier reactions. Adsorption of human γ-globulin to polystyrene latex particles. J Immunol 86:338-344.

Pankowsky DA, Ziats NP, Topham NS, Ratnoff OD, Anderson JM (1990) Morphologic characteristics of adsorbed human plasma proteins on vascular grafts and biomaterials. J Vasc Surg 11:599-606

Tanford C (1973) The hydrophobic effect: formation of micelles and biological membranes. John Wiley and Sons, New York. 200 pp

Tilton RD, Robertson CR, Gast AP (1990) Lateral diffusion of bovine serum albumin adsorbed at the solid-liquid interface. J Coll Interface Sci 137:192-203

Wolf LE, Lappe M, Peterson RD, Ezrailson EG (1993) Human immune response to polydimethylsiloxane (silicone): screening studies in a breast implant population. FASEB J 7:1265-1268.

Young BR, Pitt WG, Cooper SL (1988a) Protein adsorption on polymeric biomaterials. I. Adsorption isotherms. J Coll Interface Sci 124:28-43

Young BR, Pitt WG, Cooper SL (1988b) Protein adsorption on polymeric biomaterials. II. Adsorption kinetics. J Coll Interface Sci 125:246-260

Ziats NP, Pankowsky DA, Tierney BP, Ratnoff OD, Anderson JM (1990) Adsorption of Hageman factor (factor XII) and of the plasma proteins to biomedical polymers. J Lab Clin Med 116:687-696

Aspecific Immunoglobulin Binding to Hydrophobic Surfaces

C. J. van Oss and J.O. Naim[1,2]
Department of Microbiology, SUNY at Buffalo, Buffalo, NY and [1] Department of Surgery, Rochester General Hospital, Rochester, NY

Introduction

It is virtually impossible to discriminate between aspecific adsorption of immunoglobulins to hydrophobic surfaces and the putative specific binding of "anti-silicone antibodies" to such surfaces. The predicament is that hydrophobic (low energy) materials (e.g., silicones) will avidly adsorb, to their surfaces, most proteins (e.g., immunoglobulins) from an aqueous medium. Therefore the problem with developing a reliable immunoassay for the detection of putative anti-silicone antibodies is to control for the aspecfic binding of immunoglobulins. This study demonstrates that when employing an ELISA method for the detection of serum anti-silicone antibodies from a patient with an elevated IgG level, one can easily misinterpret the aspecfic binding of immunoglobulin as specific binding of anti-silicone antibodies.

Theory

Hydrophobic Interactions between Low-energy Molecules, Immersed in Water

The theory of the mechanism governing the "hydrophobic" attraction between low-energy molecules, immersed in water has long been enveloped in obfuscation. This is partly a consequence of the perceived meaning of the word "hydrophobic", and partly a result of the fact that the mechanism of hydrophobic interactions is not intuitively obvious. It should be stated from the outset that low-energy ("hydrophobic") molecules *do not fear or repel water*: they *attract* water molecules with considerable energy (from 40 to about 112 mJ/m^2); only hydrophilic molecules attract water more strongly (usually from 113 to 145 mJ/m^2). Hydrophobic interactions between low-energy molecules, immersed in water are solely imputable to the hydrogen binding [Lewis acid-base (AB)] energy of cohesion between the water molecules surrounding the low-energy molecules or particles. The polar, or Lewis acid-base free energy, ΔG_{1w1}^{AB} , of hydrogen bonding interaction between molecules (1) immersed in water (w) can be expressed as [1-4]:

$$\Delta G_{1w1}^{AB} = 4(\sqrt{\gamma_1^+ \gamma_w^-} + \sqrt{\gamma_1^- \gamma_w^+} - \sqrt{\gamma_1^+ \gamma_1^-} - \sqrt{\gamma_w^+ \gamma_w^-}) \qquad (1)$$

[2] The second author has provided expert testimony and consulting services on behalf of plaintiffs relating to silicone breast implant litigation. This work was supported by NIH grant No. AI-34597.

where γ_i^+ is the electron-acceptor and γ_i^- the electron donor parameter of the solid, or liquid, material, i.

The polar free energy, ΔG_{1w1}^{AB}, is always accompanied by a (usually fairly small) Lifshitz-van der Waals (LW) attraction:

$$\Delta G_{1W1}^{LW} = -2(\sqrt{\gamma_1^{LW}} - \sqrt{\gamma_w^{LW}})^2 \tag{2}$$

In the absence of strong electrostatic charges, the total interaction energy then is [1-4]:

$$\Delta G_{1w1}^{TOT} = \Delta G_{1w1}^{LW} + \Delta G_{1w1}^{AB} \tag{3}$$

The apolar (LW), together with the polar (γ^+ and γ^-) surface tension parameters can be determined by contact angle measurements with liquids, L, on a flat surface S, using the following version of Young's equation [1-4]:

$$(1+\cos\theta)\gamma_L = 2(\sqrt{\gamma_L^{LW}\gamma_S^{LW}} + \sqrt{\gamma_L^+\gamma_S^-} + \sqrt{\gamma_L^-\gamma_S^+}) \tag{4}$$

Where θ is the measured contact angle in degrees, and γ_L the total surface tension of the liquid used, so that:

$$\gamma_L = \gamma_L^{LW} + \gamma_L^{AB} \tag{5}$$

where:

$$\gamma_L^{AB} = 2\sqrt{\gamma_L^+\gamma_L^-} \tag{6}$$

Contact angles should be measured with at least three different liquids, of which two must be polar, using equation 4 three times, to solve for the three unknowns, $\gamma_S^{LW}, \gamma_S^+$ and γ_S^- [1-4], where subscript S represents, e.g., the hydrophobic material, 1, used in eqs. 1-3, above. The strongest hydrophobic interaction energy one normally encounters is that between completely apolar molecules such as alkanes, in water, where ΔG_{1w1}^{AB} = -102 mJ/m^2 (which is equal to the hydrogen-bonding free energy of cohesion of water: ΔG_{ww}^{AB} = -102 mJ/m^2).

Hydrophobic Interaction between a Hydrophobic surface and Hydrophilic Molecules, in Water

Hydrophobic surfaces also exert a "hydrophobic" attraction on hydrophilic molecules, in water. That attraction is not as strong as the attraction between two hydrophobic entities, in water, but it is by no means negligible.

The interaction between two different (condensed-phase) entities (1 and 2) in water (w) can be described by Dupré's equation [1-4]:

$$\Delta G_{1w2} = \gamma_{12} - \gamma_{1w} - \gamma_{2w} \tag{7}$$

where $\gamma_{ij} = -\frac{1}{2}\Delta G_{ikj}^{TOT}$ (cf. eq.3). Upon insertion of the appropriate γ_{ij}- parameters eq. 7 becomes:

$$\begin{aligned}\Delta G_{1w2} = (\sqrt{\gamma_1^{LW}} - \sqrt{\gamma_2^{LW}})^2 - (\sqrt{\gamma_1^{LW}} - \sqrt{\gamma_w^{LW}})^2 - (\sqrt{\gamma_2^{LW}} - \sqrt{\gamma_w^{LW}})^2 \\ +2[\sqrt{\gamma_w^+}(\sqrt{\gamma_1^-} + \sqrt{\gamma_2^-} - \sqrt{\gamma_w^-}) \\ +\sqrt{\gamma_w^-}(\sqrt{\gamma_1^+} + \sqrt{\gamma_2^+} - \sqrt{\gamma_w^+}) - \sqrt{\gamma_1^+\gamma_2^-} - \sqrt{\gamma_1^-\gamma_2^+}]\end{aligned} \tag{8}$$

A negative value for ΔG_{1w2} indicates a net attraction.

Methods and Materials

Surface Properties of Silicones and IgG

Contact angles were measured with different liquids on a silicone elastomer sheet (from an unused McGhan breast implant): $\theta_{\alpha\text{-bromonapthalene}} = 86.4°$; $\theta_{\text{diiodomethane}} = 93.4°$; $\theta_{\text{water}} = 111.7°$; $\theta_{\text{glycerol}} = 115.3°$; $\theta_{\text{formamide}} = 105.7°$; $\theta_{\text{ethylene glycol}} = 98.0°$. From these data, using eq. 4, the surface tension parameters for silicone (1) were obtained (in mJ/m^2): $\gamma_1^{LW} = 12$, $\gamma_1^+ = 0.016$, $\gamma_1^- = 1.72$ mJ/m^2.

From earlier measurements, the surface tension parameters for hydrated human IgG were[4,5]: $\gamma_2^{LW} = 34$; $\gamma_2^+ = 1.5$; $\gamma_2^- = 49.6$ mJ/m^2. For water[1-4] (also in mJ/m^2): $\gamma_w^{LW} = 21.8$; $\gamma_w^+ = 25.5$; $\gamma_w^- = 25.5$.

Test serum

The serum of a male patient with multiple myeloma whose total IgG was **8,740 mg/dl** was used as the test serum. The monoclonal IgG isotype from this serum was IgG1.

Control serum

The serum of a healthy male volunteer whose total IgG was **1,080 mg/dl** was used as the control serum.

Silicone antigen preparation

Silicone elastomer from an unused mammary implant shell (McGhan Medical, Santa Barbara, CA) was used as the antigen. The silicone elastomer was cleaned thoroughly with acetone and handled with gloved hands. The silicone sheeting was cut to fit snugly at the bottom of a 96 well flat bottom tissue culture treated polystyrene plate (Corning Glass Works, Corning, NY) using a skin punch biopsy tool.

ELISA Protocol

Fifty microliters of serum were diluted with 0.05% Tween in PBS (PBST), added to each well and incubated at room temperature for 2 hr. The plate was washed 3 times with water and 100 µl of blocking solution (1% BSA in PBST) were added and incubated at room temperture for 30 min. The plate was again washed 3 times and 50 µl of goat anti-human IgG (H +L) alkaline phosphatase conjugate (diluted 1:1000 in PBST) were added to each well and incubated at room temp. for 1 hr. The plate was washed 3 times with water and 100 µl of p-nitrophenyl phosphate (1mg/ml) substrate were added to each well and incubated for 20 min. The color reaction was stopped with 100 µl of 3N NaOH, the reaction solution was transferred to a clean 96 well plate and the absorbance measured at 405 nm by means of a microtiter plate reader. The results were expressed as the ratio of the OD of the test serum vs. the OD of the control serum at each dilution.

Results

Table 1 shows the relative IgG binding to silicone elastomer and polystyrene expressed as the ratio of the optical density (OD) reading at each serum dilution of the test serum vs. control serum.

Table 1. Relative IgG binding to silicone and polystyrene

Dilution	Silicone	Polystyrene
1:50	1.6*	2.8
1:100	1.9	2.8
1:200	1.2	3.1
1:400	16.7	3.1
1:800	4.5	2.3
1:1600	9.0	3.1
1:3200	1.7	2.1

*Ratio of the OD of the test serum vs. control serum.

Figures 1 and 2 shows the actual OD readings vs. the diluted serum for silicone and polystyrene.

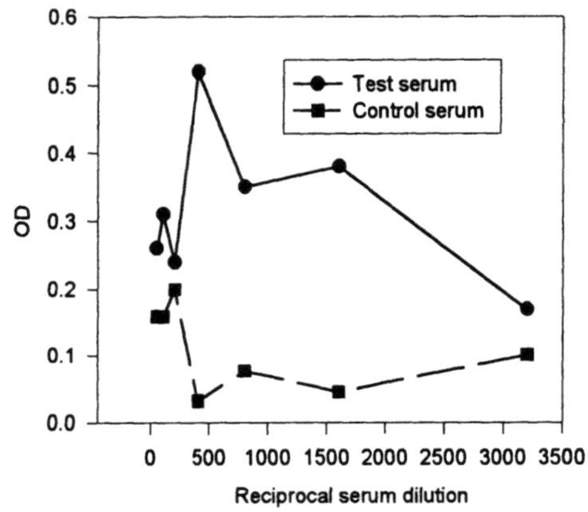

Fig. 1. IgG binding to silicone elastomer.

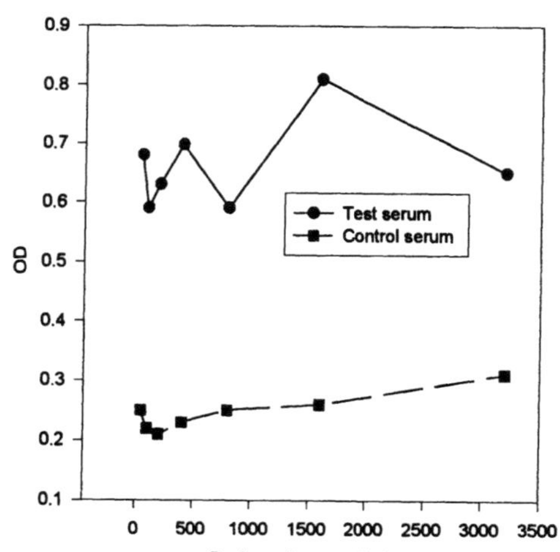

Fig. 2. IgG binding to tissue culture grade polystyrene

Discussion

From the surface properties of silicones and IgG and using eq. 8, it follows that for the interaction of human IgG (2) with silicone surfaces (1), immersed in water (w),

$$\Delta G_{1w2}^{TOT} = +2.8(\Delta G_{1w2}^{LW}) - 11.6(\Delta G_{1w2}^{AB})$$
$$= \mathbf{-8.8\ mJ/m^2}$$

It is interesting to note that there is in this case a net weak van der Waals (LW) *repulsion*, counter balanced by a much stronger "hydrophobic" (AB) *attraction*, yielding a net attraction of 8.8 mJ/m^2 . To translate that attraction into free energy per protein molecule (IgG) interacting with a silicone surface, an assumption has to be made about the contactable surface area (Sc) of the IgG molecule, attaching to silicone. It is reasonable to suppose that Sc lies somewhere between 10 and 20 nm^2 Table 2 shows the values of ΔG and the corresponding equilibrium association constant (Ka), following:

$$\Delta G_{1w2}^{TOT} \cdot Sc / kT = -\ln Ka \qquad (9)$$

Where Ka is expressed in inverse mole fractions, (one mole fraction = 0.018 L/mole) and kT = 4.04 x 10^{21} J (at 20°C). As the typical binding constants[6] (Ka) for antigen-antibody reaction range from 10^6-10^{11} L/mole, it is clear from Table 2 that the aspecific bond between IgG and silicone is at least as strong, and in most cases probably stronger, than antigen-antibody bonds.

Table 2. ΔG_{1w2}^{TOT} values for IgG adsorbing onto silicone, for contactable surface (Sc) values from 10 to 20 nm^2, in units of kT and kcal/mole, as well as the corresponding equilibrium association constants, in L/mole.

Sc (nm^2)	ΔG_{1w2} (kT)	ΔG_{1w2} (kcal/mole)	Ka[a] (L/mole)
10	-21.78	-12.6	5.2 x 10^7
12	-26.14	-15.2	4.1 x 10^9
15	-32.67	-19.0	2.8 x 10^{12}
20	-43.56	-25.3	1.5 x 10^{17}

[a] 1 L/mole = 0.018 (mole fractions) $^{-1}$.

There are a few rules that apply to the aspecific adsorption of proteins from aqueous solutions:

1. As can be seen from most Langmuir-type adsorption isotherms, the higher the protein concentration, the stronger the adsorption; see, e.g., MacRitchie[7].

2. Less hydrophophilic proteins adsorb more strongly onto hydrophobic surfaces than more hydrophilic proteins[7,8].

3. The proteins with the lowest surface potential (i.e., proteins close to their isoelectric point) adsorb more strongly, even to uncharged hydrophobic surfaces, than more charged proteins[7,9]. It should be noted that IgG is the serum protein with the lowest surface potential (hence its original designation as γ- globulin).

Two more points that pertain especially to human IgG:

4. The Fc moiety is the most hydrophobic part of IgG; Fab chains are much more hydrophilic than Fc[10].

5. Judging by the fact that only IgG1 and IgG3 adsorb onto polystyrene particles from whole serum[8,11], it may be concluded that IgG1 and IgG3 are more hydrophobic than IgG2 and IgG4[8]. It should also be noted that (of the human IgG's) only IgG1 and IgG3 are aspecific[8] as well as specific opsonins[12], which can bind to Fc receptors on phagocytic cells.

6. IgM is more hydrophilic than IgG, and IgA is the most hydrophilic of the human immunoglobulins[10]. The extreme hydrophilicity of IgA precludes the use of reversed phase liquid chromatography for its purification. To purify IgA salt mediated hydrophobic chromatography has to be resorted to[13].

Conclusion

In view of the fact that IgG aspecifically binds to silicone surfaces with a high binding energy, the possibility of specific antibody formation to silicones (and other low energy molecules) can be ruled out. This is because when *all* Ig moieties on B cells can bind to low-energy (hydrophobic) molecules, particles or surfaces, there is no selection for the emergence of any paratope that is *specific* for a given low-energy epitope. Thus it is not possible for specific anti-hydrophobic antibodies to be selectively elicited. There also is no need for them, because all Ig's (and most other proteins) bind to hydrophobic molecules anyway.

References

1. van Oss, C.J., R.J. Good and M.K. Chaudhury. (1988) Additive and non-additive surface tension components and the interpretation of contact angles. Langmuir 4: 884-891.
2. van Oss, C.J., M.K. Chaudhury and R.J. Good. (1988) Interfacial Lifshitz-van der Waals and polar interactions in macroscopic systems. Chem. Rev. 88: 927-941.
3. van Oss, C.J. (1993) Acid-base interfacial interactions in aqueous media. Colloids Surfaces A-78: 1-49.
4. van Oss, C.J. (1994) *Interfacial Forces in Aqueous Media*, Marcel Dekker, New York.
5. van Oss, C.J., R.J. Good and M.K. Chandhury. (1986) Solubility of proteins. J. Protein Chem. 5:385-405.
6. van Regenmortel, M.H.V. and A. Azimzadeh. (1994) Determination of antibody affinity. in: *Immunochemistry*, C.J. van Oss and M.H.V. van Regenmortel, Eds., Marcel Dekker, New York, pp. 805-828.
7. MacRitchie, F.(1972) The adsorption of proteins at the solid liquid interface. J. Colloid Interface Sci. 38:484-488.
8. Absolom, D.R., C.J. van Oss, W. Zingg and A.W. Neumann. (1982) Phagocytosis as a surface phenomenon: opsonization by aspecific adsorption of IgG as a function of bacterial hydrophobicity. RES-J. Reticuloendothelial Soc. 31:59-70.
9. van Oss, C.J. and J.M. Singer. (1966) The binding of immune globulins and other proteins by polystyrene latex particles. RES-J. Reticuloendothelial Soc. 3:29-40.
10. van Oss, C.J., C.F. Gillman and A.W. Neumann. (1975) *Phagocytic Engulfment and Cell Adhesiveness*. Marcel Dekker, New York, pp. 37-39.

11. Weening, R.S., D. Roos, C.M.R. Weemaes, J.W.T. Homan-Müller and M.L.J. van Schaik. (1976) Defective initiation of the metabolic stimulation of phagocytizing granulocytes: a new congenital defect. J. Lab Clin. Med. 88:757-768.
12. Nisonoff, A., J.E. Hopper and S.B. Spring. (1975) *The Antibody Molecule*. Academic Press, New York, pp. 96-97.
13. Doellgast, G.J. and A.G. Plaut. (1976) Purification of human IgA by salt-mediated hydrophobic chromatography. Immunochem. 13:135-139.

Cytotoxicity and Membrane Damage *in vitro* by Inclusion Complexes Between γ-Cyclodextrin and Siloxanes

K. Felix [1, 2], S. Janz [2], J. Pitha [3], J. A. Williams [4], E. B. Mushinski [2], G. W. Bornkamm [1] and M. Potter [2]

[1] Institut für Klinische Molekularbiologie und Tumorgenetik, Hämatologikum, GSF, München, Germany, [2] Laboratory of Genetics, NCI, NIH, Bethesda, MD, [3] Macromolecular Chemistry Section, NIA, NIH, Baltimore, MD, [4] Laboratory of Immunology, FDA, NIH, Bethesda, MD

Abstract

Inclusion complexes of γ-cyclodextrin and octamethylcyclotetrasiloxane (D4), decamethyltetrasiloxane (M10TS), and 1,3,5,7-tetramethyltetravinylcyclotetrasiloxane (TMTV-D4) were prepared to compare the cytotoxic effects of siloxanes *in vitro*. In these preparations, the hydrophobic siloxanes are surrounded by a hydrophilic shell of eight circularly linked D-glucose molecules (γ-cyclodextrin), and upon contact with plasma membranes the siloxane molecule can intercalate into the lipid bilayer of the cell membrane. XRPC24, 2-11 plasmacytoma, CH12.LX lymphoma and P388D1 macrophage-like cells were used as indicator cells in toxicity assays. Using an MTT tetrazolium reduction to formazan test, a colorimetric method to determine the number of viable cells, the 50% minimal lethal doses (CD_{50}) for the siloxane compounds were found to range from 30 to 50 μM. Sublethal doses (e.g., 15 μM and lower) resulted in the loss of lactate dehydrogenase (LDH) and glutathione (GSH) from the cytosolic compartment of the target cells and thus indicated cytotoxicity.Treatment of macrophages with siloxanes resulted in a higher production of interleukin-6 (IL-6) than was exhibited by untreated macrophages. The B9 cell bioassay of these treated cells showed as much as a 10 fold higher production (500 U/ml) of IL-6 than did the untreated cells. The degree of increase was dependent on the compound and concentration used. The results of this study show that low molecular weight siloxanes produce lethal effects on B-lymphocyte derived target cells *in vitro* and permeabilize the plasma membranes at lower sublethal concentrations.

Introduction

Our knowledge on the biochemistry of silicone and organosilicone compounds such as siloxanes is limited. The fate of ingested siloxanes, their *in vivo* degradation and bioavailability are but a few areas that require further elucidation. Silicones are being used ubiquitously, and they are commonly available as fluids, oils, rubbers or resins. Silicone compounds have also reached the food sector, e.g. as antifoams, the pharmaceutical industry, e.g. as estrogen analogs (LeVier et al., 1978) and certain medical specialties, e.g. in eye and plastic surgery (for overview see Arkles, 1983) and have thereby triggered an increasing attention to the interaction between silicone compounds and the human body. That increased awareness is best exemplified by the recent considerable controversy over the alleged long-term inertness of silicone implants, particularly breast implants. Since pathological alterations of the connective tissue, allergic disorders and autoimmune diseases such as rheumatoid arthritis, scleroderma, and lupus erythematosus have all been described in association with silicone-based breast implants (reviewied in Bridges and Vasey, 1993), a search for a cause-effect relationship has been triggered. In studies on the stability of silicone gels *in vivo*, it has been suggested that the polymeric structure of the silicone implant deteriorates with age and that low molecular siloxanes are continuously being released from the gel matrix. This process occurs in addition to a phenomenon commonly referred to as "bleeding", whereby other low molecular weight siloxane fluids that are used in the preparation of the gel leak through its elastomer shell. The siloxane compounds have been shown to penetrate the adjacent tissues, migrate to remote sites, and encounter the immune system. Octamethylcylotetrasiloxane and vinyl siloxanes are low molecular weight siloxanes and potentially part of the gel bleed. In order to gain a better understanding of the biological significance of these siloxanes, we investigated the action of octamethylcyclotetrasiloxane, decamethyltetrasiloxane and tetramethyl-tetravinylcyclotetrasiloxane on B-cell lymphoma lines, peritoneal macrophages and P388D1.

Results and Discussion

The three siloxanes that were selected as model compounds for this study are very hydrophobic. Therefore, the addition of pure siloxanes to aqueous cell culture media is not useful, since an immediate phase separation would prevent any interaction between cultured cells and siloxanes. To overcome this problem, the siloxanes were complexed with γ-cyclodextrin, a cyclic 1-4 linked glucose octamer that provides a conical structure with a hydrophilic surface and a lipophilic inner space which can accomodate small lipophilic compounds and thereby form stable, so-called host-guest inclusion complexes (Pitha et al., 1988, Szejtli, 1989). It needs to be pointed out that γ-cyclodextrin itself is non-toxic and biologically inert. Upon contact with the lipid phase of plasma membranes, the siloxanes partition from the cyclodextrin complex into the lipid bilayer and are thus incorporated into living cells. We prepared inclusion complexes between γ-cyclodextrin and octamethylcyclotetrasiloxane (D4), decamethyltetrasiloxane (M10TS) and 1,3,5,7-tetravinyltetramethyl-cyclotetrasiloxane (TVTM-D4) to test the cytotoxic effects of these siloxanes. XRPC 24 and 2-11 plasmacytoma, CH12.LX lymphoma and P388D1 macrophage-like cells were employed as indicator cell lines.

The MTT proliferation test (Promega, Madison, WI) was used to measure toxicity in XRPC 24 (Moav et al., 1986), 2-11 (Shacter et al., 1990) and CH12.LX cells (Wakatsuki and Strober, 1993). The results of these experiments are summerized in Fig. 1. The MTT test is based on the reduction of a tetrazolium salt to a formazan product by active mitochondrial enzymes. The 50% minimal lethal doses (CD_{50}) for TVTM-D4 and M10TS were dependent of the cell line used and found to range from 30 to 50 µmoles/l. It is noteworthy, however, that 2-11 and CH12.LX cells tend to form small clusters *in vitro*. Therefore, the siloxanes can probably act on the outside layer of the cluster more readily than on cells in the center of the cluster, and this situation might result in underestimating the true toxicity of siloxanes on these cells. D4 was clearly less toxic than M10TS and produced a similar dose response curve for all three cell lines. The vinyl substituted siloxane was much more potent than the methyl substituted compounds (D4 and M10TS).

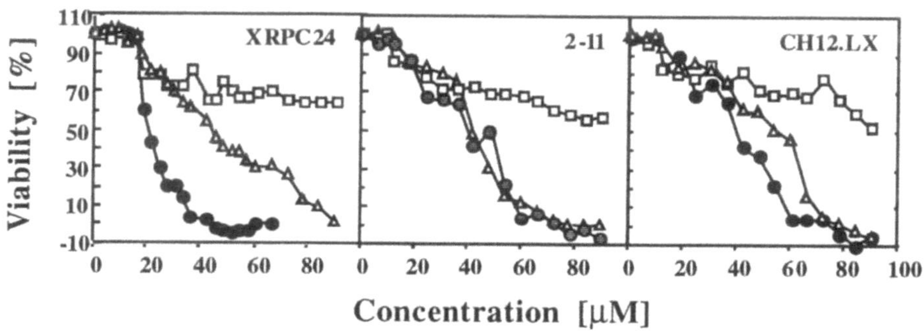

Fig. 1 MTT viability test in XRPC24, 2-11 and CH12.LX cells incubated for 24 h with different siloxanes. Filled circles, tetramethyltetravinylcyclotetrasiloxane; open triangles, decamethyltetrasiloxane; open squares, octamethylcyclotetrasiloxane. The cell cultures (3 x 10^5 cells/ml) were exposed to inclusion complexes between γ–cyclodexrin and the three siloxanes. The cells were then tested for viability using the MTT proliferation assay. Data are expressed as mean values from three independent experiments.

P388D1 cells were approximately 3 times less sensitive to TMTV-D4, D4 and M10TS than the B-lymphocyte derived tumor cells. After addition of γ-cylcodextrin siloxane complexes, P388D1 cells rapidly cleared the culture medium of the complexes, and this was accompanied by a visible increase in the size of the cytoplasmic vacuoles in these cells. We have made preliminary attempts to study the fate of tetravinyl-D4, D4 and M10TS in macrophages by GC/MS analysis. Our preliminary data indicate that these compounds probably accumulate in the cell membranes (data not shown). They do not bind to the free proteins in the culture medium to any appreciable extent. During siloxane treatment, P388D1 cells were observed under the microscope. As soon as 4 h after exposure to the highest concentration of siloxanes tested, changes in the membrane structure and the shape of the cells were observed. This reflected toxicity as confirmed by another assay that measures the release of lactate dehydrogenase (LDH). LDH is a cytosolic enzyme that can only be released after permeabilisation or disruption of the cell membrane. Fig. 2 shows that relatively low, sublethal doses (e.g., 15 μM and lower) resulted in a striking loss of LDH.

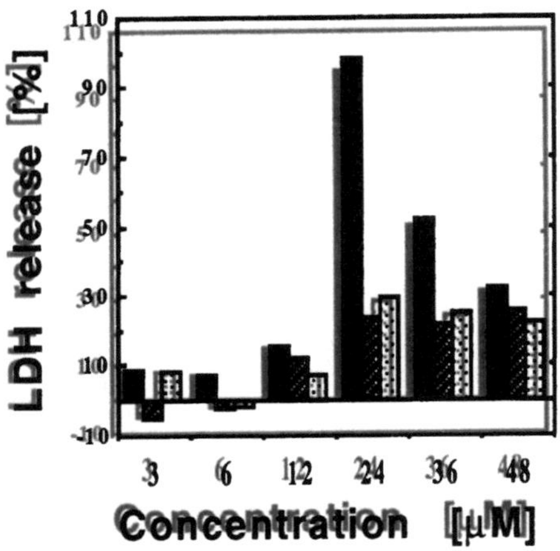

Fig 2: LDH release cytotoxicity assay. Filled columns, tetramethyltetravinylcyclotetrasiloxane; striped columns, decamethyltetrasiloxane; dotted columns, octamethylcyclotetrasiloxane. Release of LDH from XRPC24 cells exposed for 24 h to different siloxanes. LDH in culture supernatants was measured with a 30-minute coupled enzymatic assay which result in the conversion of a tetrazolium salt into a red formazan product measured at λ 490 nm.

We corraborated the LDH results by measuring the loss of glutathione (GSH), an important cytosolic compound that functions as the major intracellular antioxidant/detoxificant and also plays an important role in the control of the redox balance of the cell. Employing an enzymatic cycling test for the determination of total GSH (Tietze, 1969), we monitored the intracellular GSH levels after adding a dose range of siloxane compounds (Fig. 3).

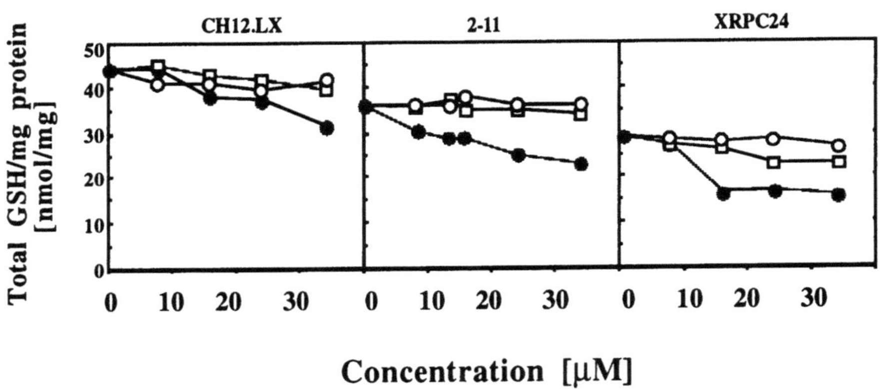

Fig. 3 Intracellular glutathione levels in CH12.LX, 2-11 and XRPC24 cells exposed to siloxanes. Open squares, decamethyltetrasiloxane; open circles, octamethylcyclotetrasiloxane; filled circles, tetramethyltetravinylcyclotetrasiloxane. The cells (3 x 10^5 cells/ml) were treated for 24 h and then assesed for total GSH and protein by the methods described by Tietze and Lowry, respectively.

Similar to the loss of LDH, sublethal concentrations of siloxanes resulted also in a slight drop of GSH and the largest effects were seen with TMTMD4. Whether the decrease in GSH is related to siloxane-induced permeabilization of cell membranes or is a consequence of its utilization for the detoxification of siloxanes is at present unclear and warrents further mechanistic studies. At any rate, the loss of GSH after treatment with siloxanes is likely to be of great physiological significance, since cytoplasmic depletion of GSH invariably results in the shift of the oxidative balance of the cell to the prooxidative state which in turn is followed by cellular damage in the form of lipid peroxidation, DNA damage or protein modification. It is noteworthy that the vinyl substituted siloxane (TMTV-D4) was consistently more toxic in all target cell lines tested than the methyl substituted siloxanes. The reason for this effect is currently unclear but could be related to the *in vitro* oxidation of the vinyl groups to more reactive moieties. Similar reactions have been shown to occur in photoscission and photooxidation processes in which the vinyl substituents were converted to silanols, carboxylic acids and esters (Lacoste and Israëli, 1993).

In another experiment we examined the effect of siloxanes on mouse macrophages by measuring the production of interleukin-6 (IL-6), an important growth factor for B-lymphocytes in mouse and man (Kishimoto,1989). In this assay, murine peritoneal macrophages were exposed to siloxanes *in vitro* for 20 h. To quantify the levels of the cytokine the culture supernatants were harvested and tested with the B9 cell bioassay (Shacter et al., 1992). The amounts of IL-6 that were secreted in response to siloxanes are given in (Table 1).

Table 1: Production of IL-6 by macrophages after a 20 hour exposure to siloxanes

Name of silicone compounds	Silicone compound [µM]				
	0	6	12	45	90
control [a]	56 [b]	-	-	-	-
cyclodextrin [c]	33	-	-	-	-
LPS [d]	8740	-	-	-	-
D4	-	28	40	135	246
TMTVD4	-	66	128	308	600
M10TS	-	59	89	337	616

[a] Macrophages (1.2 x 10^6/ml) without treatment

[b] IL-6 levels were determined with a bioassay employing IL-6 dependent B-9 hybridoma cells and are thus given in B-9 units/ml. Macrophages (1.2 x 10^6/ml) were exposed *in vitro* for 20 h to inclusion complexes between silicone compounds and γ-cyclodextrin. Then, the supernatant was tested for IL-6 levels.

[c] Macrophages (1.2 x 10^6/ml) exposed to γ-cyclodextrin (200 µg/ml)

[d] Macrophages (1.2 x 10^6/ml) stimulated with 1 µg/ml LPS

The production of IL-6 showed an approximately 10-fold increase in the presence of siloxanes as compared to negative controls including the one with γ-cyclodextrin only. However, the siloxane-induced increase in IL-6 production was moderate in comparison to the maximal IL-6 response that can be triggered by the addition of lipopolysaccharides (LPS) to macrophages. The relatively low levels of IL-6 after siloxane treatment could still be significant for the survival and proliferation of B-cells or the development of plasmacytomas (Nordan and Potter 1986).

In summary, the results of this *in vitro* study indicate that siloxanes in the 25 to

50 μmolar range are toxic to B-lymphoma and plasmacytoma cells such as CH12.LX, XRPC24 and 2-11 as well as macrophage-like P388D1 cells. The complexation of siloxanes with γ-cyclodextrin proved to be a useful method to study the toxic effects of hydrophobic siloxanes in cultured mammalian cells. The putative mechanism of toxicity as assessed by the MTT, LDH and loss of GSH tests is the intercalation of siloxane compounds into the cell membranes. One consequence of that incorporation is the leakage of ions and other cytosolic compounds from the cell resulting in the disturbance of the membrane potential, the deregulation of calcium homeostasis and the imbalance in the redox status of the cells. The concomitant shift to the prooxidative state may also affect the genomic stability of the cell, a hypothesis that is currently being investigated in our lab.

Acknowledgements

Parts of this study have been aided by a grant to K. F. from the Mildred-Scheel-Stiftung der Deutschen Krebshilfe. We are grateful to Drs. Hank Fales and Katy Zhang from the Lab. of Biophysical Chemistry, NHLBI, NIH for GC/MS analysis and to Dr. Emily Shacter from the Lab. of Immunology, FDA, NIH for help with IL-6 determinations.

References

Arkes B (1983) Look what you can make out of silicone. Chemtech 13: 542-555

Bridges AJ, Vasey FB (1993) Silicone breast implants. History, Safety, and potential Complications. Arch Intern Med 153: 2639-2644

Kishimoto T (1989) The biology of interleukin 6. Blood 74: 1-10

Lacoste J, Israëli Y (1993) Photooxidation of silicones. Polymer reprints 33: (1) 127-128

LeVier RR, Chandler ML, Wendel SR (1978) The pharmacology of silanes and siloxanes. In Biochemistry of silicon and related problems. Ed.Bendz G Lindquist I, Plenum Press, New York, pp 473-514

Moav B, Horowitz M, Cohen JB, Rechavi G, Eliyahu E, Oren M, Givol D (1986) Gene 48: 297-300

Nordan RP, Potter M (1986) A macrophage-derived factor required by plasmacytomas for survival and proliferation in vitro. Science 233: 566-569

Pitha J, Irie T, Sklar P, Nye J (1988) Drug solubilizers to aid pharmacologists; amorphous cyclodextrin derivates. Life Sciences 43: 493-502

Shacter E, Lopez RL, Beecham EJ, Janz S (1990) DNA damage induced by phorbol ester-stimulated neutrophils is augmented by extracellular cofactors. Role of histidine and metals. J Biol Chem 265: 6693-6699

Shacter E, Arzadon GK, Williams J (1992) Elevation of interleukin-6 in response to a chronic inflammatory stimulus in mice: Inhibiton by indomethacin. Blood 80: 194-202

Szejtli J (1989) Downstream processing using cyclodextrins. TIBTECH 7: 170-174

Tietze F (1969) Enzymatic method for quantitative determination of nanogram amounts of total and oxidized glutathione. Analyt Biochem 27: 502-522
Wakatsuki Y, Strober W (1993) Effects of downregulation of germline transcripts on immunoglobulin a isotope differentiation. J Exp Med 178: 129-138

The authors have not been involved in litigations nor do they recieve support from the silicone industry.

Adjuvancy of Silicones

Induction of Type II Collagen Arthritis in the DA Rat Using Silicone Gel as Adjuvant

J. O. Naim[1,2,3,4], K. M. L. Ippolito[1], R. J. Lanzafame[1,2], and C. J. van Oss[3]
[1]Department of Surgery, Rochester General Hospital, Rochester, NY and [2]The University of Rochester, School of Medicine and Dentistry, Rochester, NY and [3]Department of Microbiology, SUNY at Buffalo, Buffalo, NY

Abstract

The Dark Agouti (DA) rat has been shown recently to have a high susceptibility for developing arthritis when challenged with either heterologous or homologous collagen II mixed with mineral oil, or with mineral oil challenge alone. This study determined the arthritogenic potential of silicone gel by either mixing it with bovine collagen II (BII) or by injecting silicone gel alone in DA rats. The incidence of collagen induced arthritis was as follows: PBS group- 0/10, silicone gel group- 4/10, and IFA group- 8/9. Anti-BII antibodies were formed in most of the rats treated with either silicone gel or IFA and these groups of rats showed a positive DTH reaction. The PBS treated rats were negative for both anti-BII antibodies and DTH reaction. The incidence of arthritis formation in rats injected with silicone gel alone was 0/10, while the IFA injected rats showed an incidence of 8/10. Silicone gel taken from a commercial breast implant thus is capable of mediating collagen induced arthritis in the DA rat. However, silicone gel alone does not appear to be arthritogenic.

Introduction

The relative safety of silicone breast implants still remains a controversial issue. Many case reports that have appeared in the literature have shown an association of connective tissue types of diseases (i.e., scleroderma, rheumatoid arthritis, polymyositis, systemic lupus erythematosus, *etc.*) with silicone breast implants [1-3]. Unfortunately, most of these case reports have studied too small a population of women with implants for any reliable conclusion to be reached. Recently, a study by Gabriel *et al.* [4] studied 749 case subjects with silicone implants and found no apparent association between silicone breast implants and connective diseases or other disorders studied. Their study, although it is one of the most comprehensive to date, failed to take into account the population of women with documented rupture of their

[4] The first author has provided expert testimony and consulting services on behalf of plaintiffs relating to silicone breast implant litigation. This work was supported by NIH grant No. AI-34597.

silicone gel implants [4A]. We have found that silicone gel is a potent humoral adjuvant capable of inducing autoantibodies in rats, whereas the much lower molecular weight silicone oil, as well as the solid elastomer sheeting possess little or no adjuvant properites [5,6]. Therefore, clinical data from a population of women who are exposed to free silicone-gel, either by rupture of their implants or free injection, needs to be investigated before any conclusion regarding breast implants and their association with disease can be reached [4A].

Since our discovery that silicone gel behaves as a humoral adjuvant, we began a series of animal experiments which were designed to test whether silicone gel can mediate an autoimmune disease via its adjuvant properties. Our first experiment attempted to induce thyroiditis by immunizing Wistar rats with a mixture of silicone gel and rat thyroglobulin (Tg) [6]. This preparation failed to cause thyroiditis. We did however elicit anti-thyroglobulin antibodies in rats that were immunized with a silicone gel and rat Tg mixture. Our next experiment investigated the induction of type II collagen arthritis in Lewis rats using bovine collagen II (BII) mixed with silicone gel [7]. This study failed to demonstrate the induction of arthritis, despite the formation of anti-BII antibodies and a mild cell-mediated immune response to BII.

The Dark Agouti (DA) rat has been described as having a high susceptibilty to the development of arthritis when challenged with either heterologous or homologous collagen II mixed with mineral oil [8,11], or with mineral oil challenge alone [12]. Thus, the DA rat may afford a more sensitive animal model for testing the propensity of silicone gel to induce immunologically mediated arthritis. This investigation was undertaken to determine the arthritogenic potential of silicone gel alone or in combination with BII in DA rats.

Materials and Methods

Silicone gel was taken from an unused sterile McGhan silicone mammary implant (McGhan Medical, Santa Barbara, CA) and was prepared as described previously [5]. Briefly, silicone-gel was mixed with Dow Corning 360 Medical Fluid (20 cs silicone oil) (Dow Corning, Midland, MI) in a 1:1 ratio using a tissue homogenizer to facilitate mixing.

I. Type II Collagen Induced Arthritis:

Thirty, 180 gm., female DA [RT^{av1}] rats (Harlan Sprague Dawley, Indianapolis, IN) were equally divided among three groups: **I** -silicone gel, **II**- phosphate buffered saline (PBS)-negative control, and **III**- Incomplete Freund's adjuvant (IFA)-positive control. A stock solution of bovine collagen II* (BII) (Sigma Chemical, St. Louis, MO) was prepared in 0.1M acetic acid to a final concentration of 10 mg/ml. Each rat was injected at the base of the tail with 6 μg of BII (mixed with an equal volume of adjuvant) in 50 μl of PBS. Each animal was observed periodically for paw swelling, beginning at 7 days post-primary immunization. Both the hindpaws and forepaws were scored by the criteria reported by Cremer [10]: 1+, isolated ankle involvement; 2+, involvement of ankle and proximal 1/2 of the tarsal joint; 3+,

* This bovine collagen II is designated in the 1995 Sigma catalog as product No. C-7806 using the recognized classification for type II collagen.

involvement of ankle and the entire tarsal joint down to the metatarsal joints; 4+, involvement of entire paw, including the digits. The maximum score for each paw was totaled and was reported as the "maximum arthritis index" (MAI) for each rat, where the maximum MAI score was 16.

Rats in the silicone gel and PBS groups were given a booster immunization, identical to the primary immunization, at day 45. Only the non-arthritic rats in the IFA group received a booster immunization. Each animal was test bled via tail amputation at 21, 59 and 89 days post-primary immunization. A delayed type hypersensitivity (DTH) test was performed on all of the rats beginning on day 18 post-primary immunization according to the method of Larsson [11]. Briefly, 10 μg of BII in 20 μl of PBS was injected intradermally into the pinna of one ear (test), while the opposite ear (control) received 20 μl of PBS. Six, 24 and 48 hours after the BII challenge, the change in ear thickness (test ear thickness minus the control ear thickness) was measured using a micrometer caliper (MTI Corp., Paramus, NJ).

All rat sera were serially diluted and assayed in duplicate for anti-BII antibodies using an indirect ELISA. Each well of a 96 well microtiter plate was pre-coated with 50 μl of BII (10 μg/ml) and left overnight at 4°C. The plates were then blocked with 1% BSA in 0.05% Tween in PBS (PBST). Fifty microliters of pre-diluted rat serum were added to each well and incubated at room temperature for 2 hours. Fifty microliters of alkaline phosphatase conjugated goat anti-rat IgG (USB, Cleveland, OH) (diluted 1:500 in PBST) were added to each well and incubated at room temperature for 1 hr. One hunderd microliters of alkaline phosphatase substrate solution (1 mg/ml in diethanolamine-HCL buffer, pH 9.8) were added to each well and incubated in the dark for 30 min. The enzyme-substrate reaction was stopped at 30 min. by adding 50 μl of 3 N NaOH. The absorbance, at 405 nm, for each well was read on a Bio-Tek EL340 microplate reader (Bio-Tek Instruments, Inc, Winooski, Vt.). The data were analyzed with Kineticalc enzyme immunoassay application software version 2.12 (Bio-Tek Instruments, Inc.) in a titer mode. The best fit for the data was determined with a 4 parameter fit, and the titer threshold was set at 0.5. Under these conditons, the serum dilution producing an optical density at 405 nm of 0.5, corrected for background, was reported as the endpoint.

All rats were sacrificed at 89 days post-primary immunization. At the time of sacrifice, a sample of the afflicted paw joints was harvested from each animal and was placed in formalin for histopathological assessment. The joints were decalcified, sectioned at 6μm thickness and stained with hematoxylin and eosin (H&E). The histological samples were observed in a blind manner by a consulting pathologist (ZMT).

II. Silicone Gel Induction of Arthritis

Twenty, 180 gm., female DA [$RT1^{avl}$] rats (Harlan Sprague Dawley, Indianapolis, IN) were divided into two groups. Group I rats were injected at the base of the tail with 200 μl of silicone gel and group II rats were injected at the base of the tail with 200 μl IFA. The rats were observed for paw swelling once per week beginning the first week after injection. A DTH test for cell-mediated immunity against BII collagen was performed 18 days post-injection on each rat as described earlier. All the rats were sacrificed 69 days post-injection and at the same time a blood sample was taken from each animal. The sera were treated and assayed for anti-BII collagen as was described earlier.

Results

Figure 1 shows the incidence of arthritis and Fig. 2 shows the mean maximal arthritic index (MAI) for all the rats that were injected with BII and adjuvant. None of the PBS negative control rats exhibited any evidence of arthritis. One rat in the IFA positive control group died of unknown causes several days after the primary immunization. This rat was excluded from the IFA group data analysis leaving nine rats in the group, of which eight rats developed an arthritis. Four rats in the silicone gel group developed arthritis. The incidence of arthritis formation in the silicone gel group was statistically significant when compared to the PBS control group and not significant when compared to the IFA group of rats. Swelling and erythema were first seen to affect the hind paws. The macroscopic disease for those afflicted rats followed a chronic course which was similar to findings reported previously for homologous collagen induced arthritis [11]. The histopathology of the afflicted joints from rats in both the silicone gel or the IFA group showed the same type of cartilage and bone erosions with formation of pannus tissue overlying the cartilage. These are the classical pathological findings of afflicted joints from rats with collagen-induced arthritis that has been reported previously by Caulfield *et al.* [18].

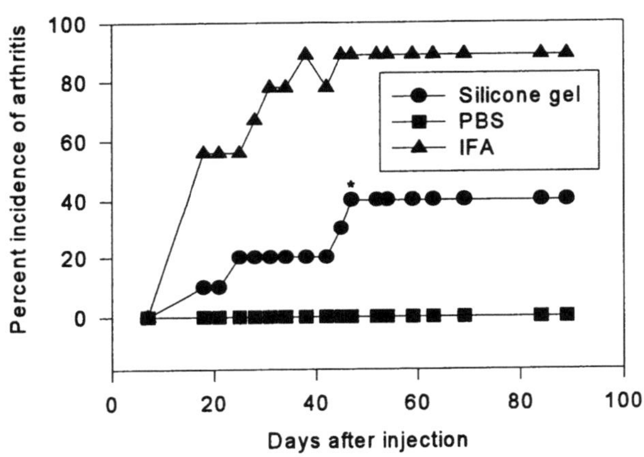

Fig 1. The incidence of arthritis in DA rats injected with BII. *$p < 0.05$ vs PBS and $p > 0.05$ vs IFA group as analyzed by Fisher's Exact test.

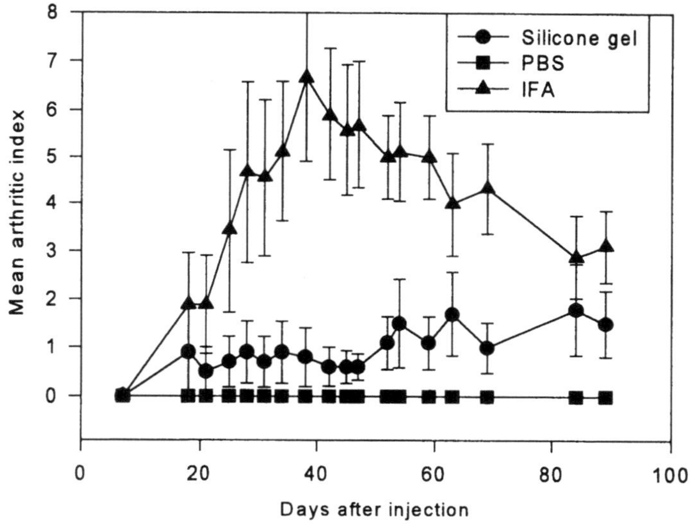

Fig 2. The mean maximal arthritic index (MAI) in DA rats injected with BII. Error bars indicate the SEM. PBS and silicone gel rats received a booster injection after 45 days.

Table 1 shows the serum antibody response to BII from all rats tested. At 21 days after the primary injection a slight amount of antibody was detected in the silicone gel and IFA group of rats. This low antibody response was most likely due to the low dose of collagen (6μg) that was injected. Nevertheless, none of the PBS treated rats produced detectable antibody. After administering a booster injection to the rats in the silicone gel and PBS group, the silicone gel treated rats showed a rise in their titers, whereas the PBS rats continued to show no detectable antibody. We chose not to administer a booster injection to the IFA group of rats at 45 days after the primary immunization because eight of nine rats had already developed a moderate to severe arthritis. Since we did not boost these animals, their anti-BII antibody titers were barely detectable at 59 and 89 days.

Table 1. Anti-BII collagen antibodies from DA rats

Groups	21 Days	59 Days	89 Days
Silicone gel	18±32[a]	90±103*	59±74
PBS	0	0*	0
IFA	33±56	7±20	11±32

[a] Mean serum antibody titer at 0.5 O.D. ± SEM. * Rats boosted 45 days post primary immunization.

Figure 3 shows the DTH test results begining 18 days after the primary immunization. Notice that the ear swelling at six hours was very slight in all of the rats indicating that immune complexes had not formed. By 24 and 48 hours, a clear positive DTH response was seen for all the rats in the silicone gel and IFA group, whereas none of the PBS treated rats showed a positive response. Note that the commercial preparation of BII, which we used (Sigma Chemical Co., St Louis, MO) contained trace amounts of pepsin as analyzed by SDS-polyacrylamide gel electrophoresis (PAGE). Vingsbo *et al.* [20] have shown that Lewis rats immunized with a crude preparation of rat collagen II (RTII), which contains pepsin, developed a strong T cell response against pepsin and weaker response against purified RTII. Therefore, it is likely that our DTH test measured cell-mediated immunity against BII-pepsin complexes.

The results from the attempted induction of arthritis by administering adjuvant alone experiment is presented in Table 2. Eight of ten rats in the IFA group developed a moderate arthritis, whereas none of the silicone gel rats developed any macroscopic signs of arthritis. Both groups of animals were negative for both anti-BII antibodies and DTH response against BII (data not shown).

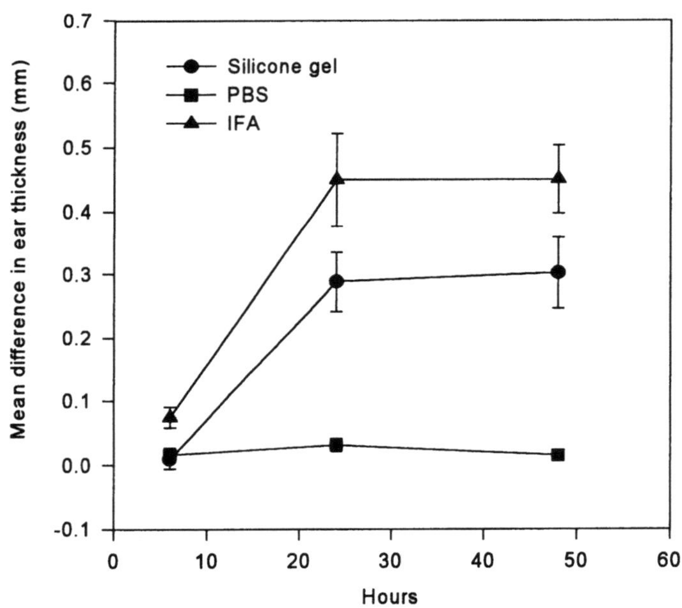

Fig 3. Delayed type hypersensitivity test of a BII-pepsin complex 18 days post primary immunization. Error bars indicate the SEM.

Table 2. The incidence of arthritis and mean maximal arthritic index (MAI) in DA rats injected with adjuvant alone

	Silicone Gel		IFA	
Days	MAI	Incidence	MAI	Incidence
7	0	0/10	0	0/10
12	0	0/10	1.9±0.62*	7/10
20	0	0/10	4.1±1.37	8/10[a]
28	0	0/10	4.4±1.63	7/10
35	0	0/10	4.2±1.41	7/10
46	0	0/10	2.7±0.91	6/10

[a] $p < 0.01$ vs silicone gel group by Fishers Exact test. *Mean ± SEM.

Discussion

Silicone gel from commercial breast implants has been shown previously by our laboratory to be a potent humoral adjuvant. The results from this study now demonstrates, for the first time, that silicone gel acting as an adjuvant, when mixed with BII, can induce arthritis in the DA rat. Our data also suggests that silicone gel can induce cell-mediated immunity against BII-pepsin complexes in DA rats. These findings are in contrast to our previous work in which we used Lewis rats for collagen induced arthritis experiments [7]. In the Lewis rats, silicone gel did not promote the onset of arthritis nor did it promote cell-mediated immunity against BII-pepsin complexes, after a single immunization. It has been demonstrated by Stuart *et al.* [13] and Trentham *et al.* [14] that collagen induced arthritis, in rats, is accompanied by a strong humoral [13] and cellular [14] immune response to collagen. Even though the amount of anti-BII antibody formation was low in this experiment, it is likely that the clinical arthritis observed in the DA rats was mediated by both cellular immunity and anti-BII antibodies which may have cross reacted with native type II collagen. Conversely, Griffiths *et al.* [15] reported that an immune responsiveness to homologous and heterologous type II collagen may not always lead to clinical arthritis in rats. This would explain in part why after boosting with silicone gel and BII, we observed a significant rise in anti-BII antibodies but no further increase in the incidence of arthritis .

The results from the experiment with adjuvant alone indicate that silicone gel does not appear capable of mediating an adjuvant arthritis, in contrast with what was observed with IFA in DA rats. Chang [16] reported that silicone gel mixed with or without heat-killed *Mycobacterium tuberculosis* was also unable to elicit arthritis when injected into Lewis rats. The induction of adjuvant arthritis with mineral oil alone is a more recent discovery which seems to be only possible in the DA rat [8,9]. However, Chang *et al.* [19] have demonstrated that adjuvant arthritis can be elicted in Lewis rats with N,N-dioctadecyl-N',N'-bis(2-hydroxyethyl) propanediamine (CP-20961) suspended in mineral oil. The pathogenesis of oil/chemical induced arthritis in DA rats is not fully understood. However recent evidence has suggested that the arthritis is T cell mediated and not mediated by serum components [12]. Thus the DA rat is a sensitive model for studying the pathogenesis of autoimmune arthritis which is inducible with various chemicals i.e., mineral oil, Arlacel® A (an emulsifier with mono-oleate as its major component, which is used in IFA) and Pristane (2,6,10,14,-tetramethylpentadecane) [9]. The DA rat would therefore serve as an appropriate model for further tests of various components found in silicone mammary implants (i.e. silicone oils and very low molecular weight octamethylcyclotetrasiloxanes) for their arthritogenic potential.

In conclusion, silicone gel taken from a commercial breast implant which was homogenized with 20 cs silicone oil and mixed with bovine collagen II, is capable of mediating collagen induced arthritis in the DA rat. However, silicone gel alone does not appear to be arthritogenic. Given the fact that silicone gel from a mammary implant is capable of mediating a disease in DA rats, and that definitive epidemiological data for showing a direct linkage of disease to women with leaking silicone breast implants may still be years away from being reported, further testing of the propensity of silicone compounds to cause adverse reactions in various animal models including the DA rat seems warranted.

Acknowledgments

We wish to thank Dr. Zygmunt Tomkiewicz, Chief of Pathology, and the Department of Pathology at The Rochester General Hospital for preparing and reviewing all our histopathological samples.

References

1. Sergott, T. J., J.P. Limoli, C.M. Baldwin Jr, and D.R. Laub. (1986) Human adjuvant disease, possible autoimmune disease after silicone implantation: a review of the literature case studies, and speculation for the future. Plast. Recontr. Surg. 78:104-114.
2. Spiera, H. Scleroderma after silicone augmentation mammoplasty. 1988. JAMA. 260:236-238
3. K.C. Shestak, R.J. Restifo, M.J. Wheatley, and D.J. Smith. (1992) The silicone-gel implant controveresy: Knowns and unknowns about implants. in: Perspectives in General Surgery, vol. 3,, B.A. Levine (Ed.). Quality Medical Publishing, St. Louis, MO. p. 26
4. Gabriel, S.E., W.M. O'Fallon, L.T. Kurland, C.M. Beard, J.E. Woods, and J. Melton. (1994) Risk of connective-tissue diseases and other disorders after breast implantation. NEJM. 330:1697-1702

4A. Naim, J.O., R.J. Lanzafame, and C.J. van Oss. (1994) [Letter]. NEJM. 331(18):1232

5. Naim,J.O., R.J. Lanzafame, and C.J. van Oss. (1993) The effect of silicone-gel on antibody formation in rats. Immunol. Invest. 22(2):151-161
6. Naim, J.O., C. J. van Oss, and R.J. Lanzafame. (1993) The induction of auto-antibodies to thyroglobulin in rats with silicone gel as adjuvant. Surgical. Forum, Vol. XLIV:676-678
7. Naim, J.O., R.J. Lanzafame, and C.J. van Oss. (1995) The effect of silicone-gel on the immune response. J. Biomaterials Science Polymer Edition. in press.
8. M. M. Griffiths, M. A. Cremer, D. S. Harper, S. McCall and G. Cannon. (1992) Immunogenetics of collagen induced arthritis in rats: Both MHC and non-MHC gene products determine the epitope specificity of immune response to bovine and chick type II collagens. J. Immunol. 149:309-316

9. Kleinau, S., H. Erlandsson, R. Holmdahl and L. Klareskog. (1991) Adjuvant oils induce arthritis in the DA rat. I. Characterization of the disease and evidence for immunological involvement. J. Autoimmunity, 4:871-880
10. M. Cremer. (1988) Type II collagen induced arthritis in rats. in: Handbook of Animal Models for the Rheumatic Diseases, R.A. Greenwald and H.S. Diamond, eds. Vol. I. CRC Press, Boca Raton, FL. p17
11. P. Larsson, S. Kleinau, R. Holmdahl, L. Klareskog. (1990) Homologous type II collagen-induced arthritis in rats: Characterization of the disease and demonstration of clinically distinct forms of arthritis in two strains of rats after immunization with the same collagen preparation. Arthritis Rheum., 33 (5):693-701
12. R. Holmdahl, T.J. Goldschmidt, S. Kleinau, C. Kvick, and R. Jonsson. (1992) Arthritis induced in rats with adjuvant oil is a genetically restricted, αβ T-cell dependent autoimmune disease. Immunology, 76:197-202
13. J.M. Stuart, M.A. Cremer, A.S. Townes, and A.H. Kang. (1982) Type II collagen-induced arthritis in rats: Passive transfer with serum and evidence that IgG anti-collagen antibodies can cause arthritis. J. Exp. Med. 155:1-16
14. D.E. Trentham, R.A. Dynesius, and J.R. David. (1978) Passive transfer by cells of type II collagen-induced arthritis in rats. J. Clin. Invest. 62:359-366
15. M.M. Griffiths and C.W. DeWitt. (1984) Genetic control of collagen-induced arthritis in rats: The immune response to type II collagen among susceptible and resistant strains and evidence for multiple gene control. J. Immunol. 132:2830-2836
16. Y. Chang. (1993) Adjuvanticity and arthritogenicity of silicone. Plast. Reconstr. Surg. 92:469-473.
17. S. Kleinau and L. Klareskog. (1993) Oil-induced arthritis in DA rats: Passive transfer by T cells but not with serum. J. Autoimmunity 6:449-458
18. J.P. Caulfield, A. Hein, R. Dynesius-Trentham, and D.E. Trentham. (1982) Morphologic demonstration of two stages in the deveolopment of type II collagen-induced arthritis. Lab. Invest. 46:321-343
19. Y. Chang, C. M. Pearson and C. Abe. (1980) Adjuvant Polyarthritis IV. Induction by a synthetic adjuvant: Immunologic, Histopathologic, and other studies. Arthritis and Rheumatism, 23:62-71.
20. C. Vingsbo, P. Larsson, M. Andersson, and R. Holmdahl. (1993) Association of pepsin with type II collagen (CII) breaks control of CII autoimmunity and triggers development of arthritis in rats. Scand. J. Immunol. 37:337-342

The Adjuvancy of Silicones: Dependency on Compartmentalization

P.C. Klykken[1] and K.L. White, Jr.[2]
[1]Dow Corning Corporation
[2]Medical College of Virginia/Virginia Commonwealth University

Studies have been conducted in mice (B6C3F1) and rats (Sprague Dawley, Fischer 344) to investigate the adjuvancy potential of silicone mammary gel and the low molecular weight silicone fluid, octamethylcyclotetrasiloxane (D4). Dependent on the experimental conditions employed, a divergent data profile emerges. If the antigen (bovine serum albumin, BSA) is emulsified with either the gel or the D4 prior to intramuscular immunization, an amplified anti-BSA IgG antibody response, as measured by multipoint ELISA methodology, is noted over the 8 week measurement period. In parallel studies, a variety of non-silicone personal care ingredients (lanolin, white mineral oil, isopropyl palmitate) were also capable of amplifying this humoral response relative to the non-adjuvant phosphate buffered saline control. These observations are consistent with the empirical knowledge that hydrophobic substances tend to augment immune responses. However, under conditions in which the antigen is not blended with the silicone prior to immunization, normal immune responses are noted. In short (10 day) and long (180 day) term gel implant studies, the optimal IgM and IgG antibody responses, as determined in the antibody forming cell assay, were equivalent between the gel implanted and control animals. Moreover, under similar exposure conditions, no adjuvancy was noted in the three Host Resistance models (B16F10 Melanoma, *Listeria monocytogenes*, and *Streptococcus pneumoniae*) tested. Antibody forming cell studies conducted after 28 days of oral or inhalation exposure to D4 have also yielded responses similar to the non-silicone exposed vehicle controls. Collectively, these data suggest that in the absence of premixing the antigen with the silicone test material, there does not appear to be any silicone induced adjuvant response.

Introduction

In the field of immunology, the term "adjuvant" has been widely used to describe substances which have the ability to enhance immune responses, without necessarily exhibiting antigenicity themselves. Recent publications using different animal models have focused on the ability of silicone gel, when co-administered with antigen, to serve as an adjuvant in both cell-mediated and humoral immune responses. Chang (1993) has reported that implant-grade silicone gel is ineffective in amplifying a cell-mediated response to EL_4 cells in Lewis rats, and unable to elicit or amplify a *Mycobacterium tuberculosis*-induced response in a rat arthritic model. In contrast, the work of Naim *et al.* (1993) demonstrated that mechanically sheared mammary gel blended with a low viscosity 20 cs polydimethylsiloxane (PDMS) fluid can amplify an antibody response to bovine serum albumin (BSA) in Sprague Dawley rats. Collectively, these data are consistent with earlier Dow Corning laboratory efforts which focused on the adjuvancy potential of various silicone materials.

The studies reported herein were conducted at both facilities and utilized multiple types of exposure regimens to examine the adjuvanticity issue: intramuscular injection of emulsified silicone-antigen test preparations, and administration of the silicone and antigen into separate anatomical compartments. In addition to Sprague Dawley rats, adjuvant effects were also evaluated employing multiple exposure regimens in B6C3F1 mice and Fischer 344 rats. The silicone materials under study include silicone gel derived from Dow Corning mammary implant devices and the low molecular weight silicone fluid octamethylcyclotetrasiloxane, which is commonly referred to as D4 (see Lane and Burns, Chapter 1, Silica, Silicon and Silicones...Unraveling the Mystery).

Materials and Methods

Animals: Female B6C3F1 mice (C57BL/6 X C3HHeN), female Sprague Dawley rats, and female Fischer 344 rats were purchased from Charles River Breeding Laboratories. Upon arrival, animals were quarantined for at least 1 week prior to use. Mice used in these studies were between 8 and 10 weeks old at the start of an experiment while the rats were between 6-8 weeks of age. Mice were housed 4 - 5 per cage in plastic boxes containing sawdust bedding, and rats were individually housed in hanging wire cages. Animals were given free access to food and tap water. In accordance with NIH guidelines, the appropriate environmental conditions (12 hour light/dark cycle, 68-78°F, 30-70% humidity) were maintained at both facilities.

Test Materials: The following Dow Corning materials were used to prepare the silicone test materials: Q7-2159A Gel contained within Silastic® II mammary implants, mammary gel bleed derived from Silastic® I mammary implants by centrifugation, and an analytical standard of D4. Mouse D4 studies conducted at MCV/VCU utilized D4 obtained from Hules America. The non-silicone materials included Klearol white mineral oil (Witco Manufacturing), isopropyl palmitate (CasChem, Inc.), glycerin USP/FCC (Fisher Scientific) and lanolin USP (Fisher Scientific). Other control materials included Freund's complete adjuvant (Sigma), corn oil (Mazola), Dulbecco's phosphate buffered saline (Mediatech), sterile, non-pyrogenic saline (Baxter), cyclophosphamide (Sigma), *C. parvum* (Sigma) and cobra venom factor (Cappel).

Preparation and Administration of Test Materials: In the mouse implantation studies, silicone gel was administered subcutaneously in the lower left ventral quadrant. The gel material, 1 ml, was injected using a Harvard infusion pump with a 5 ml syringe and a 20 guage needle. Mice were anesthetized with sodium pentabarbital (55 mg/kg i.v.) during administration. Flexible collodion USP was used to seal the needle insertion site in the skin. In the rat oral gavage studies, D4 was administered in a corn oil vehicle and in the inhalation studies D4 was delivered with room air in a stainless steel whole body exposure unit.

For the adjuvancy studies, the gel was taken from a breast implant device and mechanically sheared using a Brinkman Polytron® homogenizer. Test materials were triturated with the BSA stock (0.33 mg/ml) at equal volumes (1:1) using 10-cc glass syringes connected either with a 3-way stop cock (lanolin) or an 18 guage emulsifying needle (all other test materials). Female Sprague Dawley rats received a single 0.3 ml injection of the appropriate triturated test material in the left thigh musculature while mice received a 0.2 ml injection of the appropriate test material.

Anti-BSA ELISA: Serum samples from rats were prepared from blood collected from each animal at 2, 4, 6 and 8 weeks post-immunization and stored at -80°C until assayed. Serum from naive, non-injected littermates served as the baseline control. Mice were evaluated on weeks 4, 7 and 12 weeks post-immununization.

An ELISA (enzyme-linked immunosorbent assay) for anti-BSA IgG antibody was conducted using a multipoint data analysis. BSA prepared at 40μg/ml in phosphate buffered saline (PBS) was added to microtiter plates and allowed to sit overnight at 4°C. Following a wash step, plates were blocked with (PBS/0.05% Tween 20). After a second wash, ten, 2-fold dilutions of the serum samples prepared in blocking buffer were added and incubated for 1.5 hrs. The plates were then washed, the appropriate dilution of rabbit anti-rat IgG (H&L) (Southern Biotechnology) or rabbit anti-mouse IgG (Accurate) enzyme conjugated antibody added, and then incubated an additional 1.5 hrs. Chromogen enzyme substrate, 2,2'-azino-bis(3-ethylbenzthiazoline-6-sulfonic acid), was added after the final wash step. The reaction was stopped after 45 minutes by the addition of oxalic acid and optical density (O.D.) readings were recorded at 405 nm.

The ELISA data was evaluated using a multipoint analysis procedure. Ten serial dilutions were prepared for each sample and the log of the O.D. readings were plotted against the log of the serum dilitions. The linear region of the curve was identified for each sample and the antibody titer was defined as the reciprocal of the serum dilution which would yield an O.D. reading of 0.5 as determined by the linear regression.

Antibody Forming Cell Response: The primary IgM and IgG responses to sheep erythrocytes (sRBC) were enumerated using a modified hemolytic plaque assay. Animals were sensitized with $2x10^8$ sRBC (rats) or $7.5x10^7$ sRBC (mice). The optimum IgM response occurred 4 days after immunization and the optimum IgG response occurred 5 days after immunization. The IgG and IgM responses were measured as described previously (Bradley *et al.*, 1994a,b).

Statistical Analysis: The antibody titers and antibody forming cell response data were initially tested for homogeneity of variances using the Bartlett's Chi Square Test. Homogeneous data were evaluated by a parametric one-way analysis of variance. When significant differences occurred, treatment groups were compared to the appropriate control group using the Dunnett's t Test. Non-homogeneous data were evaluated using a non-parametric analysis of variance. When significant differences occurred, treatment groups were compared to the non-adjuvant control group using the Wilcoxon Rank Test. Mortality data were evaluated using the Fisher's Exact Chi Square Test. P values of 0.05 or less which were considered statistically significant compared to the non-adjuvant control are indicated in the figures with an asterisk (*). In the mouse studies 8-12 animals per group were used and 9-10 animals per group were used in the rat studies.

Results

Effect of Gel and D4 on the serum antibody titers to BSA: As shown in the left panel of Fig. 1, administration of BSA thoroughly mixed with either FCA, mammary gel, or D4 resulted in an enhanced antibody response in female Sprague Dawley rats. By Week 4, all groups responded with serum IgG antibody titers to BSA which were statistically greater than the non-adjuvant control animals. The mammary gel bleed test group did not differ from the PBS non-adjuvant control group at any of the time points evaluated.

Shown in the right panel of Fig. 1 is the response of B6C3F1 female mice administered BSA mixed with either FCA, mammary gel, or D4. As was observed with the Sprague Dawley rats, the mice which received either FCA, mammary gel or D4 had an enhanced IgG antibody response to BSA compared to the PBS non-adjuvant control mice. Statistical significance was observed at each time point beginning with Week 4.

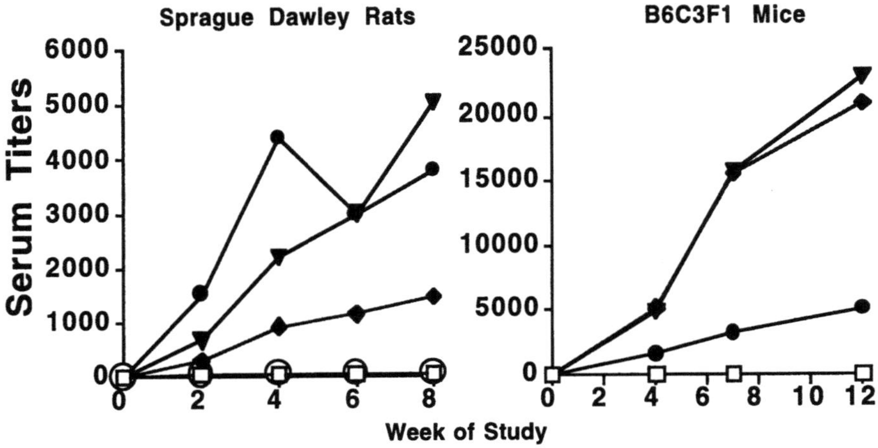

Fig. 1. BSA serum titers in Sprague Dawley rats and B6C3F1 mice implanted with gel bleed (open circles), gel (filled triangles), PBS (open squares), FCA (filled diamonds) and D4 (filled circles).

Effect of Non-Silicone Materials on Serum Antibody Titers to BSA: Shown in Fig. 2 are the results of Sprague Dawley rats administered BSA mixed with PBS, FCA or non-silicone materials which included white mineral oil, isopropyl palmitate, glycerin or lanolin. With the exception of the water soluble glycerin, each of the non-silicone materials produced an enhanced IgG antibody response to BSA compared to the PBS non-adjuvant controls. As was observed with the silicone materials, statistically significant differences were observed at each time point beginning at Week 4 for the FCA, white mineral oil, and the isopropyl palmitate treated animals. The antibody titer to BSA in the lanolin treated animals did not reach the level of statistical significance until Week 6 of the study. At all time points, animals administered BSA mixed with glycerin had antibody responses which were less than or equal to that of the PBS non-adjuvant control animals.

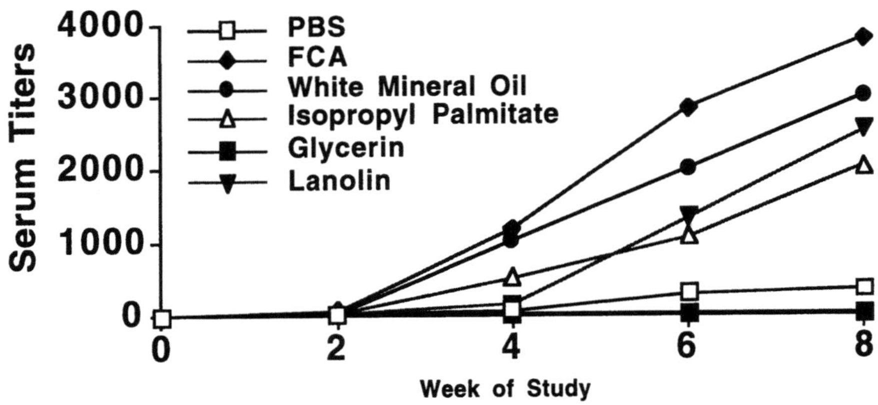

Fig. 2. BSA serum titers in Sprague Dawley rats treated with non-silicone materials.

Antibody Forming Cell (AFC) Response of B6C3F1 Implanted with Silicone Mammary Gel: Shown in Fig. 3 are the results of the IgM and IgG antibody forming cell response in female B6C3F1 implanted with silicone mammary gel for either 10 or 180 days. These data are adapted from the works of Bradley *et al.*, 1994a,b. In this study the animals were implanted with the silicone mammary gel in the mammary region and the antigen, sheep erythrocytes, was administered as an intravenous injection. Shown in the 10 day exposure panel (left) are the results of the IgM and IgG antibody forming cell response, evaluated on the peak response days. No significant difference was observed in the IgM response between the animals which received the PBS vehicle (VH) and those implanted with the silicone mammary gel. Similarly, there was no difference in the IgG response between the vehicle and mammary gel implanted animals. The positive control, cyclophosphamide (CPS, 25 mg/kg) markedly decreased both the IgG and IgM response to sheep erythrocytes.

In the right panel are the results following 180 day exposure to the vehicle or silicone mammary gel material. As was observed in the 10 day study, neither the IgM nor the IgG antibody forming cell response of animals implanted with the silicone mammary gel differed from the vehicle control animals.

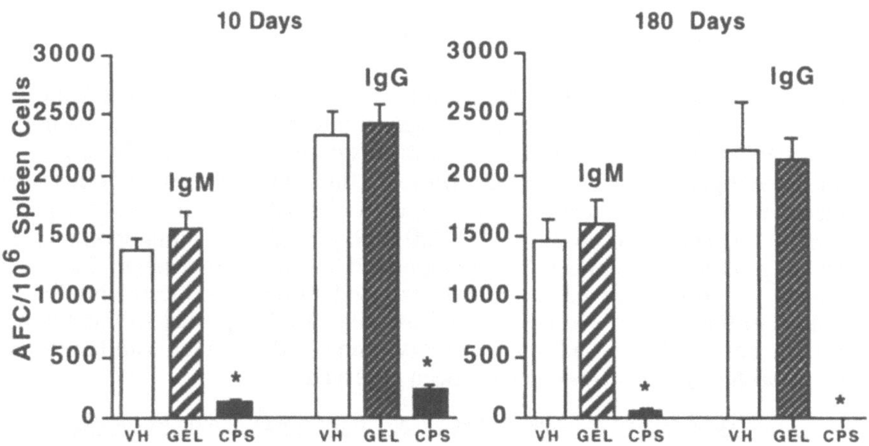

Fig. 3. AFC response in B6C3F1 mice implanted with silicone gel. Peak response days for the IgM and IgG were 4 and 5 days post sRBC immunization respectively.

Antibody Forming Cell (AFC) Response of Female Fischer 344 Rats Treated for 28 Days with D4 by Oral Gavage or Inhalation: Shown in Fig. 4 are the results of IgM antibody forming cell response of female Fischer 344 rats treated for 28 days with D4. In the left panel are the results when the animals received the D4 by oral gavage. As in the murine AFC study, the sheep erythrocyte antigen was administered by intravenous injection. No significant differences were detected between the vehicle (corn oil) animals and any of the test groups which received D4. Treatment with the positive CPS (25 mg/kg) control produced a significant decrease in the IgM antibody forming cell response to sheep erythrocytes. The right panel shows the antibody forming cell response of animals exposed to one of five doses of D4 by inhalation. As noted, no significant difference was observed in the IgM antibody forming cell response between the room air vehicle control and any of the dose levels of D4 administered. CPS (25 mg/kg) produced the expected decrease in the antibody forming cell response.

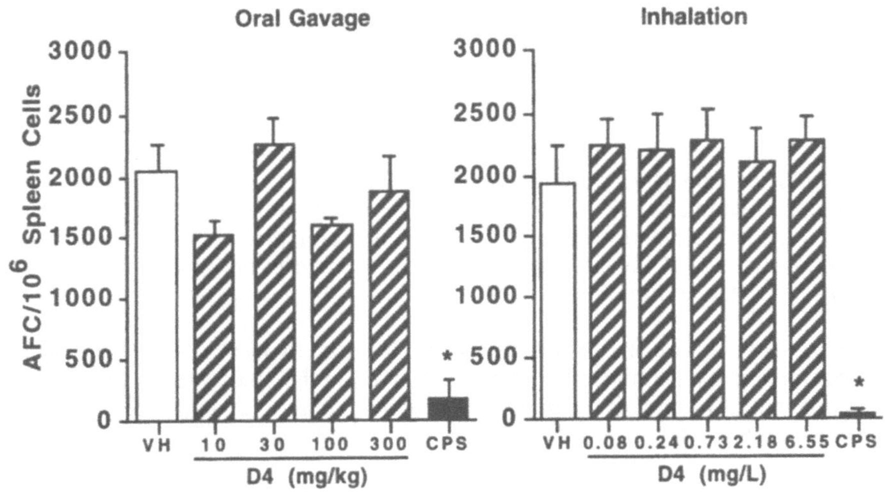

Fig. 4. IgM AFC response in Fischer 344 rats treated with D4.

Effect of Gel and D4 on Host Resistance: Shown in Tables 1 and 2 are the effects of exposure to silicone mammary gel on host resistance in three pathogen model systems. In Table 1 are shown the results of an extensive study conducted with the pathogen *Listeria monocytogenes.* In this study three time points were evaluated with five challenge levels of the microbial pathogen at each time point. The immunosuppressive control CPS (200 mg/kg) and the immunopotentiating control *C. parvum* (35 mg/kg) were incorporated into the study design. Increased resistance was not observed in animals exposed to the silicone mammary gel compared to the vehicle (saline) control animals. Had exposure to the silicone mammary gel resulted in adjuvant activity, enhanced survival, similar to that observed with *C. parvum*, should have been observed.

Table 1. Absence of silicone gel induced effect on host resistance to *Listeria monocytogenes*

Day	Treatment	Challenge A	Challenge B	Challenge C	Challenge D	Challenge E
		4.6×10^4	9.1×10^4	1.8×10^5	3.7×10^5	9.1×10^5
10	Vehicle	3/10[a]	7/10	7/10	9/10	10/10
	Gel	4/10	6/10	8/10	7/10	8/10
	C. parvum				0	0
	CPS	9/10	9/10			
		1.9×10^4	5.6×10^4	1.7×10^5	5.6×10^5	1.7×10^6
45	Vehicle	0/10	3/10	1/10	3/10	9/10
	Gel	0/10	1/10	8/10	8/9	10/10
	C. parvum				1/10	1/10
	CPS	1/10	7/10			
		4.1×10^4	1.2×10^5	3.3×10^5	8.2×10^5	2.5×10^6
90	Vehicle	2/10	2/10	4/10	4/10	7/10
	Gel	1/10	3/10	5/10	8/10	8/10
	C. parvum				0/10	1/9
	CPS	7/10	9/10			

[a]Values represent number dead/number on study.

The data presented in Table 2 have been adapted from the studies of Bradley *et al*, 1994a,b. In each of the host resistance models, two or more challenge levels of the pathogen were utilized. As reported in Table 2, exposure to silicone mammary gel for either 10 or 180 days failed to alter host resistance to the bacterial pathogens *Streptococcus pneumoniae* and *Listeria monocytogenes*. Additionally, in animals challenged with graded doses of B16F10 melanoma cells, no significant difference in tumor burden was noted between the gel implanted and saline control animals. Treatment with the positive controls CPS (200 mg/kg) or cobra venom factor (CVF, 100 ACU/kg) decreased host resistance in the different pathogen models.

Table 2. Absence of host resistance effects following 10 day or 180 day silicone gel exposure

Day	Organism	Treatment	Challenge A	Challenge B	Challenge C
			1.4×10^7	2.8×10^7	
10	*Strep. pneumoniae*	Vehicle	0/12[a]	9/12	
		Gel	0/12	8/12	
		CVF	12/12	12/12	
			1.2×10^4	3×10^4	5×10^4
	Listeria monocytogenes	Vehicle	4/10	7/12	10./10
		Gel	2/10	0/12	10/10
		CPS	12/12	12/12	10/10
			1×10^5	3×10^5	
	B16F10 Melanoma	Vehicle	2886 ± 233[b]	6812 ± 670	
		Gel	2711 ± 232	6267 ± 899	
		CPS	3172 ± 335	7312 ± 688	
			7.3×10^6	1.5×10^7	
180	*Strep. pneumoniae*	Vehicle	3/11	4/12	
		Gel	6/12	4/12	
		CVF	12/12	12/12	
			7.8×10^3	1.5×10^4	
	Listeria monocytogenes	Vehicle	0/12	8/12	
		Gel	1/12	9/12	
		CPS	12/12	12/12	
			1×10^5	3×10^5	
	B16F10 Melanoma	Vehicle	1466 ± 200	4724 ± 493	
		Gel	1151 ± 92	5391 ± 421	
		CPS	2815 ± 232	12600 ± 1327	

[a]Values represent number dead/number on study
[b]Values represent mean ± se cpm/lung

Discussion:

Substances which are known to possess adjuvanticity are diverse and include synthetic polymers, polyanions, liposomes, surfactants, and products of microorganisms (Warren, 1992). The studies reported herein confirm and extend the published observations of Naim *et al.* (1993) that silicone mammary gel can also function as an adjuvant under the appropriate experimental conditions. Emulsified preparations of sheared mammary gel with or without the addition of a 20 cs viscosity PDMS fluid are capable of eliciting a potent adjuvant response relative to the Freund's complete adjuvant positive control. The low molecular weight silicone fluid D4, and other non-silicone personal care ingredients are also able to function as adjuvants and amplify a humoral response when injected intramuscularly with the BSA antigen. In contrast, and of note from a risk assessment perspective, the laboratory preparation of mammary gel bleed (silicone fluid which has migrated through the mammary implant shell) did not elicit an adjuvant response under these experimental conditions.

To ascertain whether the mammary gel or D4 can act as an adjuvant and non-specifically augment an immune response when the antigen is not mixed with the silicone, animals were pre-exposed for various periods of time to intact, unadulterated silicone test material prior to challenging with a known antigen. Under these exposure conditions, which may better approximate the clinical setting, there is no apparent evidence of an elevated antibody response to the sRBC antigen. In addition, no enhanced host resistance to a *Listeria monocytogenes, Streptococcus pneumoniae* or a B16F10 melanoma tumor challenge was observed in silicone gel implanted animals.

The larger question is whether adjuvanticity elicited by a silicone or non-silicone material can be linked to disease. Studies to date with incomplete Freund's adjuvant (IFA) have demonstrated that the test material is oncogenic in mice, but only in a line of male Swiss mice. The adjuvant did not produce malignancies in female Swiss mice, nor in other mice strains (Murray *et al.*, 1972). In humans, no differences have been noted with respect to neoplasia, allergic diseases or collagen diseases, more than 30 years since a mineral oil-adjuvanted influenza vaccine was administered intramuscularly to approximately 18,000 military recruits (Beebe *et al.* 1969 and Page *et al.* 1993).

Consistent with the IFA experience, the emerging epidemiological data suggests that there is no increased risk of connective tissue disease in silicone breast-implanted women (Gott and Tinkler, 1994).

Disclosure: P. Klykken has served as an expert witness on behalf of Dow Corning Corporation. K. White has served as a consultant to other breast implant device manufacturers and has received grant support from Dow Corning Corporation.

References

Beebe GW, Simon AK, Vivona S (1972) Long-term mortality follow-up of Army recruits who received adjuvant influenza virus vaccine in 1951-1953. Am J Epidemiol 95:337-346

Bradley SG, Munson AE, McCay JA, Brown RD, Musgrove DL, Wilson S, Stern M, Luster MI, White KL, Jr. (1994a) Subchronic 10 day imunotoxicity of polydimethylsiloxane (silicone) fluid, gel and elastomer and polyurethane disks in female B6C3F1 mice. Drug Chem Toxicol 17:175-220

Bradley SG, White, KL, Jr., McCay JA, Brown RD, Musgrove DL, Wilson S, Stern M, Luster MI, Munson AE (1994b) Immunotoxicity of 180 day exposure to polydimethylsiloxane (siloxane) fluid, gel and elastomer and polyurethane disks in female B6C3F1 mice. Drug Chem Toxicol 17:221-269

Chang Y-H (1993) Adjuvanticity and arthritogenicity of silicone. Plast Reconstr Surg 92:469-473

Gott DM, Tinkler JJB (1994) Evaluation of evidence for an association between the implantation of silicones and connective tissue disease. Medical Devices Directorate Report, UK Department of Health, 14 Russell Square, London.

Murray R, Cohen P, Hardegree MC (1972) Mineral oil adjuvants: biological and chemical studies. Ann Allergy 30:146-151

Naim JO, Lanzafame RJ, van Oss CJ (1993) The adjuvant effect of silicone-gel on antibody formation in rats. Immuno Invest 22:151-161

Page WF, Norman JE, Benenson AS (1993) Long-term follow-up of Army recruits immunized with Freund's incomplete adjuvanted vaccine. Vaccine Res 2:141-149

Warren HS (1992) Adjuvants. In: Roitt IM (ed) Encyclopedia of Immunology. Academic Press, London, pp 28-30

The Adjuvant Effect of Silicone Gel and Silicone Elastomer Particles in Rats

S. L. Hill, M. G Landavere, and N. R. Rose

The Johns Hopkins University, School of Medicine, Department of Pathology & School of Hygiene and Public Health, Department of Molecular Microbiology and Immunology
720 Rutland Avenue, Ross Building 664G, Baltimore, Maryland 21205

Abstract

This study examines the adjuvant properties of silicone oil, silicone gel and silicone elastomer using a foreign antigen, bovine serum albumin (BSA). Seventy male Harlan Sprague-Dawley rats, approximately 250 grams each, were divided into 7 groups: A- incomplete Freund's adjuvant (IFA) with BSA; B- silicone oil with BSA; C- IFA/silicone oil with BSA; D- 50% silicone gel/50% silicone oil with BSA; E- silicone oil/1000 micron elastomer particles with BSA; F- silicone oil/500 micron elastomer particles with BSA; G- saline with BSA. Rats were implanted intramuscularly with mixtures or emulsions of the above described treatment materials. Cardiac punctures were performed on days 0, 14, 28, 42, and 55. Serum IgG antibody response to BSA was determined by enzyme-linked immunosorbent assay (ELISA). Rats were sacrificed on day 55 and sections of the injection sites were collected and stained for histopathologic evaluation. The results demonstrated that silicone gel functions as a potent immunologic adjuvant as measured by a heightened IgG antibody response to BSA. In contrast silicone elastomer particles have no apparent adjuvant effect as determined by the low anti-BSA antibody levels in these treatment groups throughout the course of the study. Histologically, silicone gel and silicone elastomer elicit a moderate to severe "foreign body" granulomatous inflammatory response at the injection site. Silicone oil elicits mild or no local inflammatory response.

Disclosure: This study was supported by a grant from the Mentor Corporation. Dr. Rose has served as an expert witness on behalf of defendents in legal proceedings involving silicone breast implants.

Introduction

An adjuvant can be defined as a substance that enhances the immune response to an antigen. Weak antigens may be rendered more immunogenic when administered with an adjuvant. The heightened immune response may take the form of antibody or cell-mediated immunity, or both. Considerable controversy has developed as to the potential adjuvant properties of components of silicone implants; namely, silicone oil, silicone gel and silicone elastomer. In an investigation by Naim et al., silicone gel from a breast prosthesis (McGhan Medical Corporation) mixed with silicone oil (Dow Corning 360 Fluid, 20 centistoke) acted as an immunological adjuvant as measured by a heightened IgG antibody response to BSA in rats [1]. This group additionally examined the adjuvanticity of silicone oils of varying molecular weights in a similar experimental system [2]. Testing with four different Dow Corning 360 Medical silicone oils of increasing molecular weight they found that only rats immunized with the highest molecular weight oil (M.W. -60,000, 12,500 cs) showed a significant increase in anti-BSA antibodies.

The purpose of the present study was to examine the adjuvant properities of silicone gel in association with a foreign antigen as measured by a heightened IgG antibody response to BSA, confirming the results of Naim et al. [1] as well as Klykken et al. (personal communication). Additionally, we evaluated the adjuvant properties of silicone elastomer particles in rats. The findings confirm that silicone gel but not silicone oil acts as a potent adjuvant in this experimental model but further indicate that silicone elastomer particles have no apparent adjuvant effect.

Materials and Methods

Materials

BSA, phosphate buffered saline (PBS), IFA, dimethylpolysiloxane (silicone oil, 20 cs), and p-Nitrophenyl Phosphate substrate solution were purchased from Sigma Chemical Company (St. Louis, MO). Silicone gel was obtained from a sterile Siltex Low Bleed Gel-filled Mammary Prosthesis provided by Mentor Corporation (Lot #84522). Silicone elastomer particles were provided by Mentor Corporation. Two groups of particles, 500 micron and 1000 micron, were generated by Metuchen Analytical Laboratory. Briefly, three mammary prosthesis (Siltex Saline-filled Mammary Prosthesis with Mentor Leaf Valve, Cat#354-2835M, Lot#

79456) were pulverized using a Wylie Mill and liquid nitrogen. Two particle sizes were generated, 500 micron (30-35 mesh) and 1000 micron (16-18 mesh).

Animals

Seventy male Sprague-Dawley rats (Harlan, Indianapolis, IN), weighing approximately 250 grams each, were randomized, quarantined for one week and individually ear notched for identification. They were housed 2-3 rats per plastic cage. Rats had free access to standard Purina rodent chow and water (municipal source). Approved animal care and housing practices were followed, as mandated by the Johns Hopkins University Animal Care and Use Committee. Groups of 10 animals were divided into the following experimental groups: A- IFA with BSA; B- silicone oil with BSA; C- IFA/silicone oil with BSA; D- 50% silicone gel/50% silicone oil with BSA; E- silicone oil/1000 micron silicone elastomer particles with BSA; F- silicone oil/500 micron silicone elastomer particles with BSA; and G- saline with BSA. Blood samples were collected by intracardiac puncture on days 0, 14, 28, 42, and 55. Each animal was anesthetized by inhalation of methoxyflurane (Metafane) and restrained in dorsal recumbency. A 5/8" 25 g needle was introduced through the diaghram into the chest cavity and right cardiac ventricular chamber. Approximately 1 ml of blood was withdrawn, allowed to clot at 4^0 C, sera collected and stored at -70^0C until tested for anti-BSA IgG antibody. Body weights were determined upon receipt, at randomization and weekly throughout the study. All animals were sacrificed on day 55 of the study, except group G (saline with BSA) which was sacrificed on day 35.

Immunization

Each animal was anesthetized by inhalation by methoxyflurane (Metafane). The left caudal thigh area was shaved and a 1.5 cm incision was made extending into the underlying muscle fascia. Using a 1 ml sterile glass pipet, 0.3 ml of the appropriate test article was delivered into the caudal thigh muscle incision. Animals receiving elastomer particles had particles placed into the incision site using a glass rod subsequent to the instillation of the emulsion. Skin incisions were closed using 2-3 stainless steel autoclips.

Test Procedure

Group A: an appropriate volume of IFA was mixed with an equal volume of 0.34 mg/ml BSA stock solution. An emulsion was produced by trituration between two connected 10 cc borosilicate glass syringes. Group B: an appropriate volume of dimethylpolysiloxane 20 cs was mixed with an equal volume of BSA stock solution and generation of an emulsion was attempted by trituration as described above. Group C: an equal volume of IFA and silicone oil was mixed. Subsequently, an equal volume of BSA stock solution was added. Generation of an emulsion was attempted by trituration. Group D: an appropriate amount of silicone gel obtained from a silicone breast implant was placed in a pre-weighed glass container. The fluidity of the silicone gel was enhanced by homogenization using an Omni homogenizer fitted with a 7 mm generator probe. After 6-8 cycles of homogenization, an equal volume of silicone oil (dimethylpolysiloxane, 20 cs, Sigma Chemical Company) was added. The mixture was rehomogenized with an additional 6-8 cycles. An equal volume of BSA stock solution was added and generation of an emulsion attempted by trituration between two borosilicate glass syringes. Group E: an appropriate volume of silicone oil was weighed and an equivalent weight of 1000 micron elastomer particles weighed and stored in glass tubes until impalntation. BSA at twice the volume of silicone oil was added to the silicone oil and an emulsion made as described above. The emulsion was delivered to the implantation site followed by the addition of the elastomer particles. Group F: test article preparation was indentical to that described for group E, except that 500 micron silicone elastomer particles were used. Group G: equal volumes of normal saline solution (0.9% NaCl) and BSA stock solution were mixed and injected into left caudal thigh muscles. Table 1 summarizes the various treatment groups.

Table 1. Treatment Groups

Group	Treatment
A*	IFA with BSA
B	Silicone oil with BSA
C	IFA/silicone oil with BSA
D	50% silicone gel/50% silicone oil with BSA
E	Silicone oil/1000 micron elastomer particles with BSA
F	Silicone oil/500 micron elastomer particles with BSA

* Each test group consisted of ten rats.

Anti-BSA IgG ELISA

Serum samples were thawed immediately prior to use. Anti-BSA IgG titers were determined by ELISA. Dynateck Immunolon 2, 96 well microtiter plates were coated with 50 ul of BSA solution (10 ug/ml) in carbonate buffer (pH 9.6). Plates were sealed with plastic wrap and incubated overnight at 4^0C, then plates washed with 0.05% Tween-20 in PBS (wash solution) using a Skatron 300 automatic plate washer. Plates were subsequently blocked by adding 100 ul of wash solution for 30 minutes and the wash solution was decanted. One hundred microliters of each serum sample into 1:250 dilution in wash solution were tested in triplicate. Plates were incubated for two hours at room temperature, then washed three times with wash solution. Alkaline phosphatase-conjugated, affinity-purified goat anti-rat IgG, 100 ul, diluted 1:10,000 in wash solution was added to each well and incubated for 1 hour. Plates were washed three times, 100 ul of alkaline phosphatase substrate solution, p-nitrophenyl phosphate (1 mg/ml in diethanolamine-HCl buffer, pH 9.8) added, and plates incubated in the dark. The reactions were read at 30 minutes after substrate addition with a microtiter reader (Dynateck MR600) at 450 nm. The antibody response was computed by adjusting the optical density (O.D.) readings using a standard adjustment formula to compensate for interplate variation. The adjustment formula sets up a relationship between the positive and negative controls run on each plate and the O.D. for each sample. The use of the same positive and negative controls for every plate allows the comparison of O.D. values from different plates. This formula is as follows:

100/(Positive control- Negative control) = X/Sample O.D. reading

In all cases the positive control was the arbitrarily chosen sample A8 at day 42 and the negative control was A8 at day 0.

Histopathology
At the time of sacrifice (day 55, Groups A-F), tissue at the implantation site (left caudal thigh) and control site (right caudal thigh) was removed from each rat and placed into separate vials containing 10% neutral buffered formalin. Tissues were paraffin embedded and tissue sections stained with hematoxylin and eosin for light microscopic examination. Slides were read in blinded fashion and inflammatory infiltrate graded as: mild (<5% of tissue section involved and absence of well formed granulomas; Grade 1), moderate (5-10% tissue section involvement; Grade 2), or severe (>10% tissue section involvement with well formed granulomas; Grade 3).

Statistical analysis
Anti-BSA IgG level and histopathologic lesion variations between treatment groups were evaluated by ANOVA (Tukey) analysis. The mean rat weight and standard deviation for each time point was determined for each treatment group. The mean rat weigh change and standard deviation for each test group was also determined.

Results

Figure 1 represents the adjuvant effects of the various test materials on anti-BSA antibody production. The injection of BSA with phosphate buffered saline (Group G) produced only a low titer of antibodies on day 14, indicating that BSA alone is poorly immunogenic in rats. The silicone gel/silicone oil combination acted as a potent adjuvant and, in fact, had greater adjuvant properties than IFA. Silicone oil (Group B) and silicone elastomer particles (Groups E and F) did not differ from Group G (saline), indicating that these test materials do not have adjuvant activity under conditions of these experiments.

Figure 1

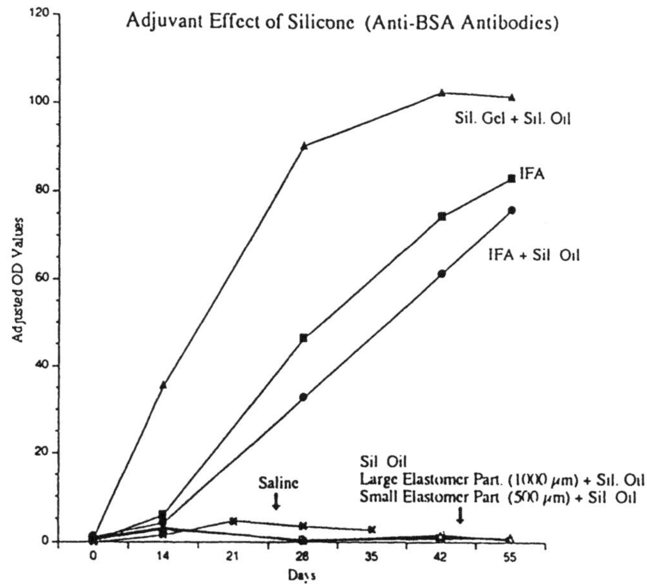

Table 2 shows the adjusted anti-BSA antibody levels for groups A-F. Values for group G show no significant elevation in anti-BSA antibody throughout the course of the study (data not shown).

Table 2. Adjusted BSA antibody levels in the 6 groups of rats. Data are expressed as mean± SD. (Adjustment formula for interplate variation: 100/ (positive - negative control) = x/ OD reading)

Groups	n*	Day 1	n	Day 14	n	Day 28	n	Day 42	n	Day 55
A	9	.289 (.270)	10	5.95 (4.200)	10	46.34 (36.253)	10	71.41 (39.879)	10	83.02 (32.237)
B	10	.517 (.240)	8	2.82 (1.499)	9	.333 (.280)	9	1.18 (.659)	9	795 (.401)
C	10	1.150 (.180)	8	4.00 (2.487)	9	32.78 (26.959)	9	61.30 (21.837)	8	75.97 (19.082)
D	10	.618 (.566)	10	35.40 (16.560)	10	90.60 (11.725)	10	102.82(20.832)	10	101.80 (10.387)
E	10	.284 (.410)	8	2.52 (.506)	10	.323(.250)	10	.568 (.749)	10	.986(.520)
F	10	.893 (.319)	8	3.19 (1.565)	10	.172 (.169)	10	1.59 (1.227)	10	.326 (.241)

* n represents the number of samples tested per group.
Variation in numbers within a group may be due to either animal death or insufficient sample.

Statistical analysis revealed that there were minor differences in anti-BSA antibody levels between various treatment groups at day 0 (before treatment). These levels probably represent pre-existing "natural" antibody to BSA. These differences are presumably due to chance during randomization. Day 14, 21 (p<0.0001)and 28 (p=0.0005) data show that there is a statistically significant elevation of anti-BSA antibody levels between silicone gel/silicone oil treated animals and all other treatment groups (Fig.2). This finding indicates that silicone gel is a more potent and faster acting adjuvant than IFA. Paired t-Test evaluating day1 vs. day 14 rise in anti-BSA antibody level reveals a significant increase in antibody in IFA (p=0.0034), silicone oil (p=0.0007), silicone gel/silicone oil (p<0.0001), and silicone elastomer (p=0.0063). Silicone oil and silicone elastomer levels were comparible to saline treated animals. In subsequent evaluations (days 42 and 55) the silicone gel/silicone oil combination is comparable to that of IFA and both are significantly elevated as compared to silicone oil and silicone elastomer implanted animals (Fig.3). Anti-BSA antibody levels appear to peak at day 42 in silicone gel/silicone oil treatment group, but continue to rise in the IFA treatment group.

Figure 4 represents average group weights over time. It shows a continued increase in body weight for all groups at the time points examined and indicates that there is no significant difference in weights between the treatment groups. The animals were in good general health and that there was adequate intake of food throughout the course of the study.

Figure 2

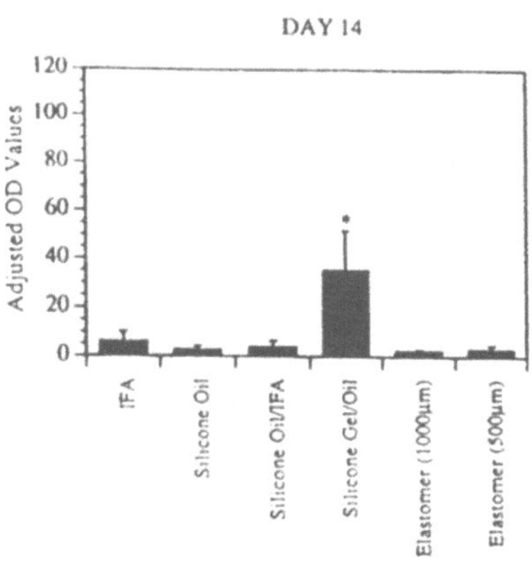

* Significant rise in anti-BSA antibodies as compared to all other treatment groups ($p = < 0.0001$)

Figure 3

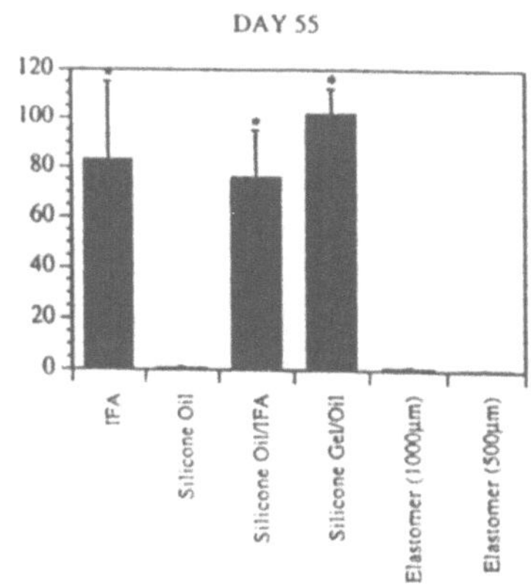

*These groups are not statistically significant to each other ($p = > 0.05$), but are significant to all other groups ($p = < 0.0001$)

Histopathologic evaluation of the left caudal thigh muscle implantation sites was accompanied by examination of the right caudal thigh muscle for each animal. The average histopathologic grades for each group are represented in Table 3. Light microscopic evaluation revealed moderate to severe inflammation only on the left in rats treated with IFA (Group A), IFA + silicone oil (Group C), and silicone gel/ silicone oil (Group D). There was mild to moderate inflammatory infiltrates in left caudal thigh muscles of animals implanted with silicone elastomer particles. The infiltrate appeared to be more intense in animals treated with 500 micron particles versus those treated with 1000 micron elastomer particles. We attribute this finding to the greater surface area of the 500 micron particles. Animals implanted with silicone oil showed minimal inflammatory infiltrates. The right caudal thigh muscle sections from all animals showed no significant cellular infiltrate.

Table 3. Histopathologic Grade

Group	Treatment	n	Mean ± SD[a]
A	IFA + BSA	10	2.1 ± 0.74
B	SO[b] + BSA	9	1.2 ± 0.44
C	SO + IFA + BSA	8	2.1 ± 0.83
D	SG[c] + SO + BSA	10	2.1 ± 0.57
E	500 u SE[d] + SO+ BSA	10	1.3 ± 0.48
F	1000 u SE + SO + BSA	10	1.9 ± 0.57

[a] Standard deviation, [b] silicone oil, [c] silicone gel, [d] silicone elastomer particles.

Figure 4. Average Weights for all Treatment Groups.

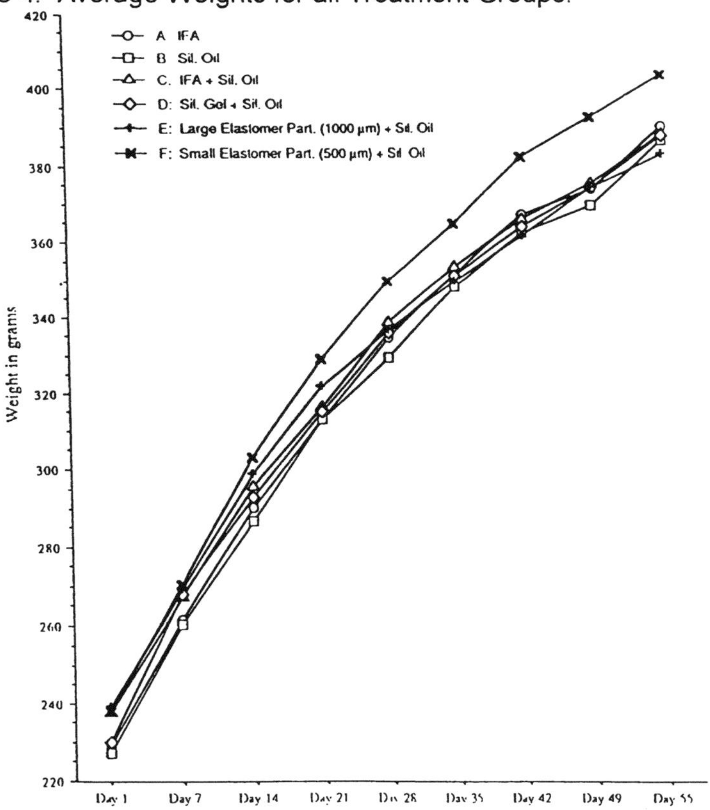

Silicone oil treated animals (Group B) show a significantly less inflammatory than IFA (Group A), IFA + silicone oil (Group C) and silicone gel/ silicone oil (Group D) implanted rats. There is, however, no significant difference in the histopathologic grades between silicone oil and both groups of silicone elastomer treated animals. Additionally, there is no significant difference in the average histopathologic grades between groups implanted with IFA, IFA/ silicone oil, or silicone gel/ silicone oil and those receiving silicone elastomer particles (Fig. 5). Silicone elastomer particles elicit a mild local inflammatory infiltrate. IFA (Fig. 6) and silicone/IFA treated animals (Groups A and C) exhibited moderate to severe inflammatory infiltrates involving the epimysium and frequent extension into the underlying muscle bundle. Lesions were characterized by well formed granulomas with multinucleated giant cells and scattered aggregates of epitheliod macrophages surrounded by dense infiltrates of lymphocytes, plasma cells, neutrophils and occasional eosinophils. Silicone oil treated animals (Group B) showed minimal inflammatory infiltrates. Occasional multinucleated giant cells and vacuolation were seen within the subcuticular tissue, epimysium or underlying muscle bundle, but there was little evidence of an accompaying lymphoplasmacytic infiltrate. Well formed granulomas were observed in animals treated with silicone gel/ silicone oil

Fig. 5 Histopathologic Grades

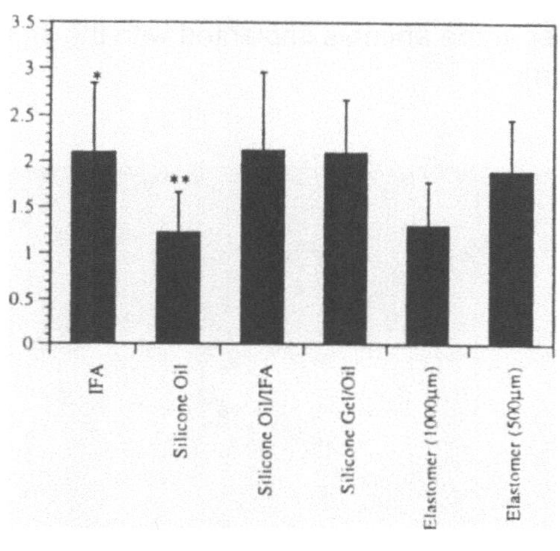

* IFA treated animals have a statistically significant greater histopathologic grade as compared to silicone oil treated rats ($p < 0.05$)

** Silicone oil implantation results in a significantly lower inflammatory responce ($p<0.05$) as compared to IFA/Silicone oil and silicone gel treated animals as determined by the Tukey-Kramer multiple comparisons test mixture (Group D). The granulomas with centralized clear vacuoles, located in the subcutis and epimysium and extending into the underlying muscle, were frequently lined by a thick layer of foamy macrophages surrounded by a dense infiltrate of lymphocytes and plasma cells interrupted by small aggregates of epitheliod macrophages and occasional multinucleated giant cells. Isolated vacuoles were seen scattered throughout the dense cellular infiltrate (Fig. 7a). Polarizing light revealed non-polarizing flat gray globular material, presumably silicone, within macrophages and extracellular vacuoles (Fig. 7b). Both groups of rats treated with silicone elastomer (Groups E and F) exhibited cellular infiltrates at the sight of implantation. Lesions were characterized by irregular to coalescing clear vacuoles containing gray- white refractile irregular shaped particles (elastomer particles). The walls of these vacuoles were composed of loose fibrous connective tissue with infiltrates of lymphocytes, plasma cells, neutrophils, and occasional eosinophils. Vacuoles were frequently lined by a single layer of macrophages with intermittent aggregates of multinucleated giant cells (Fig. 8a). Upon polarization, large irregular fragments of elastomer failed to polarize. However, thin spiculated fragments within macrophages did polarize (Fig. 8b). It has been speculated previously that these sharp spicules represent silica [3]. The extracellular elastomer particles were frequently found to be out of the plane of section. The intensity of the cellular infiltrate was higher in the animals implanted with the small elastomer pieces (500 micron).

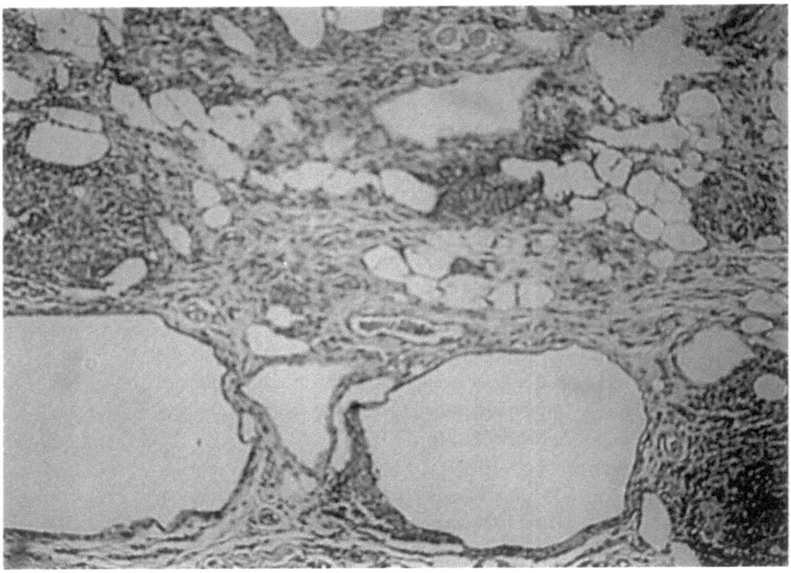

Figure 6. IFA + BSA (100x). Multiple granulomas with clear centralized vacuoles surrounded by thin rim of macrophages. Surrounding subcuticular tissue has numerous small vacuoles and aggregates of lymphocytes, plasma cells, neutrophils and occasional eosinophils.

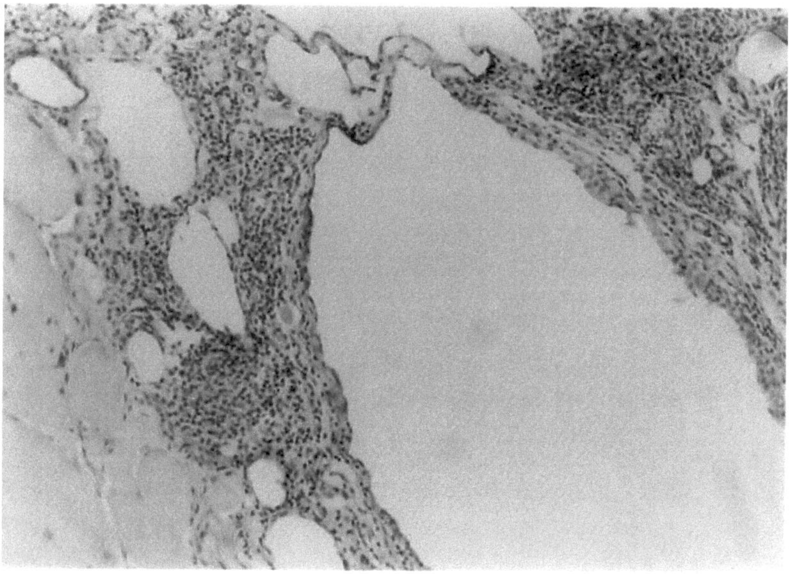

Figure 7a. Silicone oil + IFA + BSA (100x). Multiple variably sized vacuoles lined occasionally by flattened macrophages Surrounded by moderate infiltrate of lymphocytes, plasma cells and occasional neutrophils.

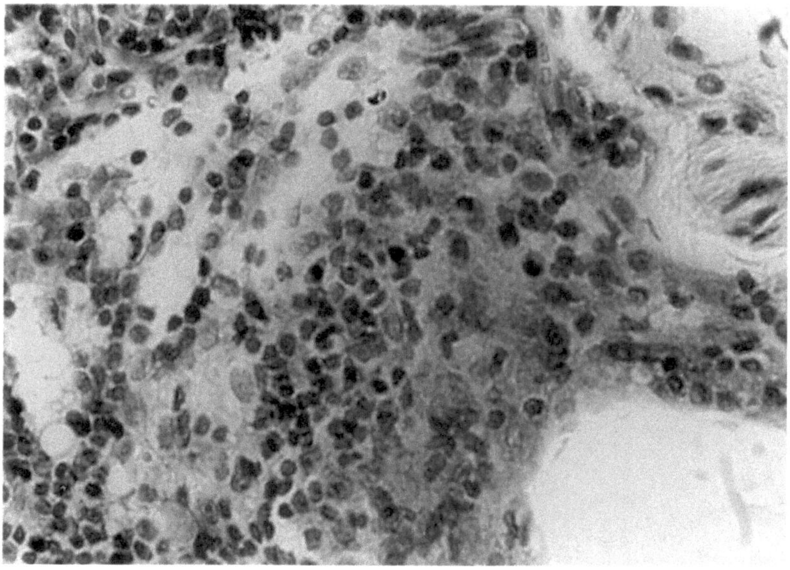

Figure 7b. Silicone oil + IFA + BSA (400x). Granuloma with centralized clear vacuole surrounded by multiple layers of epitheliod macrophages and occasional multinucleated giant cells. This is rimmed by moderate infiltrate of lymphocytes and vacuoles containing a light gray globular material.

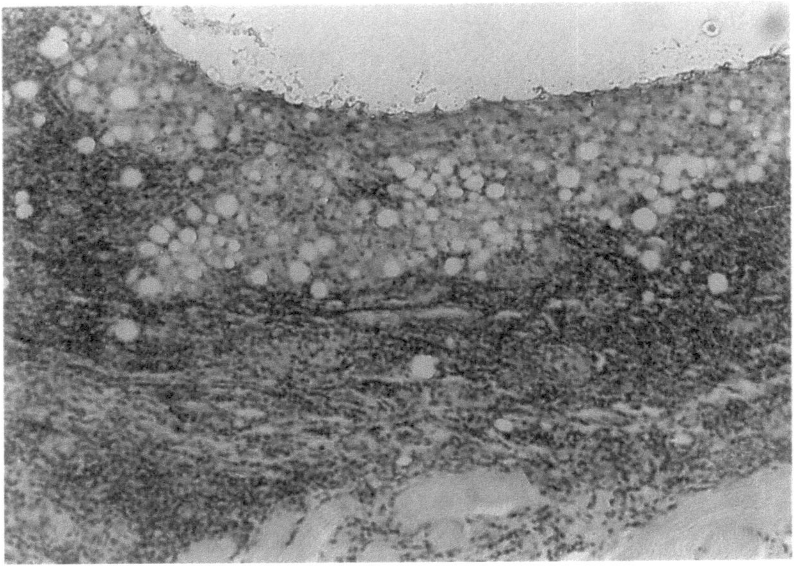

Figure 8a. Silicone gel/Silicone oil + BSA (100x). Large well formed granuloma with centralized clear vacuole rimmed by thick layer of foamy macrophages containing numerous intra- and extracellular vacuoles. This is surrounded by thick layer of lymphocytes and plasma cells with intermittent satellite granulomas consisting of small aggregates of epitheliod macrophages. Inflammatory infiltrated extends into underlying skeletal muscle.

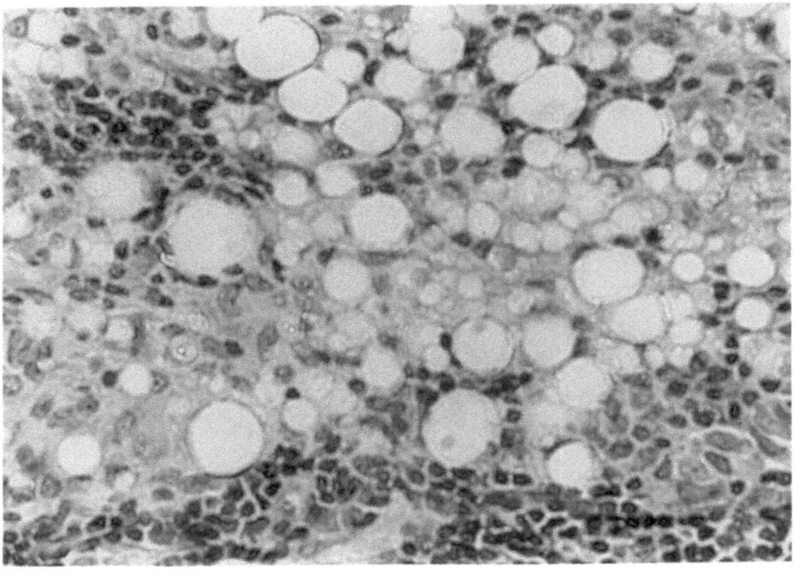

Figure 8b. Silicone gel/Silicone oil + BSA (400x). High power magnification of foamy macrophage layer. Numerous vacuoles contain grayish-green globular material slightly retracted from vacuole wall. Vacuoles are both intra- and extracellular.

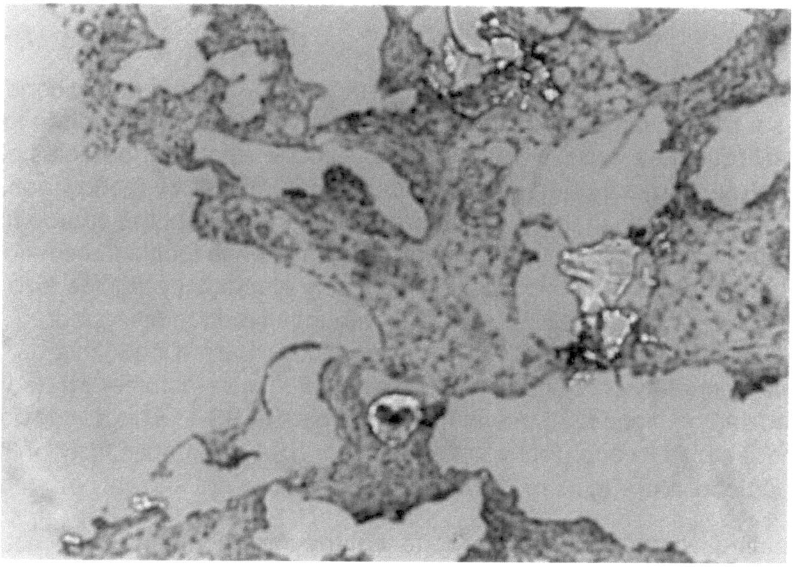

Figure 9a. 500 micron Silicone elastomer + BSA (100x). Multiple to coalescing vacuoles containing irregular refractile particles (silicone elastomer) within the subcuticular tissue surrounded by loose fibrous connective tissue infiltrated by lymphocytes and plasma cells.

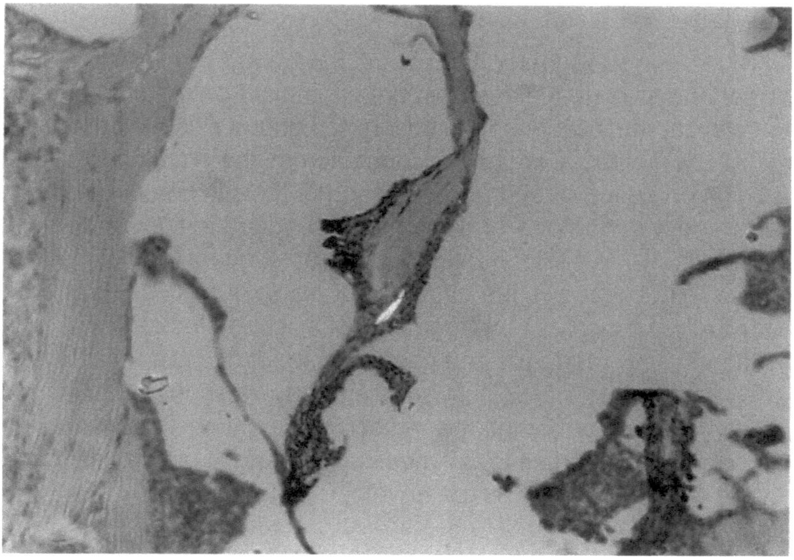

Figure 9b. 500 micron Silicone elastomer + BSA (100 x, polarizing lense). Multiple coalescing vacuoles containing irregular refractile non-polarizing particle and a polarizing spicule within macrophage layer lining a vacuole. Inflammatory inflitrate entraps a skeletal muscle myocyte.

Discussion

The findings of this experiment confirm that silicone gel but not silicone oil acts as a potent immunologic adjuvant as measured by a heightened IgG antibody response to BSA. Furthermore, silicone elastomer particles had no apparent adjuvant effect in this model as determined by the low anti-BSA antibody levels in these treatment groups throughout the course of the study. Additionally, silicone gel elicited an intense local inflammatory response at the sight of implantation. Silicone elastomer particles also induced a local mixed cellular infiltrate, with inflammation being more intense in animals implanted with small particles. Surprisingly, this infiltrate frequently contained many plasma cells, but elastomer treated rats showed no significant rise in IgG antibodies to BSA. This suggests that the B cells are apparently not specific for BSA. The specificity of the immunoglobulin products of the infiltrating B cells is not known.

Our findings support previous reports that the intensity of the cellular response increases with the molecular weight of the silicone polymer [4]. This was found for silicone oil and silicone gel. However, in this study silicone elastomer, highest in molecular weight, tended to elicit an inflammatory response greater than silicone oil, but less than silicone gel/ silicone oil mixture. The inflammatory response did not correspond with adjuvant potency.

Concern has been raised as to the potential adjuvant properties of silicone gel and silicone elastomer in breast implant patients and the potential clinical ramifications of exposure to various silicone products. Leakage of low molecular weight silicones across the envelope appears to be a common event. Some fragmentation of the silicone envelope has been observed with particles of elastomer embedded in the surrounding fibrous capsule. Unlike silicone gel, our results suggest that low molecular weight linear silicone oil does not possess adjuvant properties. The study further indicates that fragments of silicone elastomer may elicit a local inflammatory response and contribute to fibrogenesis, but do not show adjuvanticity in our model. In another study, described in this volume, we have found that the low molecular weight cyclic siloxane, D4, also has adjuvant properties in the mouse. The extent of diffusion of these cyclic compounds across the envelope is not known.

The patients at greatest risk of exposure to silicone gel are those who have experienced rupture of their mammary prosthesis. However, slow leakage of cyclic compounds may occur without rupture. Both of these populations may induce a heightened humoral immune response to foreign antigens. Whether they could initiate an immune response to self-antigens is not known. The development of autoimmune disease, moreover, requires multiple immune events, such as adequate antigen presentation, activation of self-reactive T cells to induce cell-mediated immunity, reversal of anergy, vulnerability of the target organ and genetic predisposition. The identification of circulating autoantibodies alone does not necessarily indicate the occurrence of autoimmune disease. In fact, in the normal population, the level of circulating autoantibodies tends to increase with increasing age. These studies, therefore, do not address the potential of silicone compounds to induce autoimmune disease.

Future studies will examine the potential mechanism of the adjuvanticity of silicone gel. The silicone gel/silicone oil mixture gives evidence of a heightened IgG antibody response to BSA and therefore suggests that silicone gel may serve as a depot and allow for slow release of antigen. We will test various methods of trituration/homogenization to optimize the adjuvant properties with BSA. Additionally, we will examine the potential of silicone gel to act as an adjuvant in the induction of autoimmune disease in genetically susceptible animals.

References

1. Naim JO, Lanzafame RJ (1993) The Adjuvant Effect of Silicone-Gel on Antibody Formation in rats. Immunological Invest., 22 (2), 151-161.
2. Naim JO, Ippolito KML, Lanzafame RJ (1995) The Effect of Molecular weight and Gel Preparation on Humoral Adjuvancy of Silicone oils and Silicone gels. Immunological Invest., 24(3), 537-547.
3. Raso DS, Greene WB, Vesely JJ, Willingham MC (1994) Light Microscopy Techniques for the Demonstration of Silicone Gel. Arch Pathol Lab Med 118, 984-987.
4. Picha GJ, Goldstein JA (1991) Analysis of the Soft-Tissue Response to Components Used in the Manufacture of Breast Implants: Rat Animal Model. Plastic and Reconstructive Surg. 87 (3), 490-500.

Silicone Gel and Octamethylcyclotetrasiloxane Potentiate Antibody Production to Bovine Serum Albumin in Mice

J. J. Nicholson III[1], G. E. Wong[2], C. G. Frondoza[1,3], and N. R. Rose[1,4][1]
Johns Hopkins University, Departments of Molecular Microbiology and Immunology[1], Biology[2], Orthopaedic Surgery[3], and Pathology[4]

Abstract

Earlier studies, in the rat, have shown that silicone gel acts as a potent adjuvant for antibody production against bovine serum albumin (BSA). The purpose of the present study is to determine whether components of the silicone breast implant (silicone oil, silicone gel, and octamethylcyclotetrasiloxane [D4]) potentiate the antibody response to BSA in mice. Groups of ten A/J mice received a single subcutaneous injection of 0.1 ml of BSA emulsified with the following: a) silicone preparations, b) incomplete Freund's adjuvant, or c) saline alone. Antibodies to BSA were measured using an enzyme-linked immunosorbant assay. The results indicate that both D4 and the silicone gel potentiate antibody production to BSA in mice. Known adjuvants have been shown to induce autoimmune syndromes in animal models. Whether silicones can act in a similar mechanism is still unclear.

Introduction

For over forty years it has been speculated that some component(s) of mammary implants act as adjuvants interacting with autologous antigens to induce autoimmune disease-like syndromes in women with silicone breast implants.[2] Since the 1960s, over one hundred cases of silicone breast implant recipients were reported to exhibit autoimmune-like syndromes. The authors speculated that the development of autoimmune syndromes in these women was associated with exposure to the silicone implants. Whether or not silicone from breast implants plays a role in the pathogenesis of autoimmune disorders is not clear, but several investigators have proposed that the silicone could do so by acting as an adjuvant.[2,3,4] In 1964, Miyoshi et al. described the occurrence of connective tissue disease-like syndromes in patients whose breasts had been injected directly several years earlier with a paraffin or impure silicone-related substance.[5] Miyoshi speculated that the injected foreign material played a role as an adjuvant in the pathogenesis of these syndromes. These syndromes, referred to as human adjuvant disease, resembled the development of polyarthritis in rats following injection of complete Freund's adjuvant.[6,7,8]

To determine if silicones are able to induce autoimmune disease, it would be informative to first evaluate whether or not silicone can act as an adjuvant. In 1993, Naim et al. showed that silicone gel acts as a potent adjuvant, enhancing the antigenicity of bovine serum albumin (BSA) in Sprague Dawley rats.[9] Naim tested silicone oil and gel, but did not examine the low molecular weight residual cyclic prepolymer that is found in the gel-filled implant. It is well documented that low molecular weight silicone "bleeds" through even the "low-bleed" implant envelopes[.10] This strongly suggests that breast implant recipients are exposed to the low molecular weight residual pre-polymer of octamethylcyclotetrasiloxane(D4). We used a mouse model to analyze the adjuvant effect of silicones on antibody production. As a basis for comparison we injected a well-known, potent adjuvant: incomplete Freund's adjuvant (IFA).[11] The purpose of the present study is to determine whether components of the silicone breast implant (silicone oil, silicone gel, and D4) potentiate antibody response to BSA in A/J mice.

Materials & Methods

Experimental Groups

Seven groups of ten, 6 to 8 week old male A/J mice (Jackson Laboratories Bar Harbor, ME) were injected with 0.1 ml of BSA (250 μg/ml) emulsified with the following: Group 1- phosphate buffer solution, pH 7.2 (PBS); Group II- 20 cs silicone oil (Sigma Co., Lot# 112H0513); Group III- 50% silicone gel-oil homogenized mixture; Group IV- IFA(Sigma Co., Lot# 102H0347); Group V- IFA mixed with an equal volume of silicone oil; Group VI- D4 (Dow Corning, Lot# LL044530); and Group VII- IFA mixed with an equal volume of D4. LeVier's protocol for dealing with silicone gel implants

(Mentor, Silatex® Low Bleed Gel-filled Mammary Prosthesis, Lot# 84522) was followed.[12].

Determination of antibody production to BSA by ELISA:

The mice were bled via retro-orbital plexus, under Metaphane narcosis, at 0, 15, 30, 45, 60, 75, and 90 days after immunization. Standard enzyme linked immunosorbent assays (ELISA) were performed to determine the antibody levels (serum diluted 1:1000 with PBS, pH 7.2) to BSA.[13] We used Immunolon 96 well microtitration plates (Dynatek, Alexandria, VA), alkaline phosphatase conjugated affinity pure goat anti-mouse HC & LC specific IgG(Sigma Co., Lot# 063H8930), para Nitrophenyl Phosphate substrate (Sigma Co., Lot# 054H8911), and mouse monoclonal anti-BSA IgG (Sigma Co., Lot #123H4812). The optical density (O.D.) was read at 405 nm with a microtiter plate reader (Vmax, Molecular Devices).

Statistical Analysis

ANOVA was analyzed using StatView IV (Abacus Concepts, Inc.). A Fisher Test was utilized to determine the statistical significance of data between the groups. This test was utilized to generate p-values at a 5% significance level.

Results

Figure 1 presents the antibody response for each group. Injection of BSA mixed with PBS elicited a low level of response that peaked on day 45, followed by a decline to baseline by day 90. As expected, we found that IFA significantly ($p<0.0001$) enhanced the antibody production to BSA, compared with the PBS control group. In comparison to the PBS controls, the 50% silicone gel-oil emulsion significantly ($p<0.0001$) enhanced the production of BSA antibodies. In contrast to the silicone gel-oil emulsion, the silicone oil alone did not significantly ($p>0.250$) enhance antibody levels against the BSA. Antibody levels in mice injected with D4 elicited significantly ($p<0.0001$) higher antibody levels to the BSA, than the PBS control group. An injection containing silicone oil, IFA, and BSA yielded significantly higher antibody levels than IFA alone on post-immunization days 45 and 90 ($p=0.0316$ and $p=0.0403$, respectively) The mice that were immunized with IFA and D4 in combination had the greatest enhancement of antibody production when compared to the PBS control, although this was not statistically significant ($p=0.112$) when compared with the group receiving IFA alone.

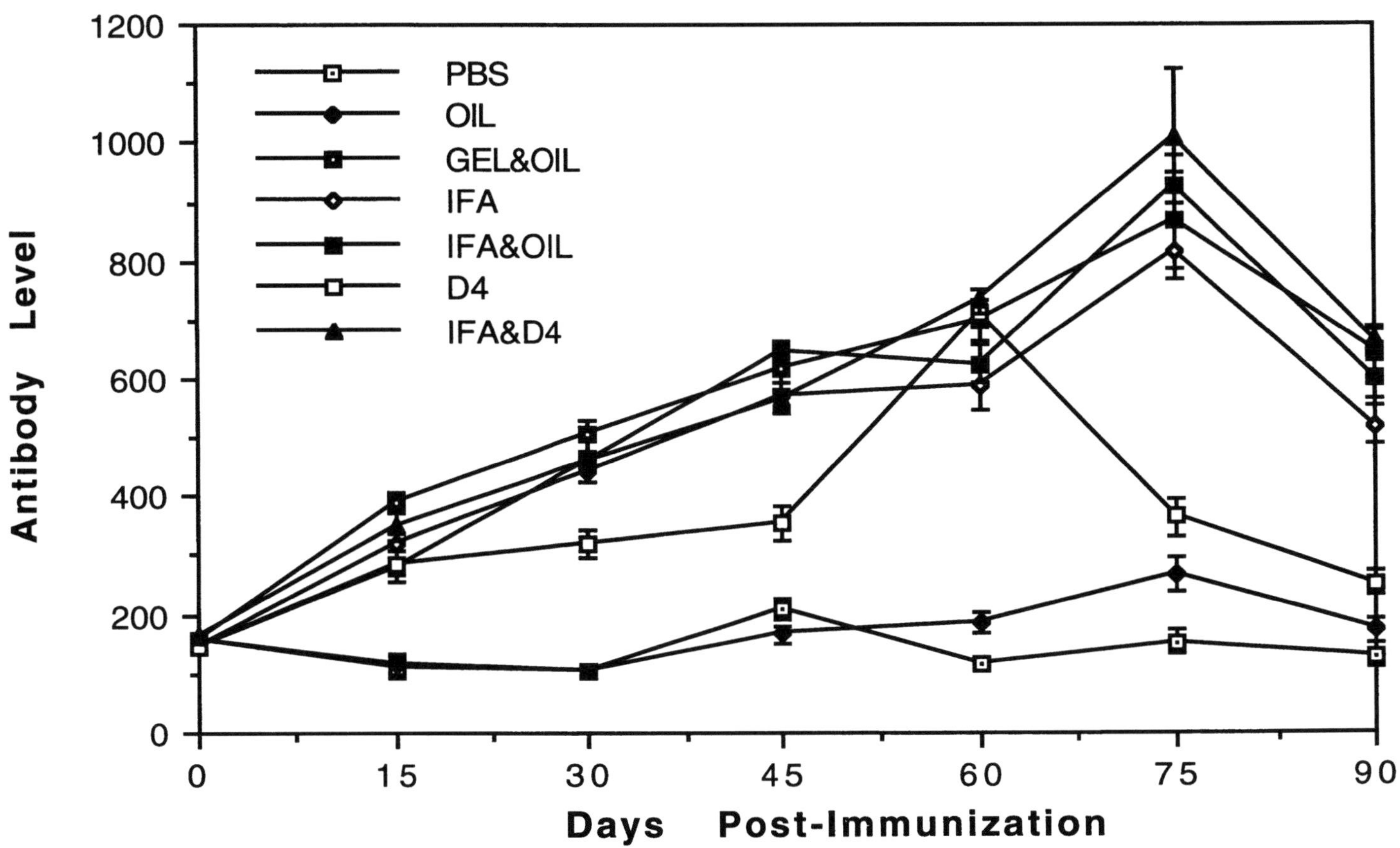

Fig. 1 Average time course of anti-BSA antibody production for each group of ten mice. (Error bars= ±SEM)

Discussion

The major findings of the present study are that both silicone gel and the low molecular weight D4 potentiate antibody response to BSA in mice. As previously stated, adjuvants have been shown to produce autoimmune disease in animal models, without requiring the co-administration of a specific self antigen. The best known example of such an adjuvant is complete Freund's adjuvant (CFA), which contains mineral oil emulsified with heat-killed tubercle bacilli. In 1956, Pearson described reproducible generalized or focal arthritis, synovitis, periostitis and tendonitis after a single intradermal injection of CFA alone in rats.[7,8] He called this disease adjuvant arthritis. Similar adjuvant-induced arthritis has been found to occur in MRL-lpr mice.[14]

There is a great controversy over what is responsible for induction of adjuvant-induced arthritis in the animals. One current view is that a mycobacterium 65kDa protein, a member of the heat shock family of proteins, is the causative agent of adjuvant-induced arthritis.[15,16] The administration of the oil vehicle alone or a suspension of the acid-fast microorganism in saline failed to induce arthritis.[17,18] Other studies suggest that the mycobacterium is not needed. Kleinau et al. observed that percutaneous exposure to IFA, adjuvant oil minus the bacterium, caused arthritis in DA rats.[19] Nonspecific stimulation of the immune system may result in a breakdown of tolerance to self-molecules, which could progress to an autoimmune disease.

Adjuvants are known to elicit a battery of cytokines. The arthritic effects of CFA were blocked when IL-1 antibodies were administered to the animals.[20] In addition, IL-1 alone was observed to induce arthritis in rats.[20] It is possible that the syndromes reported in breast implant patients are cytokine-mediated. Since the mechanism by which Freund's adjuvant induced adjuvant arthritis remains undefined, we cannot be certain that the silicone could not act in a similar manner to induce autoimmune syndrome.

We have verified that silicone gel acts as an adjuvant in mice as well as rats[9]. This finding strengthens the possibility that it might also act as an adjuvant in other animals, including humans. Although silicone gel exerts a higher and more sustained adjuvant effect on antibody production than D4, it could be argued that the low molecular weight D4 is clinically a more important adjuvant. It is known that low molecular weight silicones, such as D4, are able to "leach" through the implant envelope.[10] In contrast, the high molecular weight, high viscosity, and complex branching of the silicone gel would render it less likely to diffuse through the implant envelope into the surrounding tissues.

Although silicone gel and D4 potentiated the antibody response to a foreign antigen, it still must be determined whether or not they potentiate antibody response to self antigens. Experiments testing self antigens are underway.

References

1. Dr. Rose has served as expert witness on behalf of defendants in several legal proceedings involving silicone breast implants. He has also served as consultant for Mentor Corporation, a manufacturer of breast implants.
2. Vasey FB, Havice DL, Bocsnegra TS, et al (1994) Clinical and immunologic findings in fifty consecutive women with silicone breast implants and connective tissue disease. Semin Arthritis Rheum 24 (1 Suppl 1):22-28
3. Sahn EE, Garen PD, Silver, et al. (1990) Scleroderma following augmentation mammoplasty: report of case and review of the literature. Arch Dermatol 126:1198-1202
4. Shons AR, Schubert W (1992) Silicone breast implants and immune disease. Ann Plast Surg 28:491-499
5. Miyoshi K, Miyaoki T, Kobayashi Y, et al. (1962) Hypergammaglobulinemia by prolonged adjuvanticity in man: disorders developed after augmentation mammoplasty. Jap Med J: 2122, 9-14
6. Miyoshi K, Miyaoki T, Kobayashi Y (1973) Adjuvant disease in man. Clin Immunol 5: 785-794
7. Pearson CM (1956) Development of arthritis, periarthritis, and periostitis in rats given adjuvants. Proc Soc Exp Med 91: 95-100
8. Pearson CM, Wood FD (1981) Studies of polyarthritis and other lesions induced in rats by injection of mycobacterial adjuvant. I. General clinical and pathological characteristics and some modifying factors. Arthritis Rheum 2: 440-459
9. Naim JO, Lanzafame, van Oss CJ (1993) The adjuvant effect of silicone gel on antibody formation in rats. Immunol Invest 22: 151
10. Wilkerson P (1992) Report presented before the General and Plastic Surgery Device Evaluation Panel, FDA, Bethesda, MD, February 1992
11. Roitt IM (1994) Essential immunology. Blackwell Scientific Publications, Boston
12. LeVier RR. Discussion of: Semple JL, Narini PP, Hay JB (193) Preparation techniques for silicone gel in the evaluation of its in vivo effects. Plast Reconstr Surg 92(5):979-81
13. Rose NR, Freidman H, Fahey JL, Eds (1986) Manual of clinical laboratory immunology. 3rd Ed. American Society for Microbiology, Washington, D.C.
14. Ratkay LG, Zhang L, Tonzetich J, Waterfield JD (1993) Complete Freund's adjuvantinduces an earlier and more severe arthritis in MRL-lpr mice. Journal of Immunol 151(9):5081-7
15. Lopez-Guerrero JA, Lopez-Bote JP, Ortiz MA, et al (1993) Modulation of adjuvant arthritis in Lewis rats by recombinant vaccinia virus expressing the human 60-kiladalton heat shock protein. Infect Immun 61(10):4225-31
16. van Eden W (1991) Heat-shock proteins as immunogenic bacterial antigens with the potential to induce and regulate autoimmune arthritis. Immunol Rev 121:5-28
17. Koga T, Pearson CM, Narita T, Kotani S (1973) Polyarthrities induced in the rats with cell walls from several bacteria and two streptomyces species. Proc Soc Exp Biol Med 143: 824
18. Whitehouse MW, Orr KJ, Beck FWJ, Pearson CM (1974) Freund's adjuvants: relationship of arthritogenicity and adjuvanticity in rats to vehicle composition. Immunol 27: 311
19. Kleinau S, Erlandsson H, Klareskog L (1994) Percutaneous exposure of adjuvant oil causes arthritis in DA rats. Clin Exp Immunol 96: 281-284.
20. Perretti M, Mudridge KG, Becherucci C, Parente L (1991) Evidence that interleukin-1 and lipoxygenase metabolites mediate the lethal effect of complete Freund's adjuvant in adrenalectomized rats. Lymphokine Cytokine Res 10 (4): 239-43

Macrophages, Polyreactive and Antilipid Antibodies

Fibrogenic and Other Biological Effects of Silica

Anthony C. Allison
Dawa Corporation, Belmont, CA 94002

Introduction

Crystalline silica, silicon dioxide (SiO_2), has a simple chemical structure but potent biological effects. The structures of different crystalline and amorphous forms of silica and related molecules are reviewed by Heaney and Banfield (1993) and their biological effects are reviewed by Guthrie (1992). The commonest form is quartz, although other tetrahedral crystalline forms of silica (tridymite, crystobalite) have comparable effects. In contrast, stishovite is an octahedral form of crystalline silica, produced under conditions of high temperature and pressure. It is biologically inert, like titanium dioxide (rutile). Silica dust exposure during the mining and smelting of metal ores has long been known to produce pulmonary fibrosis (silicosis or phthisis) and to increase the incidence of tuberculosis (Collis, 1919). In some countries, such as the People's Republic of China, large numbers of occupationally exposed workers are showing progressive impairment of lung function. It is desirable to clarify the underlying pathogenesis and, if possible, control it.

The carcinogenic effects of silica are less dramatic than those of asbestos, which induces a unique type of cancer (mesothelioma), as well as increasing the incidence of adenocarcinomas, especially in cigarette smokers. However, epidemiological evidence strongly suggests that chronic silicosis predisposes to an increased lung cancer risk, which is due either to high silica exposure or to the fibrotic process or to both factors (Goldsmith, 1994).

The fibrogenic effects of silica are easily reproduced in experimental animals, such as rats and mice, which has facilitated analysis of the underlying molecular and cell biology, as well as genetic differences in responses. In fact silica provides a convenient probe for studying the process of fibrogenesis, which is important not only in the lungs (in silicosis, following irradiation and bleomycin treatment and spontaneous) but also in the liver (cirrhosis), skin (scleroderma and keloid formation) and the peritoneal and pelvic cavities (adhesions, intestinal obstruction and infertility). Collagen deposition in arterial walls also occurs in atherosclerosis.

Although the biological effects of crystalline silica are more potent than those of the many amorphous forms of silica, the latter can be fibrogenic and carcinogenic. Silicones presumably elicit fibrosis and other tissue reactions by similar mechanisms. Again, genetic differences in individuals exposed to comparable amounts of silicones might influence the magnitude and nature of tissue responses. In this paper the mechanisms by which silica induces fibrotic responses, and likely mediators, are reviewed. Evidence will be presented that this response is lymphocyte-independent. However, a strong granulomatous reaction, including collagen deposition, can also be elicited by responses of T-lymphocytes to antigens (e.g. schistosome egg antigens), or by a toxic chemical such as bleomycin. If silicones are eliciting immune responses, they could produce tissue reactions, including fibrosis and contracture around breast implants, by an analogous mechanism.

Collaboration of Macrophages and Fibroblasts in Silica-induced Fibrogenesis

Following inhalation into the lungs, silica particles are rapidly engulfed by alveolar and interstitial macrophages, which are therefore the first cells involved in the process. Pulmonary fibroblasts do not normally take up crystalline silica particles greater than about 1 µM, but their numbers are markedly increased following silica exposure, and collagen synthesis is also greatly augmented, as shown not only by histology, but also by measurement of tissue hydroxyproline levels. This led us to study effects of silica on cultured macrophages and to suggest that macrophages and fibroblasts collaborate in silica-induced fibrogenesis (Allison et al., 1966). According to an updated version of this hypothesis, silica induces the production by macrophages of factors that stimulate the recruitment and proliferation of fibroblasts and their differentiation into collagen-synthesizing cells. In response to the macrophage-produced mitogenic factor fibroblasts proliferate. In response to another macrophage-produced factor the expression in fibroblasts of procollagen genes is increased. Procollagen mRNAs are then efficiently translated; procollagen is synthesized, and undergoes proteolytic processing to form collagen; and finally collagen is cross-linked and deposited, together with other intercellular matrix constituents (e.g. proteoglycan, fibronectin, and tenascin).

That macrophages and fibroblasts collaborate in fibrogenesis by a mechanism not involving cellular contact is demonstrated by a simple experiment (Allison et al., 1977). Diffusion chambers - plastic rings with 0.8 µM diameter millipore filters cemented to both sides - have been used to place cells in confined situations in the body, usually the peritoneal cavity. Cells and particles above 1 µM in diameter cannot escape from intact chambers, as verified by appropriate controls, but proteins and other macromolecules diffuse readily into or out of the chambers. As shown in fig. 1A, we found that when silica particles and macrophages were placed in diffusion chambers in the peritoneal cavities of mice, they elicited proliferation of fibroblasts and collagen deposition in the parietal and visceral peritoneum (Allison et al., 1977). Silica particles alone, or macrophages alone, in the diffusion chambers did not elicit a fibrogenic response. It was concluded that silica induces macrophages to release a factor or factors stimulating the recruitment and proliferation of fibroblasts and their differentiation into collagen-synthesizing cells. We now know that there are several candidate cytokines for roles in the mediation of these effects (table 1), and evidence identifying the most important is reviewed below.

Table 1. Cytokines produced by macrophages and CD4$^+$ T-lymphocytes with effects on fibroblasts

Effect on fibroblasts	Cytokine	Producing cell	Reference
Chemotaxis	TGF-β	Macrophage	Postlethwaite et al. (1994)
	IL-4	Lymphocyte	Postlethwaite & Sayer (1991)
Mitogenic	TNF-α	Macrophage	Piguet et al. (1990a,b)
	IL-1	Macrophage	Schmidt et al. (1984)
	PDGF	Macrophage	Ross et al. (1986)
	FGF	Macrophage	Folkman & Klagsbrun (1987)
	Fibrosin	Lymphocyte	Prakash et al. (1995)
Induction of collagen synthesis	TGF-β	Macrophage	Ignotz & Massague (1986)
	IL-4	Lymphocyte	Postlethwaite et al. (1992)

In these experiments there was no sign of a lymphocytic infiltrate around the diffusion chambers, suggesting that lymphocytes do not participate in silica-mediated fibrogenesis. In fact, the fibrogenic effects of silica are not markedly affected by the absence of T-lymphocytes (Hubbard, 1989). This contrasts with the requirement of T-lymphocytes to increase lung TNF-α mRNA and the development of pulmonary fibrosis following exposure to the drug bleomycin (Piguet et al., 1989), which occurs by the lymphocyte-dependent mechanism discussed in the next section.

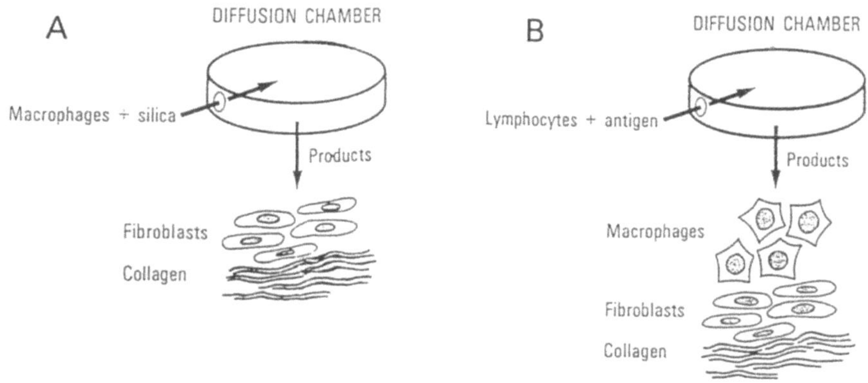

Fig. 1. Diagram of experiments with diffusion chambers.

A different experimental approach led to similar conclusions (Stark et al., 1988). Quartz was injected into one hind footpad of mice, and the popliteal lymph nodes (PLN) were recovered 40, 90 and 180 days later. The PLN of the drainage chain showed a comparable progressive enlargement (up to a factor of 200) in all 6 mouse strains tested. However, morphometric measurements of the fibrotic areas in the PLN showed marked strain differences. For example, after 180 days 11% of the cross-sectional area of PLNs was collagen in BALB/c mice, but only 0.3% in DBA-2 (both $H\text{-}2^d$). A comparison of BALB/c nu/nu and +/nu mice showed that quartz-induced fibrosis does not require T-cells. The authors suggest that SiO_2 is not an antigen, that the lymphoproliferative effects of silica can be separated from its fibrogenic effect, and that MHC molecules and T-cells do not have a major influence on the latter. They conclude: "That leaves macrophages, which are activated by silica and known to produce fibrogenic cytokines, and fibroblasts, which respond to these cytokines, as the most likely candidate cells expressing the genetic difference described".

In view of the remarkable difference in fibrogenic effects of silica in various mouse strains, it is likely that women will show individual differences in tissue responses to silica and silicones released from breast implants.

Collaborations of Lymphocytes, Macrophages, Mast Cells, Platelets and Fibroblasts in Antigen-induced and Bleomycin-induced Fibrogenesis

We extended the diffusion chamber experiments to model lymphocyte-dependent fibrogenesis occurring, for example, around schistosome eggs and in tuberculous lesions (Allison et al., 1977). Sensitized T-lymphocytes and antigen were placed in the chambers (Fig. 1B). These were found to elicit, around the chambers, a potent granulomatous response, with many macrophages, new blood vessel formation, peripheral immigration of fibroblasts, and deposition of collagen.

It is now known that $CD4^+$ lymphocytes activate macrophages. These release mature TGF-β which, together with IL-4 produced by activated $CD4^+$ T-cells, is chemotactic for fibroblasts (Postlethwaite et al., 1994; Postlethwaite and Sayer, 1991). These cytokines are thought to be mediators of the recruitment of fibroblasts into granulomatous lesions. Activated macrophages produce TNF-α, which is mitogenic for fibroblasts (Piguet et al., 1990a,b). A product of activated $CD4^+$ lymphocytes which stimulates proliferation of fibroblasts is the recently cloned fibrosin (Prakash et al., 1995), TGF-β and IL-4 induce the synthesis of collagen by fibroblasts (Ignotz and Massague, 1986; Postlethwaite et al., 1992).

Two other cell types come into the picture. Claman (1990) has drawn attention to the presence in the skin of experimental animals with chronic graft-versus-host disease of numerous mast cells, including a relatively high proportion of degranulated cells. Presumably cytokines released from the GVH reaction stimulate the production and activation of mast cells. IL-3 is a critical lymphokine in mast-cell production (Ihle et al., 1983). Among the cytokines released by mast cells are TNF-α (Gordon and Galli, 1990), which could stimulate the proliferation of fibroblasts, and IL-4 (Burd, 1995), which could induce procollagen gene expression in these cells (Postlethwaite et al., 1992). Mast cells are abundant in situations where excess collagen is produced (Claman, 1990).

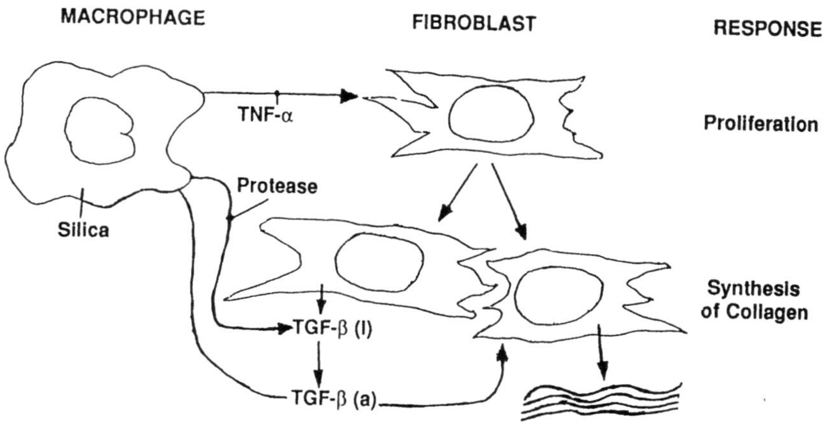

Fig. 2. Diagram illustrating the mitogenic effect of TNF-α on fibroblasts and the induction by active TGF-β (a) of collagen synthesis in fibroblasts. TGF-α (l) is the latent form of the cytokine.

Piguet and Vesin (1994) have drawn attention to bleomycin-induced trapping of blood platelets in the lungs of mice. The effects of antibodies suggested that CD11a on platelets interacts with CD54 induced on alveolar endothelium to mediate such trapping, which was correlated with fibrogenesis. Platelets contain abundant PDGF, which stimulates proliferation of fibroblasts, and TGF-β, which induces procollagen gene expression. However, bleomycin-induced pulmonary fibrosis is not greatly influenced by thrombocytopenia (Evans et al., 1990; Piguet and Vesin, 1994). Hence the relative contribution of platelets, as compared with other cell types, to fibrogenesis is not yet established.

Effects of Silica on Cultured Macrophages

We found (Allison et al., 1966) that quartz and other tetrahedral silica crystals of respirable size (0.5-5 μM) are highly cytotoxic for macrophage cultures. In fact, we recommended that silica be used to deplete macrophages *in vivo*, a procedure that became widely used (Kagan and Hartman, 1984) before it was replaced by the better method of Van Rooijen and Sanders (1994). However, macrophages tolerate smaller amounts of silica, which activates them to secrete factors stimulating the proliferation of fibroblasts (Heppleston and Styles, 1967), as we had predicted (Allison et al., 1966).

Another remarkable change in cultured macrophages produced by tolerated amounts of silica is abrogation of their capacity to restrict the multiplication of intracellular bacteria. We found that in control macrophages a virulent strain of Mycobacterium tuberculosis (H37RV) multiplied freely whereas an avirulent strain (H37RA) did not; in the presence of silica both strains grew equally well (Allison and Hart, 1988). Thus the well-known epidemiological finding that silicotic humans are predisposed to tuberculosis (Collis, 1919) is explained at the level of the macrophage-silica interaction, without necessary involvement of lymphocytes.

The cellular basis of this silica-augmented susceptibility is unknown. Transgenic mouse experiments have shown that TNF-α and IFN-γ prevent the growth of bacteria within macrophages (Aggarwal and Puri, 1995), and perhaps responses to these, or other cytokines with similar effects, are eliminated by silica.

The cytotoxicity of silica was correlated with its capacity to disrupt the membranes of secondary lysosomes in macrophages, shown histochemically by release of marker enzymes (Allison et al., 1966). The mechanism by which silica exerts effects on lysosomal and other membranes requires consideration.

Physico-Chemical Properties of Silica in Relation to its Biological Effects

It is remarkable that an inorganic compound with the simple structure of silicon dioxide, which does not form covalent bonds with biological molecules, or catalyse bond formation or breakage, should have such potent *in vivo* effects. We drew attention to a possible mechanism: the capacity of the unionized silanol groups on silica to form hydrogen bonds with phosphate ester groups of phospholipids and amide groups of proteins (Nash et al., 1966). Briefly, there are two classes of hydrogen bonding compounds. The larger group comprises hydrogen acceptors such as ethers, ketones and other compounds with active lone-pair electrons on oxygen or nitrogen. The smaller class comprises hydrogen donors, of which only phenols are important among organic compounds, and silicic and tannic acids among inorganic compounds. The latter can interact with hydrogen acceptors such as phosphate ester groups of phospholipids and amide groups of proteins, as shown by model experiments (Nash et al., 1966). For example:

$$\equiv\text{Si–OH} + \text{O=N–} \rightarrow \equiv\text{Si–OH}\cdots\cdots\text{O=N–}$$

$$\equiv\text{Si–OH} + \text{O=P}\equiv \rightarrow \equiv\text{Si-OH}\cdots\cdots\text{O=P}\equiv$$

$$\equiv\text{Si–OH} + \text{NH=} \rightarrow \equiv\text{Si–OH}\cdots\cdots\text{NH=}$$

This has been widely accepted as a general model for interactions of silica with biological macromolecules (Bendz and Lindquist, 1978; Shi et al., 1989; Mao et al., 1994).

On the surface of tetrahedral silica crystals is a rigid array of unionized silanol groups that can function as hydrogen donors. By forming hydrogen bonds with phosphate ester groups of phospholipids they can distort membrane structure. Silica crystals were found to increase the permeability of entrapped ions through the phospholipid bilayers of liposomes (Weissmann and Rita, 1972). Silica is also hemolytic (Nash et al., 1966).

Support for our proposed mechanism for the biological effects of silica came from the observation that polyvinylpyridine-N-oxide protects erythrocytes from hemolysis and macrophages from silica toxicity. The basic unit, pyridine-N-oxide, has an oxygen atom with a high negative charge which is able to form strong hydrogen bonds but not abstract hydrogen from water to form ions. The polymer had previously been shown to suppress the formation of collagen in animals exposed to silica (Schlipköter et al., 1963).

Interactions of silica with lipoprotein and protein films are well known, and silica particles adsorb proteins and denature them. In fact, a protein coat on silica particles inhibits cell lysis and delays lysosomal disruption until the protein is digested in secondary lysosomes.

The mechanism by which silica induces the production of cytokines by macrophages is unknown. However, three possible mechanisms can be suggested. Because of interactions with membrane enzymes and lipids, silica could trigger lipid-based signal-transduction systems, such as the activation of phospholipase C with production of inositol phosphates and phosphatidyl glycerol. Alternatively, silica could crosslink or otherwise activate receptor proteins in the membranes of endocytic vacuoles, thereby triggering signal transduction systems. A third possibility arises from the fact that silica can generate oxygen radicals (Shi et al., 1994) which could activate transcription factors augmenting TNF-α gene expression (Allison et al., 1995).

TNF-α is the Principal Factor Produced by Macrophages Stimulating Proliferation of Fibroblasts in Silicosis

The production by activated macrophages of mature TGF-β is discussed in the next section. Since TGF-β is chemotactic for fibroblasts (Postlethwaite et al., 1991) and is present in silicotic nodules (Williams et al., 1993) it could mediate recruitment of fibroblasts into the nodule, where they proliferate.

Several products of activated macrophages have mitogenic effects on fibroblasts. These include interleukin-1 (Schmidt et al., 1984), platelet-derived growth factors (Ross et al., 1986) and basic fibroblast growth factor (Folkman and Klagsbrun, 1987). However, the most important mediator of fibroblast proliferation in silicosis appears to be TNF-α (Piguet et al., 1990a). These authors found that a single intratracheal installation of silica in mice led to a marked increase in the level of lung TNF-α messenger RNA which lasted for more than 70 days, while, there were no obvious changes in the amounts of messenger RNAs for IL-1 or TGF-β. TNF mRNA was shown by *in situ* hybridization to be present in macrophages, and TNF was localized in these cells by immunocytochemistry. As shown in Fig. 3, silica-induced collagen deposition was almost completely prevented by anti-TNF antibody, and was significantly increased by continuous infusion of mouse recombinant TNF-α (Piguet et al., 1990a). The same authors also showed that in non-silicotic animals subcutaneous release of TNF induces a focal accumulation of fibroblasts and collagen deposition (Piguet et al., 1990b).

TGF-β may be the Principal Cytokine Inducing Collagen Synthesis by Fibroblasts on Silicosis

Of the growth factors mediating fibrogenesis, transforming growth factor-β (TGF-β) appears to be particularly important. Three isoforms, TGF-β1, TGF-β2 and TGF-β, have been cloned from cDNA libraries. TGF-β1 is most fully characterized and regarded as the prototype of the TGF-β family. TGF-β1 is biologically active as a mature form, a 25 kDa homodimer linked by disulfide

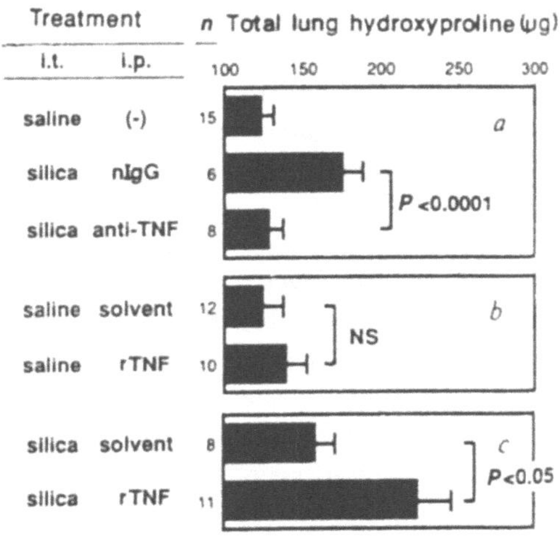

Fig. 3. Intratracheal (i.t.) infusion of silica increases lung hydroxyproline in mice, and antibody against TNF eliminates this effect whereas normal IgG does not (a). In the presence of silica, intraperitoneal (i.p.) infusion of TNF-α augments lung hydroxyproline (c), whereas in the absence of silica TNF does not have this effect (b). Courtesy of Piguet et al. (1990a) and the publishers of Nature.

bonds. A higher molecular mass precursor, produced by macrophages, fibroblasts and other cell types, is biologically inactive. This latent form of TGF-β can be processed to the mature form by exposure to proteinases or acidic conditions (e.g. in acidified endosomes). For example, activated macrophages, and fibroblasts stimulated by TNF-α, release plasminogen activators which catalyse the generation of plasmin; plasmin can convert latent TGF-β into the active form (Barnard et al., 1990). Activated macrophages themselves release mature TGF-β (Wahl et al., 1990).

TGF-β is chemotactic for fibroblasts (Postlethwaite et al., 1994). However, the major effect of TGF-β on fibroblasts is stimulation of the synthesis of collagen (Ignotz and Massague, 1986) as well as of other extracellular proteins (proteoglycan, fibronectin and tenascin - see Barnard et al., 1980).

In conditions leading to liver fibrosis (carbon tetrachloride, schistosomiasis, hepatic irradiation) increased expression of TGF-β occurs early and is maintained throughout the time of fibrogenesis (see Sanderson et al., 1995). Hepatic expression of active TGF-β in transgenic mice results in liver fibrosis (Sanderson et al., 1995). These observations suggest that TGF-β acts *in vivo* as a powerful stimulus for collagen formation during chronic tissue injury.

Williams et al. (1993) used specific antibodies to localize latent and mature (active) forms of TGF-β in the lungs of rats following quartz installation. Mature TGF-β was observed in macrophages and fibroblasts at the periphery of silicotic lesions as well as in the extracellular matrix. TGF-β was also found in type II pneumocytes. These observations support the interpretation that active TGF-β is released in silicosis and is likely to be a major mediator of the synthesis of collagen and other extracellular matrix constituents.

In lymphocyte-dependent fibrogenesis IL-4 could act synergistically with TGF-β in stimulating collagen synthesis (Postlethwaite et al., 1992).

Silica-Induced Carcinogenesis

Epidemiological evidence that silica exposure increases the risk of lung cancer in occupationally-exposed humans is reviewed by Goldsmith (1994). Crystalline silica induces tumors in rats, but not in mice and hamsters (Saffiotti et al., 1993). Differences in the responses of these rodents to silica are instructive because they point to a critical role of host factors. By extrapolation, humans might be expected the show individual differences in response to silica and silicones. A single intratracheal instillation of silica was found in rats to elicit a marked fibrogenic reaction and hyperplasia of alveolar type II cells, followed by the frequent development of lung tumors (adenocarcinomas). Mice (of three strains) showed moderate fibrosis, but no persistent epithelial cell hyperplasia and no lung tumor induction. Syrian golden hamsters showed only macrophage storage of crystalline silica dust without fibrogenesis or epithelial hyperplasia. Saffiotti et al. (1993) suggest that the high level of production of TGF-β by type II pneumocytes in silicotic rats may contribute to hyperplasia of these cells and augment cancer susceptibility.

The same authors (Mao et al., 1994) propose that crystalline silica can bind closely to DNA (presumably by hydrogen bonding to phosphate ester groups) and generate oxygen radicals that can damage DNA (Shi et al., 1994), thereby increasing risk of cancer development.

Is this Information Relevant to Silicone Breast Implants?

As discussed by others at this conference, silica is a constituent of some breast implants. Moreover silicones, when emulsified, particularly in the form of small ingestible particles coated with complement or other proteins, could induce the production of TNF-α and mature TGF-β, with consequent deposition of fibrous tissue. If an autoimmune response is elicited, fibrous tissue could be formed by the lymphocyte-dependent pathway. Marked individual differences in tissue reactions to material from breast implants would be expected.

Inhibition of Fibrogenic Responses to Silica

Inhibition of fibrogenesis induced by silica, bleomycin, irradiation and other agents would be clinically worthwhile. The question arises whether this is feasible. In view of the importance of TNF-α in fibrogenesis (Piguet et al., 1990a) one strategy is to inhibit the production or effects of TNF-α. Two classes of drugs efficiently inhibit the production of TNF-α. One of these is a group of pyridinyl-imidazole compounds which bind to a pair of protein kinases required for efficient translation of TNF-α mRNA (Lee et al., 1994). The second is a small group of antioxidants that prevent the oxidative activation of NF-κB, AP-1 and other transcription factors required for induced expression of the TNF-α gene (Eugui et al., 1994; Allison et al., 1995).

Antioxidants have the additional interesting property that they can block the induced expression of procollagen genes in fibroblasts (Houglum et al., 1991; Geesin et al., 1991). For example, the dicatechol antioxidant nordihydroguiauretic acid inhibits the production of TNF-α by activated cells of the monocyte-macrophage lineage (Eugui et al., 1994) and bleomycin-induced pulmonary fibrosis (Phan and Kunkel, 1986). The importance of oxidants in the pathogenesis of pulmonary fibrosis following inhalation of asbestos is shown by the protective effect of polyethylene glycol-conjugated catalase (Mossman et al., 1990). The well-known capacity of ionizing radiation and anthracyclines such as bleomycin to generate oxygen radicals may likewise be implicated in their fibrogenic activity. Optimizing antioxidants for inhibition of fibrogenesis is desirable.

Understanding the cell biology of fibrogenesis opens up the possibility of its pharmacological control, which could have application not only to silicosis but also to bleomycin- and radiation-induced pulmonary fibrosis, idiopathic pulmonary fibrosis, cirrhosis of the liver and adhesions in the peritoneal and pelvic cavities. Such drugs might also help to reduce tissue and pelvic reactions to materials released from breast implants in women.

References

Aggarwal BB, Puri RK (1995) Common and uncommon features of cytokines and cytokine receptors: an overview. In: Aggarwal BB, Puri RK (ed) Human cytokines: their role in disease and therapy. Blackwell Science, Oxford, pp 3-24.

Allison AC, Clark IA, Davies P (1977) Cellular interactions in fibrogenesis. Ann Rheum Dis 36, suppl 8-13.

Allison AC, Harington JS, Birbeck M (1966) An examination of the cytotoxic effects of silica on macrophages. J Exp Med 124:141-150.

Allison AC, Hart PD (1968) Potentiation by silica of the growth of Mycobacterium tuberculosis in macrophage cultures. Brit J exp Path 49:465-476.

Allison AC, Lee JC, Eugui EM (1995) Pharmacological regulation of the production of the proinflammatory cytokines TNFα and IL-1β. In: Aggarwal BB, Puri RK (eds). Human cytokines: their role in disease and therapy. Blackwell Science, Oxford, pp 689-713.

Barnard JA, Lyons RM, Moses HM (1990) The cell biology of transforming growth factor β. Biochim Biophys Acta 1032:79-87.

Burd PR (1995) Role of cytokines in mast cell functions. In: Aggarwal BB, Puri RK (ed) Human cytokines: their role in disease and therapy. Blackwell Science, Oxford, pp 87-99.

Claman HN (1990) Mast cells and fibrosis. The relevance to scleroderma. Rheumatic Disease Clinics of North America 16:141-151.

Eugui EM, De Lustro B, Rouhafza S, Ilnicka M, Lee SW, Wilhelm R, Allison AC. Some antioxidants inhibit, in a co-ordinate fashion, the production of tumor necrosis factor-α, IL-1β and IL-6 by human peripheral blood mononuclear cells. Internat Immunol 6:409-422.

Evans TW, McAnulty RJ, Rogers DF et al. (1990) Bleomycin-induced lung injury in the rat: effects of the platelet-activating factor (PAF) receptor antagonist BN52021 and platelet depletion. Env Hlth Perspect 85:65-69.

Folkman J, Klagsbrun M (1987) Angiogenic factors. Science 235:442-447.

Geesin JC, Hendricks LJ, Gordon JS, Berg RA (1991) Modulation of collagen synthesis by growth factors: the role of ascorbate-stimulated lipid peroxidation. Arch Biochem Biophys 289:6-11.

Guthrie GD (1992) Biological effects of inhaled minerals. Amer Mineral 77:225-243.

Goldsmith DF (1994) Silica exposure and pulmonary cancer. In: Savet JM (ed) Epidemiology of lung cancer. Marcel Dekker, New York, pp 245-297.

Heaney PJ, Banfield JA (1994) Structure and chemistry of silica, metal oxides and phosphates. In: Guthrie GD Jr, Mossman BT (eds) Health effects of mineral dusts. Mineralogical Society of America, Washington DC, Reviews in Mineralogy 28:185-234.

Heppleston AG, Styles JA (1967) Activity of a macrophage factor in collagen formation by silica. Nature 214:521-522.

Hubbard AK (1989) Role for T-lymphocytes in silica-induced pulmonary inflammation. Lab Invest 61:46-50.

Ihle JN, Keller J, Oroszlan S et al. (1983) Biologic properties of homogeneous interleukin-3. J Immunol 132:282-287.

Ignotz RA, Massague J (1986) Transforming growth factor-β stimulates the expression of fibronectin and collagen. J Biol Chem 261:4337-4345.

Kagan E, Hartmann DP (1984) Elimination of macrophages with silica and asbestos. Methods Enzymol 108:325-335.

Lee JC, Laydon JT, McDonnell PC et al (1994) A protein kinase involved in the regulation of inflammatory cytokine biosynthesis. Nature 372:739-746.

Mao Y, Daniel LN, Whittaker N, Saffiotti U (1994) DNA binding to crystalline silica characterized by Fourier-transform infrared spectroscopy. Environmental Health Perspectives 102, suppl 10:165-171.

Mossman BT, Marsh JP, Sesko A et al (1990) Inhibition of lung injury, inflammation, and interstitial pulmonary fibrosis by polyethylene glycol-conjugated catalase in a rapid inhalation model of asbestosis. Amer Rev Resp Dis 141:1266-1271.

Nash T, Allison AC, Harington JS (1966) Physico-chemical properties of silica in relation to its toxicity. Nature 210:259-261.

Phan SH, Kunkel SL (1986) Inhibition of bleomycin-induced pulmonary fibrosis by nordihydroguiauretic acid. Am J Pathol 124:343-352.

Piguet PF, Collart MA, Gram G, Kapanci Y, Vassali P (1989) Tumor necrosis factor/cachectin plays a key role in bleomycin-induced pneumopathy and fibrosis. J Exp Med 170:655-663.

Piguet PF, Collart MA, Gram GE, Sappino AP, Vassalli P (1990a) Requirement of tumor necrosis factor for development of silica-induced pulmonary fibrosis. Nature 344:245-247.

Piguet PF, Gram G, Vassalli P (1990b) Subcutaneous infusion of tumor necrosis factor induces local proliferation of fibroblasts, capillaries and epidermal cells, or massive tissue necrosis. Am J Path 136:1990-1998.

Piguet PF, Vesin C (1994) Pulmonary platelet trapping induced by bleomycin: correlation with fibrosis and involvement of the β2 integrins. Inter J Exp Pathol 75:321-328.

Postlethwaite AE, Sayer JM (1991) Fibroblast chemotaxis by human recombinant interleukin-4. J Clin Invest 87:2147-2152.

Postlethwaite AE, Holness MA, Kitai H, Raghow R (1992) Human fibroblasts synthesize elevated levels of extracellular matrix proteins in response to interleukin-4. J Clin Invest 90:1479-1485.

Postlethwaite AE, Raghow R, Ballou L, Sampath TK (1994) Osteogenic protein-1, a bone morphogenetic protein member of the TGF-β superfamily, shares chemotactic but not fibrogenic properties with TGF-β. J Cell Physiol 161:562-570.

Prakash S, Robbins PW, Wyler D (1995) Cloning and analysis of murine cDNA that encodes a fibrogenic lymphokine, fibrosin. Proc Natl Acad Sci USA 92:2154-2158.

Ross R, Raines EW, Bowen-Pope DF (1986) The biology of platelet-derived growth factor. Cell 46:155-169.
Saffiotti U, Daniel LN, Mao Y et al (1993) Biological studies on the carcinogenic mechanisms of quartz. In: Guthrie GD Jr, Mossman BT (eds) Mineralogical Society of America, Washington DC. Reviews in Mineralogy 28:523-544.
Schlipköter HW, Dolgner R, Brockhaus A (1963) Ein Beitrag zur Therapie der experimentellen Silikose. Deutsch Med Wschr 88:1895-1899.
Schmidt JA, Oliver CN, Lepe-Zuniga JL, Green I, Gery I (1984) Silica-stimulated monocytes release fibroblast proliferation factors identical to interleukin 1. J Clin Invest 73:1462-1472.
Shi X Mao Y, Daniel LN, Saffiotti U, Dalal NS, Vallyathan V (1994) Silica radical-induced DNA damage and lipid peroxidation. Environmental Health Perspectives 102, suppl 10:149-154.
Stark M, Zaidi S, Hilscher B, Hilscher W, Gleichmann E (1988) High- and low-responder mouse strains with respect to silica-induced fibrosis. Immunobiology 178:100-101.
Van Rooijen N, Sanders A (1994) Liposome depletion of macrophages: mechanism of action, preparation of liposomes and applications. J Immunol Methods 174:83-93.
Wahl SM, Allen JB, Wong HL, Dougherty SF, Ellingsworth LR (1990) Antagonistic and agonistic effects of transforming growth factor-β and IL-1 in rheumatoid synovium. J Immunol 145:2514-2519.
Weissmann G, Rita GA (1972) Molecular basis of gouty inflammation: interaction of monosodium urate with lysosomes and liposomes. Nature (New Biol) 240:167-172.
Williams AO, Flanders KC, Saffiotti U (1993) Immunohistochemical localization of transforming growth factor-β in rats with experimental silicosis, alveolar type II hyperplasia, and lung cancer. Am J Pathol 142:1831-1840.

Macrophages in Host Defense Mechanisms

Nico van Rooijen, Odilia L.C. Wijburg, Germie P.J.M. van den Dobbelsteen and Annemarie Sanders.

Dept. of Cell Biology & Immunology, Faculty of Medicine, Vrije Universiteit, 1081 BT Amsterdam, The Netherlands.

Macrophages and the Liposome Mediated Macrophage "Suicide" Approach

From an evolutionary point of view, macrophages form an ancient cell population, representing the main host defense mechanism until the development of the immune system. It might be speculated that, during evolution, macrophages have also acquired important functions in the regulation of humoral and cellular immune reactions and in the control of cell functions of various non-phagocytic cells. As a consequence, in mammals, macrophages may be multifunctional cells.

Selective *in vivo* depletion of macrophages is a generally accepted approach to study whether macrophages are involved in any particular biomedical control mechanism. Since the effects of the usual methods for macrophage depletion, such as treatment with silica, carrageenan, anti-macrophage antibodies etc. were neither selective nor complete, we have developed a new approach. This macrophage "suicide" technique is based on the liposome mediated intra-phagocytic delivery and accumulation of drugs that disturb the metabolism of macrophages, ultimately leading to irreversible damage and depletion (Van Rooijen and Van Nieuwmegen, 1984; Van Rooijen and Sanders, 1994). The specificity of the approach with respect to phagocytic cells of the mononuclear phagocyte system (MPS) can be explained as follows. The natural fate of liposomes is phagocytosis and once ingested by macrophages, the phospholipid bilayers of the liposomes are disrupted under the influence of lysosomal phospholipases. Since clodronate does not easily escape from the cell by crossing the cell membranes, the clodronate release from liposomes will result in an intracellular accumulation. When the clodronate concentration exceeds a treshold value, irreversible damage will be caused and the macrophage will be killed. Clodronate released in the circulation from dead macrophages or by leakage from liposomes, will not easily enter non-phagocytic cells. Moreover, it has an extremely short half life in circulation and body fluids. Therefore, other cells than macrophages are not affected by this treatment. Using this approach, the multifunctional role of macrophages in host defense reactions has been confirmed. They serve as accessory cells for the induction of humoral and cellular immune reactions against particulate antigens, are responsible for the non-immune resistance against microorganisms and grafted cells, and regulate functions of various non-phagocytic cells which participate in immune responses (see also table 1).

Macrophages as Scavengers

Macrophages are well known for their scavenger function. They are able to ingest and digest macromolecular complexes such as antigen-antibody complexes (van Oss et al., 1974), foreign invaders such as bacteria, viruses (Wijburg et al., 1995) and yeast cells (Qian et al., 1994), aged erythrocytes and remnants of affected or apoptotic cells (Fadok et al., 1992). Carbon particles that were intravenously injected 24 h after depletion of splenic macrophages by liposome encapsulated clodronate, showed a distribution pattern that was completely different from that observed in normal animals (Van Rooijen and Van Nieuwmegen, 1984). This pattern did not correspond with the localization pattern of splenic macrophages, but with that of sinus lining endothelial cells in the red pulp of the spleen. The latter cells do not phagocytose the particles, but their uptake is mediated by pinocytosis. In normal animals, sinus lining cells play a minor role in the clearance since their uptake of carbon particles is much slower than that of macrophages. However, when clearance of carbon particles from the circulation is delayed as a consequence of the depletion of macrophages from spleen and liver, exposure of the sinus lining cells to the carbon particles is prolonged and consequently, their uptake is increased. In a similar way, the relative participation of liver endothelial cells in the clearance of IgA (Bogers et al., 1991a) and IgG (Bogers et al., 1991b) immune complexes appeared to be markedly increased after depletion of liver macrophages (Kupffer cells) by liposome encapsulated clodronate. Such differences in antigen uptake in macrophage depleted mice were also observed during mouse hepatitis virus (MHV) infection. In normal mice, infection in the spleen starts in marginal metallophilic macrophages and in marginal zone macrophages. Only later in infection dendritic cells in the white pulp are infected (Wijburg et al., 1995). Macrophage depletion before infection of mice resulted in an increase in the number of dendritic cells infected with MHV. Moreover, infected dendritic cells could be detected already 24 h after infection (unpublished results, Wijburg et al.,).

Table 1. Macrophage functions in host defense mechanisms

Intracellular activity		Extracellular activity	
Function	Mechanism	Function	Mechanism
Scavenger function (clearance)	Ingestion (phagocytosis) intracellular killing of microorganisms and enzymatic digestion	Product mediated defense	Production and secretion of soluble mediators such as NO, TNFα and IL-6
Antigen (pre)processing and presentation	Processing and presentation <u>or</u> transfer of processed antigenic fragments to other accessory cells	Regulation of cellular differentiation, migration and activity	Production and secretion of cytokines such as: IL1β, IL-6, IL-10, IL-12, TNFα and chemokines

Macrophages in Non-Immune Resistance

Immunocompromised mice are widely used to maintain human cells in models of human hemopoietic and immunological processes in order to study their role and manipulability in host defense mechanisms, pathological disorders and diseases. However, in spite of the absence of functional T-cell and B-cell mediated immunological activity against the injected or engrafted human cells, the latter are not completely protected against host resistance and as a consequence, their numbers rapidly decrease to unacceptable levels. Macrophages have been postulated to play a crucial role in the rapid disappearance of injected or engrafted human cells from SCID- or NIHIII-mice. Therefore, various experiments have been performed in order to determine if selective depletion of macrophages improved the survival and functional activity of human peripheral blood leucocytes (Fraser et al., 1995) or *Plasmodium falciparum* infected human red blood cells (Badell et al., 1995) in such mice. After administration of human peripheral blood leucocytes (PBL), control SCID mice had no detectable human cells within 72 h as determined by FACS analysis. Animals that were treated with clodronate-liposomes however, maintained a large proportion of human cells in peripheral blood and spleen. After simultaneous implantation of human fetal thymic and liver tissue in SCID mice (SCID-hu Thy/Liv mice), production of phenotypically normal human T-cells into the periphery is induced for prolonged periods. However, due to the activity of macrophages, they are rapidly cleared resulting in a low degree of persistance of human cells. SCID-hu Thy/Liv mice injected with clodronate-liposomes showed a transient increase in the number of human cells in peripheral blood and a large accumulation of human cells in the white pulp compartments of the spleen. These results demonstrate that murine macrophages play a crucial role in human cell clearance, in spite of the absence of a functionally active immune system.

Selective depletion of Kupffer cells strongly enhanced tumour growth in the liver of Wag/Rij rats, that were inoculated with syngeneic CC531 colon carcinoma cells (Heuff et al., 1993). These and many other experiments have demonstrated that macrophages are also important for the non-immune resistance against tumour cells.

Macrophages as Accessory Cells in the Induction of Immunity against Particulate Antigens

Which lymphoid and non-lymphoid cells are required for the induction of an antibody response, depends on the type of antigen used for immunization. Antigens are usually divided in thymus dependent (TD) and thymus independent (TI) antigens according to whether CD4 positive helper T-lymphocytes are required for activation of B-lymphocytes to become plasma cells. It is therefore not surprising that macrophages are supposed to play a role in TD immune responses, since accessory cells are generally believed to present their processed antigens to T-lymphocytes. Because macrophages ingest particulate antigens much more avidly than non-particulate antigens, macrophages might influence immune responses against non-particulate and particulate antigens to a different extent. The macrophage "suicide" technique has been applied to investigate the requirement of macrophages in the onset of humoral immune reactions against both non-particulate and particulate TD antigens.

To study the role of splenic macrophages in antibody responses against non-particulate antigens, both clodronate-liposomes (for depletion of macrophages) and antigens were injected intravenously (see review: Van Rooijen, 1992). Antibody titers as well as numbers of antibody forming cells in the spleen were not reduced when various (TI) non-particulate antigens were given within a few days after depletion of macrophages. Also the localization pattern of antibody forming cells in the spleen was not markedly changed. In contrast, primary as well as secondary challenge of macrophage-depleted animals with non-particulate TD antigens, induced enhanced serum antibody levels as compared to responses in non-treated animals. Numbers of antibody forming cells were increased over prolonged periods of time. From these results it was concluded that macrophages are not required for the induction of an antibody response against non-particulate TD antigens. On the contrary, they seem to suppress such responses by active or passive mechanisms, e.g. competition for the antigen between macrophages and dendritic cells (see Claassen 1987, Delemarre 1990).

Sheep red blood cells (SRBC), protein antigens that had been converted from non-particulate to particulate antigens by their association with liposomes and bacterial antigens were used to study the role of macrophages in the onset of humoral immunity against particulate antigens (Delemarre et al., 1991; Su and Van Rooijen, 1989; Buiting, 1995). Contrary to responses observed after administration of non-particulate antigens to macrophage-depleted animals, macrophage depletion before administration of these particulate antigens resulted in strongly reduced antibody responses (Su and Van Rooijen, 1989; Delemarre et al., 1991; Van Rooijen, 1992; Buiting, 1995). In the experiments with liposome encapsulated antigens, both the liposomal phospholipid composition and the administration route were similar for liposome encapsulated clodronate and liposome encapsulated antigens. Therefore, clodronate and antigens were targeted to the same macrophages in the same lymphoid compartments. Consequently, problems related to possible differential targeting were minimalized. Since liposome encapsulated antigens are masked and thus prevented from recognition by surface receptors on lymphoid cells, and liposomes are avidly phagocytosed by macrophages, phagocytosis of liposomes followed by unmasking of the encapsulated antigens seems to be a logical first step in the induction of an immune response. Indeed, *in vitro* antigen presentation experiments have shown that macrophages are necessary and sufficient for antigen presentation of liposome encapsulated antigens to T-lymphocytes (Dal Monte and Szoka, 1989; Szoka, 1992). Like B-lymphocytes, dendritic cells show only a limited activity of phagocytosis. Therefore these cells were not expected to take up any appreciable amount of liposomes (Steinman, 1991).

From the experiments described here it was concluded that macrophages play a role in the induction of antibody responses against particulate antigens but not in the induction of antibody responses against non-particulate antigens. It is not likely however, that macrophages by themselves are responsible for both processing and presentation of particulate antigens. Macrophages were postulated to be involved in the induction of humoral immunity against particulate antigens, by performing a (pre)processing step. In this dual accessory cell concept, processing by macrophages is followed by transfer of the processed antigens to cells which are better equipped for antigen presentation (Van Rooijen, 1992), e.g. dendritic cells.

Evidence is accumulating that macrophages may also play a role in the induction of cytotoxic T-lymphocyte (CTL) responses in vivo. Dendritic cells are generally believed to be responsible for processing and presentation of antigens to T-lymphocytes (Austyn 1992). However, purified splenic dendritic cells, pulsed in vitro with liposomal antigen, were less effective in class I MHC mediated antigen presentation than the same cells, pulsed *in vivo* by intravenous antigen administration. This points to a difference in efficacy between antigen processing *in vivo* and *in vitro* (Huang et al., 1992). However, this difference in efficacy of antigen presentation by splenic dendritic cells can also be explained by the difference in capability of antigen uptake and presentation between freshly isolated or cultured dendritic cells. Whereas the latter proved to be very efficient in antigen presentation but hardly phagocytosed liposomal antigen, freshly isolated dendritic cells were shown to be poor presenters (Austyn, 1993). Intravenous injection of mice with liposome encapsulated clodronate, blocked the secondary CTL responses induced by liposomal ovalbumin (OVA, Huang et al., 1992; Zhou et al., 1992; Nair et al.,1995), in spite of the finding that splenic dendritic cell functions were not affected by the intravenous treatment with clodronate liposomes (Nair et al.,1995). Conclusion from these results was that after administration of liposome incorporated OVA, macrophages might well be involved in a first antigen processing step in the induction of OVA-specific CTL responses. Furthermore, addition of supernatant from OVA-liposome treated macrophages to naive dendritic cell-T cell cultures *in vitro* resulted in OVA-specific T cell responses (Nair et al., 1995). Also the induction of CTL responses by other particulate antigens such as antigens associated with cell debris, appeared to depend on the presence of macrophages as accessory cells. Treatment with silica and carrageenan, which impairs macrophage functions, completely inhibited these CTL responses and the CTL activity could be restored by transfer of macrophages via infusion (Debrick et al., 1991). It has been postulated that (pre)processing of liposomal and other particulate antigens by macrophages could be followed by transfer of the fragmented antigens to dendritic cells, as has been discussed above for the induction of antibody responses (Van Rooijen, 1992; Nair, 1995).

Macrophages as Regulators of Host Defense Mechanisms

Macrophages are well known producers of various cytokines. So, it is not surprising that there is a rapidly growing body of evidence for a role of macrophages in the regulation of functional activity of non-phagocytic cells. Hepatic natural killer cells, present in liver sinusoids, represent an organ-associated natural killer cell population, which show a higher level of activation and a different morphology when compared to peripheral blood natural killer cells. They develop as a result of an influx of the latter cells into the liver microenvironment, followed by activation or differentiation (Vanderkerken et al., 1995). After depletion of macrophages (Kupffer cells) in the liver by liposome encapsulated clodronate, numbers of hepatic natural killer cells decreased in close correlation with the depletion of Kupffer cells (Vanderkerken et al., 1995). These authors also demonstrated that Kupffer cell-conditioned medium enhanced the viability and tumour-cytotoxic activity of hepatic natural killer cells *in vitro*, as well as their adherence to liver endothelial cells. Splenic dendritic cells, placed in culture for one or more days undergo a functional transformation that equips them to activate unprimed syngeneic T cells. Dai et al. (1995) have shown that macrophages play a role in this cytokine-mediated phenomenon.

A single intratracheal dose of liposome encapsulated clodronate resulted in the elimination of alveolar macrophages from the lung, creating a model to study the *in vivo* role of alveolar macrophages in the pulmonary immune response. Results of such studies, in which thymus-dependent antigens were administered intratracheally after depletion of alveolar macrophages, showed that elimination of alveolar macrophages had a dramatic effect on the pulmonary immune response. An increase in the numbers of antibody forming cells in lung-associated lymph nodes and a prolongation of the response were found, as well as the induction of antibody forming cells in the lung tissue itself (Thepen et al., 1989). It was concluded from these results that alveolar macrophages are likely to play a role in controlling of the pulmonary immune response in a suppressive way. More recently it has been confirmed that alveolar macrophages actively suppress the antigen-presenting cell function of pulmonary dendritic cells *in vivo* (Holt et al., 1993).

Peritoneal macrophages as well as macrophages in the draining parathymic lymph nodes can be depleted by intraperitoneal administration of liposome encapsulated clodronate (Biewenga et al., 1995). This treatment resulted in an enhanced immune reaction in the parathymic lymph nodes to intraperitoneally administered antigen, as demonstrated by the increased numbers of specific antibody forming cells in the macrophage-depleted animals (Soesatyo et al., 1991). The latter results suggest that peritoneal macrophages play a regulatory role in the local humoral immune response.

References

Austyn JM (1992) Antigen uptake and presentation by dendritic leukocytes. Semin Immunol 4:227-236

Austyn JM (1993) Dendritic cells: Nature's adjuvants. NATO ASI series. Series A. Life sciences Vol. 261, pp1-10, Plenum Press

Badell E, Pasquetto V, Van Rooijen N, Druilhe P (1995) A mouse model for human malaria parasites. Parasitology Today In press

Biewenga J, Van der Ende MB, Krist LFG, Borst A, Ghufron M, Van Rooijen N (1995) Macrophage depletion and repopulation in the rat after i.p. administration of Cl_2MBP-liposomes: Depletion kinetics and accelerated repopulation of peritoneal and omental macrophages by administration of Freundš adjuvant. Cell Tissue Res 280:189-196

Bogers WMJM, Stad RK, Janssen DJ, Prins FA, Van Rooijen N, Van Es LA, Daha MR (1991a) Kupffer cell depletion in vivo results in clearance of large sized IgA aggregates in rats by liver endothelial cells. Clin Exp Immunol 85:128-136

Bogers WMJM, Stad RK, Janssen DJ, Van Rooijen N, Van Es LA, Daha MR (1991b) Kupffer cell depletion "in vivo" results in preferential elimination of IgG aggregates and immune complexes via specific Fc receptors on rat liver endothelial cells. Clin Exp Immunol 86:328-333

Buiting, AMJ (1995) Splenic macrophage subpopulations: Origin, Turnover and Functional Aspects. Academic Thesis, Vrije Universiteit, Amsterdam

Claassen E (1987) Antibody Forming Cells in the Spleen. Academic Thesis, Vrije Universiteit, Amsterdam

Dal Monte P and Szoka Jr FC (1989) Effect of liposome encapsulation on antigen presentation in vitro; comparison of presentation by peritoneal macrophages and B cell tumors. J Immunol 142:1437-1443

Dai R, Van Rooijen N, Dijkstra CD, Streilein JW (1995) Relative roles of T cells and macrophages in cytokine-mediated functional transformation of cultured splenic dendritic cells. Cell Immunol In press

Debrick JE, Campbell PA, Staerz UD (1991) Macrophages as accessory cells for class-I MHC restricted immune responses. J Immunol 147:2846-2852

Delemarre FGA (1990) The Role of Macrophages in the Humoral Immune Response in Lymph Nodes and Spleen of Mice. Academic Thesis, Vrije Universiteit, Amsterdam

Delemarre FGA, Kors N, Van Rooijen N (1991) Elimination of spleen and of lymph node macrophages and its difference in the effect on the immune response to particulate antigens. Immunobiology 182:70-78

Fadok VA, Savill JS, Haslett C, Bratton DL, Doherty DE, Campbell PA, Henson PM (1992) Different populations of macrophages use either the vitronectin receptor or the phosphatidylserine receptor to recognize and remove apoptotic cells. J Immunol 149:4029-4035

Fraser CC, Chen BP, Webb S, Van Rooijen N, Kraal G (1995) Circulation of human hemopoietic cells in SCID mice following Cl_2MDP-liposome mediated macrophage depletion. Blood In press

Heuff G, Oldenburg HSA, Boutkan H, Visser JJ, Beelen RHJ, Van Rooijen N, Dijkstra CD, Meyer S (1993) Enhanced tumour growth in the rat liver after selective elimination of Kupffer cells. Canc Immun Immunother 37:125-130

Holt PG, Oliver J, Bilyk N, McMenamin C, McMenamin PG, Kraal G, Thepen T, (1993) Downregulation of the antigen presenting cell functions of pulmonary dendritic cells in vivo by resident alveolar macrophages. J Exp Med 177:397-407.

Huang L, Reddy R, Nair SK, Zhou F, Rouse BT (1992) Liposomal delivery of soluble protein antigens for Class I MHC mediated antigen presentation. Res Immunol 143:192-196.

Nair S, Buiting AMJ, Van Rooijen N, Huang L, Rouse BT (1995) Interaction between macrophages and dendritic cells for induction of cytotoxic T lymphocyte responses. Int Immunol In press

Qian Q, Jutila MA, Van Rooijen N, Cutler JE, (1994) Elimination of mouse splenic macrophages correlates with increased susceptibility to experimental disseminеted candidiasis. J Immunol 152:5000-5008

Soesatyo M, Biewenga J, Van Rooijen N, Kors N, Sminia T (1991) The "in situ" immune response of the rat after intraperitoneal depletion of macrophages by liposome-encapsulated dichloromethylene diphosphonate. Res Immunol 142:533-540

Steinman RM (1991) The dendritic cell system and its role in immunogenicity. Annu Rev Immunol 9:271

Su D, Van Rooijen N (1989) The role of macrophages in the immunoadjuvant action of liposomes: Effects of elimination of splenic macrophages on the immune response against intravenously injected liposome associated albumin antigen. Immunology 66:466-470

Szoka FC Jr (1991) The macrophage as the principal antigen presenting cell for liposome encapsulated antigens. Res Immunol 142:186-188

Thepen T, Van Rooijen N, Kraal G (1989) Alveolar macrophage elimination in vivo is associated with an increase in pulmonary immune responses in mice. J Exp Med 170:499-509

Vanderkerken K, Bouwens L, Van Rooijen N, Van den Berg K, Baekeland M, Wisse E (1995) The role of Kupffer cells in the differentiation process of hepatic NK cells. Hepatology In press

Van Oss CJ, Gillman CF, Neumann AW (1974) Phagocytosis as a surface phenomenon. IV. The minimum size and composition of antigen-antibody complexes that can become phagocytized. Immunol Commun 3:77-84

Van Rooijen N, Van Nieuwmegen R (1984) Elimination of phagocytic cells in the spleen after intravenous injection of liposome encapsulated dichloromethylene-diphosphonate. An enzymehistochemical study. Cell Tissue Res 238:355-358

Van Rooijen N (1992) Macrophages as accessory cells in the "in vivo" humoral immune response: From processing of particulate antigens to regulation by suppression. Sem Immunol 4:237-245

Van Rooijen N, Sanders A (1994) Liposome mediated depletion of macrophages: Mechanism of action, preparation of liposomes and applications. J Immunol Meth 174:83-93

Zhou F, Rouse BT, Huang L (1992) Induction of cytotoxic T lymphocytes with protein antigen entrapped in membranous vehicles. J Immunol 149:1599-1604

Wijburg OLC, Heemskerk MHM, Sanders A, Boog CJP, Van Rooijen N (1995) Role of $CD4^+$ cytotoxic T lymphocytes in recovery from mouse hepatitis virus infection. submitted

Structure and Function of Natural Antibodies

P. Casali and E.W. Schettino
The Division of Molecular Immunology
Department of Pathology
Cornell University Medical College
New York, New York 10021-4896

Introduction

The presence of immunoglobulins (Ig) in the circulation of normal humans and animals that bind a variety of foreign antigens, such as bacterial components and products, viruses, protozoa, fungi, as well as self antigens, such as nucleic acids, phospholipids, erythrocytes, serum proteins, cellular components, insulin and thyroglobulin, has been recognized since the beginning of this century [1-9]. Because their emergence is independent of known and/or intentional immunization, these antibodies have been termed "natural antibodies". In contrast to antigen-induced antibodies, which are mainly IgG and monoreactive, a considerable proportion of natural antibodies are IgM and polyreactive, that is they bind several unrelated antigens with different affinities. Natural polyreactive and monoreactive IgG and IgA antibodies also exist [7]. The vast majority of natural antibodies, whether IgM, IgG or IgA, are produced by $CD5^+$ B cells, the predominant lymphocytes in the neonatal cell repertoire [10, 11]. Because of their broad reactivity with a variety of microbial components, these antibodies may play a major role in the primary line of defense against infections. Owing to their ability to bind self antigens, they may serve as templates for some of the high-affinity autoantibodies that emerge in patients with autoimmune disease, particularly those associated with a significant expansion of $CD5^+$ B cells [12-14].

Antigen Binding by Natural Antibodies

The interaction of antigen and antibody has long been explained in terms of a lock-and-key model, in which the specificity for antigen of the antibody binding site underlies the need for antibody diversity. In contrast to antigen-induced antibodies, which are monoreactive and antigen-specific, a major proportion of natural antibodies are polyreactive, displaying different affinities for different antigens [3, 5-9], even those very different in nature, e.g., proteins, nucleic acids, and polysaccharides. Our studies on natural polyreactive monoclonal antibodies, generated from healthy subjects, have clearly established that these antibodies bind different antigens in a dose-saturable fashion and with different efficiencies (Fig. 1) [7]. These studies have also shown that the binding of most natural polyreactive antibodies to a given antigen can be cross-inhibited by a variety of different antigens in a dose saturable fashion (Fig. 1). The ability of a polyreactive antibody to bind to multiple antigens may rely upon the recognition of: (i) identical, (ii) similar, or (iii) different epitopes in the context of different antigens (Fig. 2) [5, 15, 16].

Recognition of an identical epitope on different antigen molecules is at the basis of the long-recognized immunological phenomenon of antigen cross-reactivity.

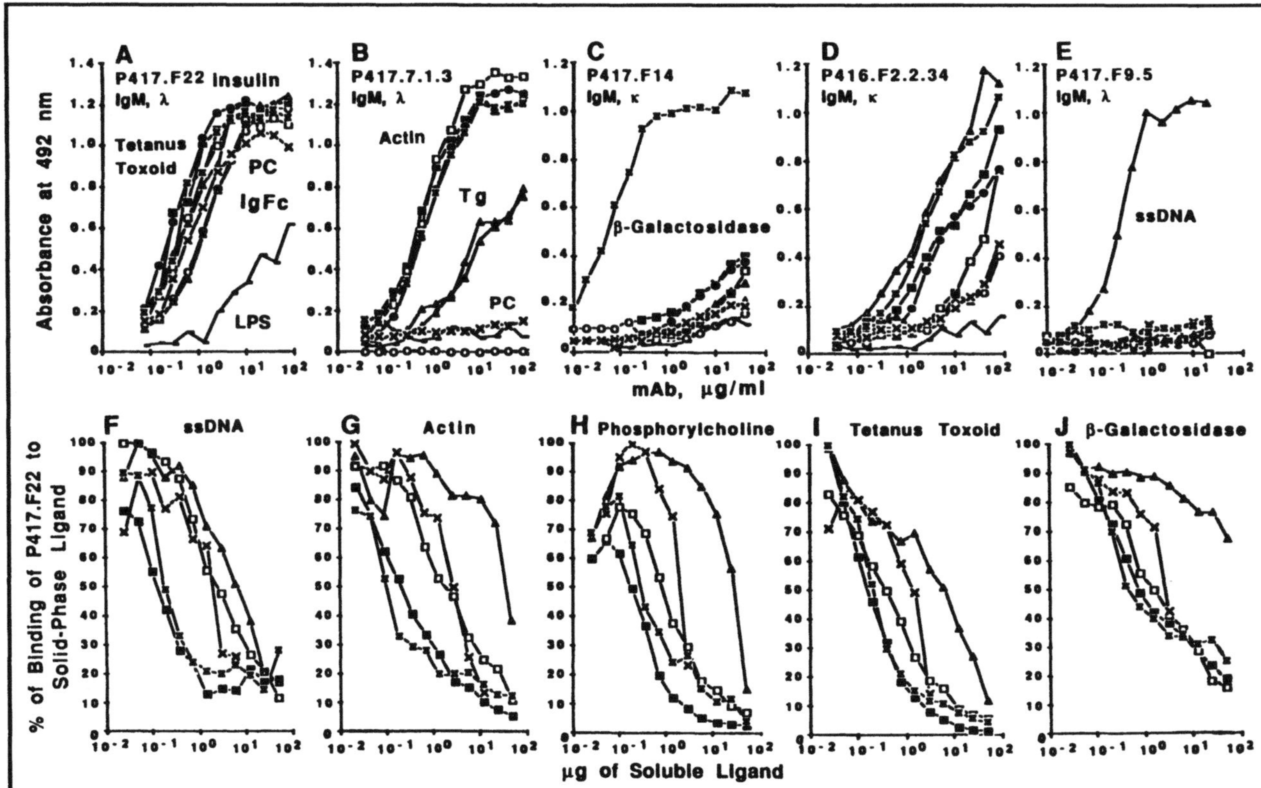

Fig. 1. A to E, dose-saturable binding of IgM monoclonal antibodies (mAbs), generated using sorted B-1b (A to C) and B-1a cells (D and E), to solid-phase ligands. Antigen-binding activity of each mAb is expressed as optical absorbance at 492 nm. F to J, dose-dependent inhibition of the binding of mAb P417.F22 to solid-phase ligands by soluble homologous or heterologous ligands. Samples of mAb P417.F22 (0.4 μg) were incubated with increasing amounts of soluble ligand. After 18 hours, mixtures were transferred to ELISA plates precoated with ssDNA (F), actin (G), phosphorylcholine (H), tetanus toxoid (I), or β-galactosidase (J). In the competitive inhibition experiments, the amount of mAb bound to the solid phase antigen is expressed as a percentage of the binding activity measured in the absence of any soluble ligand (100% of binding activity). The following antigens were used: IgG Fc fragment (o), ssDNA (Δ), insulin (●), thyroglobulin (▲), actin (❑), phosyporylcholine (X), tetanus (■), β-galactosidase (x), and LPS (-).

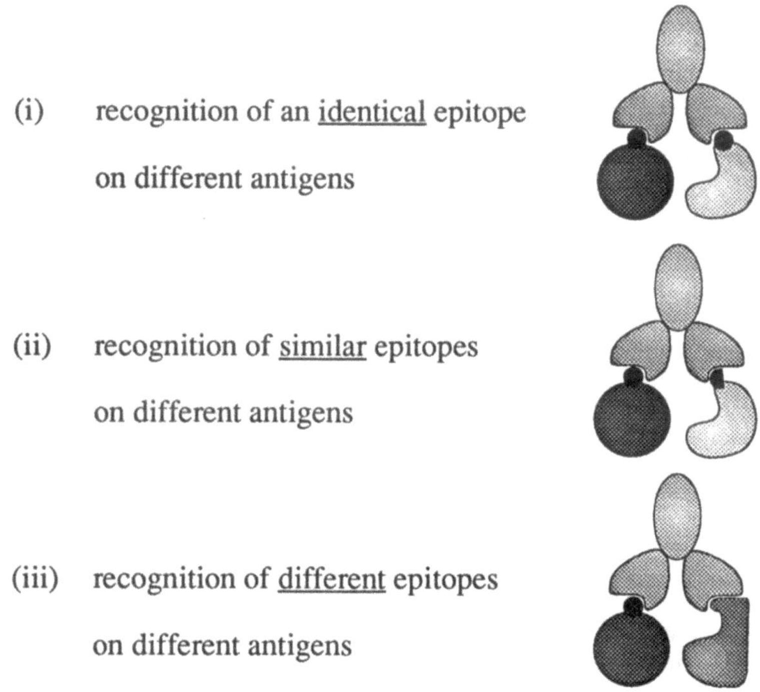

Fig. 2. The ability of antibodies to bind different antigens can rely on three discrete types of antigen recognition, i.e., recognition of: identical, similar, or different epitopes in the context of different antigens. Recognition of identical epitopes on different antigens (i), is at the basis of the classical immunological "cross-reactivity". Recognition of structurally similar epitopes on different antigens (ii), relies on the same principle, that is the binding of different antigens is inherent to structural features of the antigens. The recognition of identical (i) or similar epitopes (ii) in the context of different antigens possibly accounts for the observed polyreactivity of natural antibodies in only a few cases. In contrast to antigen-induced "specific" antibodies, natural polyreactive antibodies in general recognize antigens that are unlikely to share identical or similar epitopes, that is, natural antibodies bind different epitopes (iii). Thus, polyreactivity is a function of structures inherent to the binding cleft of the antibody and not a function of structural features shared by different antigens.

It is well established that high affinity antibodies induced by a given antigen can efficiently cross-react with another antigen. For example, the identity of a 12 amino acid epitope on *Trypanosoma cruzi* surface protein to an epitope on a protein of mammalian nerve axons [17] may lead to an anti-trypanosomal antibody-mediated neurological autoimmune disorder (chronic Chagas disease). Like the recognition of the same epitope, the recognition of similar epitopes on different antigen molecules, can result in immunological cross-reactivity among different antigens [4]. The ability of anti-DNA autoantibodies to bind appropriately spaced phosphate residues in the context of a variety of polynucleotides and phospholipids exemplifies this kind of cross-reaction [18]. In the recognition of both identical and similar epitopes on different molecules, the structural correlate(s) for immunological cross-reactivity is inherent to the antigen molecule. The antigens, however, recognized by most polyreactive antibodies are very different in nature, e.g., proteins, nucleic acids, phospholipids or polysaccharides, and are unlikely to share identical or similar epitopes. This antigenic heterogeneity suggests that natural antibody polyreactivity is mainly a function of structural features inherent to the binding cleft of the antibody and not a function of structural features shared by different antigens.

Polyreactive and monoreactive natural antibodies can display low dissociation constants (K_d) (high affinity) for certain antigens, in the same order of magnitude of those displayed by specific antibodies or autoantibodies generated through an affinity maturation process [9, 19, 20]. This feature of natural antibodies raises the issue of what functional difference exits between an unmutated natural antibody displaying a high affinity for a given antigen and an antibody with a similar high affinity induced *in vivo* by the same antigen. As recently proposed by Foote and Milstein [21], not the affinity but the rapid binding of the antigen, yielding a high on-rate or K_{on}, may constitute the feature of specific antibodies selected through hyperimmunization. Two antibodies displaying similar affinities for the same antigen can differ widely in on-rates [21]. In the course of an antibody response, the affinity maturation process may proceed throughout sequential selection of clonotypes displaying progressively high K_{on}, but, most often, similar affinity values, expressed as K_d.

Identification of the Natural Antibody-Producing Cells and Ig V_H Gene Expression

The first indication that natural antibodies are produced by a discrete B cell subset came from studies involving autoimmune NZB mice. These mice spontaneously develop autoimmune pathology and display a high proportion of Ly-1$^+$ B cells [22]. Ly-1, and its human equivalent, CD5, were first recognized as T cell markers [23, 24], and are known to contain a tyrosine phosyporylation site, a feature of many growth factor receptors [24, 25]. Ly-1$^+$ B cells from NZB [22] and normal mice [26] spontaneously produce IgM with the features of natural antibodies. Ly-1$^+$ B cells develop from pre-B cells during neonatal life, and are maintained thereafter as self-replenishing IgM$^+$ B cells, while "conventional" Ly-1$^-$ B cells develop later in life and are replenished from bone marrow surface IgM progenitors [27]. Some other features which distinguish Ly-1$^+$ B cells from their conventional Ly-1$^-$ counterparts are their unique surface Ig expression (IgM^{hi} and IgD^{lo}), their absence from the lymph nodes and bone marrow, and their abundant presence in the peritoneal cavity [26, 28]. In humans, the CD5 antigen was first identified on the surface of B lymphocytes from patients with chronic lymphocytic leukemia (CLL) [29-31]. The physiologic equivalents of neoplastic CLL CD5$^+$ B cells were identified shortly afterwards in healthy individuals [32, 33]. Characteristics such as natural antibody production, specific tissue distribution, and unique ontogenic development, distinguish CD5$^+$ from "conventional" B cells in humans, as shown for the murine Ly-1$^+$ equivalents [11, 34-37].

In contrast with the vast majority of natural antibodies, whether IgM, IgG, or IgA, which are produced by CD5$^+$ B lymphocytes, antigen-induced antibodies, such as memory IgG to tetanus toxoid, are produced by the CD5$^-$ B lymphocytes [37]. This segregation suggests functions unique to the two B lymphocytes subsets: CD5$^+$ cells are committed to the production of preimmune, natural antibodies, while CD5$^-$ B cells contain the elements that participate in secondary or tertiary high affinity responses. Evidence indicating that natural antibody production is not an exclusive property of CD5$^+$ B cells, but may also be a property of some CD5$^-$ B

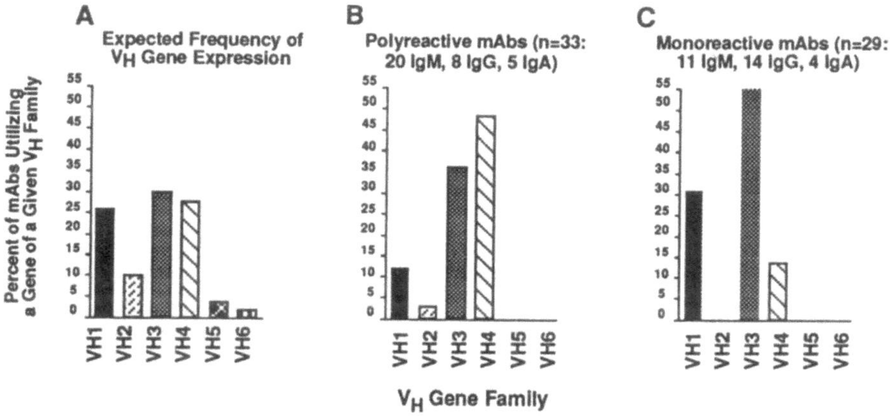

Fig. 3. Expected and actual utilization of different V_H gene families by 33 polyreactive and 29 monoreactive human monoclonal antibodies (mAbs) with different binding activities. *A*, expected frequency of V_H gene expression based on genomic V_H segment number and family complexities, as by Matsuda et al. (1993) [45] and Cook et al. (1994) [46]. *B*, V_H gene usage by 33 polyreactive mAbs. *C*, V_H gene usage by 29 monoreactive mAbs. Polyreactive and monoreactive antibodies overutilize genes of the V_H4 and V_H3 families, respectively ($p<0.05$, χ^2 goodness of fit test) Polyreactive antibodies utilize genes of the V_H4 family with a significantly higher frequency than monoreactive antibodies do ($p<0.01$, χ^2 homogeneity test).

cells [3, 13, 37, 38] was confirmed by segregating, as a discrete subset, natural antibody producing CD5$^-$ B cells from the total CD5$^-$ B cell population. The rationale for this approach was based on experiments in the mouse, suggesting that B cells, expressing at low density, the high molecular weight form of the leukocyte common antigen [39, 40], L-CA, produce antibodies with features similar to those of natural antibodies [41-43]. Our experiments showed that like CD5$^+$ B cells, CD5$^-$CD45RA^{lo} (CD45RA is the high molecular weight form of the L-CA) but not CD5$^-$CD45RA^{hi} B cells are highly enriched in IgM-producing cell precursors committed to the production of natural antibodies [7]. Because of their proposed early ontogenic emergence, CD5$^+$ B cells and their murine equivalents, have been termed B-1a cells; human CD5$^-$CD45RA^{lo} B cells, like the murine Ly-1 "sister" B cells, have been termed B-1b cells [44]. "Conventional" B lymphocytes identified in the mouse as surface Ly-1$^-$ IgM^{lo}/IgD^{hi}, and in the humans as CD5$^-$CD45RA^{hi} cells, are termed B-2 cells.

The V_H genes utilized by B-1a and B-2 cells have been hypothesized to be different, consistent with a different (early and late, respectively) ontogenic emergence of these two cell subsets. Our recent experiments [Chai et al., in preparation], examining different types of B cells sorted from the adult peripheral blood, have shown that B-1a cells overexpress genes of the V_H4 family, while "conventional" B-2 cells overexpress genes of the V_H3 family. B-1b cells express a selection of V_H genes more similar to that of B-2 than B-1a cells. Since both B-1a and B-1b cells are equally committed to the production of natural antibodies, the above findings suggest that genes of both V_H4 and V_H3 families can be associated with polyreactivity. Furthermore, the preferential utilization of the V_H3 genes by B-2 cells suggests that these V_H genes can encode not only polyreactive, but also monoreactive antigen-induced antibodies. In fact, comparison of 33 natural polyreactive human antibodies (IgM, IgG and IgA) with 29 monoreactive human antibodies (IgM, IgG and IgA), generated in our laboratory, has shown that polyreactive antibodies, with different antigen binding patterns, utilize genes of the V_H4 family at significantly higher frequency then their monoreactive counterparts (Fig. 3).

Structural Correlates for Antibody Reactivity

Polyreactive antibodies, overall, significantly overutilize genes of the V_H4 family, but they also utilize, to encode multiple antigen binding sites, the same V_H4 genes or V_H genes of other families, including the V_H3 family, and the same J_H, $V\kappa$, $V\lambda$, $J\kappa$ and/or $J\lambda$ gene segments utilized by monoreactive antigen-induced antibodies [7, 19, 47-51]. Thus, utilization of discrete V gene segments is not the strategy necessarily used by natural antibodies to encode polyreactive antigen binding sites. We explored the possibility that natural antibodies differ from their monoreactive counterparts with respect to the somatic diversification process that they may undergo, if any. Consistent with the notion that natural antibodies are generated independently of specific antigenic stimulation, the majority of genes encoding the variable regions of these (IgM) antibodies are in germline (unmutated) configuration [5]. To analyze the possibility that natural polyreactive antibodies can undergo somatic diversification, similar to that characteristic of their monoreactive antigen-induced counterparts, we analyzed the primary structure of a number of both polyreactive IgG and IgA natural antibodies. The choice of the IgG and IgA classes was dictated by the assumption that if polyreactive somatically mutated antibodies existed, these would be more numerous among IgG and IgA than IgM. Thus, selection for IgG or IgA would increase the probability of generating polyreactive mAbs with mutated V regions. The polyreactive human IgG monoclonal antibody (mAb10), generated from a healthy adult, exemplifies the features of the natural antibodies analyzed [48]. This antibody was found to be encoded by a V_H gene that represented the point-mutated form of the germline V4-39 gene template [48]. The distribution of the nucleotide substitutions, clustering in the complementarity determining regions (CDRs), and the high replacement to silent mutation (R:S) ratio, 4:1, were consistent with an antigen-selection of such mutations. These findings and those we reported elsewhere [19, 47-49, 51] support the hypothesis that natural polyreactive IgM antibody-producing cells can class switch to IgG while undergoing an antigen-directed selection process, which is underpinned by somatic hypermutation.

Having shown that natural polyreactive antibodies can undergo somatic mutation and antigen selection, we addressed the issue of whether natural polyreactive antibodies can provide the templates for antigen-induced high affinity autoantibodies characteristic of autoimmune diseases. To this end, we generated a number of polyreactive IgG and IgA mAbs by selecting for binding to DNA and other self antigens, using B cells from different patients with systemic lupus erythematosus (SLE) [49, 51]. The features of these autoantibodies are exemplified by the analysis of the polyreactive high affinity, anti-DNA, IgA mAb412.66.F1. This autoantibody utilizes a V_H gene that represents the somatically point-mutated form of the germline V3-23 gene, with R:S mutation ratios in the V_H gene CDRs of 5:0 and of 2:2 in the FRs. These structural features of high R:S mutation ratios in the CDRs and low in the FRs was shared by all other polyreactive anti-DNA autoantibodies and was consistent with an antigen-selection of such mutations. Taken together, these findings suggest that natural antibodies can undergo a somatic diversification process in the healthy human adult and can provide the templates for high affinity autoantibodies in autoimmune patients.

Having established that polyreactive natural antibodies can utilize the same V and J gene segments as monoreactive antigen-induced antibodies do, and like these antibodies, can undergo somatic diversification, we asked whether somatically generated structures, such as that of the H chain CDR3, and perhaps the L chain CDR3, can provide the correlates for polyreactivity. The structures lining the antigen binding site of an antibody molecule consist of the three heavy (H)- and the three light (L) chain CDRs [52, 53]. All six CDRs are involved in antigen binding, but the H chain CDR3 seems to play a major role, particularly in the case of large naturally occurring antigens [54]. In most natural polyreactive antibodies, the H chain CDR3 is relatively long [54, 55], possibly providing the structural basis for a large antigen-combining site. A broad antigen-combining site would allow polyreactive antibodies to accommodate a variety of dissimilar epitopes. Even if a large H chain CDR3 is critical for polyreactivity, other features of the structures lining the antigen binding site may provide the correlate for the broad ligand specificity of polyreactive antibodies. For instance, the binding cleft of some murine anti-DNA antibodies contains a preponderance of basic arginine residues, enabling the formation of salt bridges with negatively charged antigens, such as DNA, RNA, and oligonucleotides [56, 57]. Such an ionic interaction between arginine and nucleic acid phosphate may be an important factor determining the characteristic features of not only naturally occurring antibodies to DNA found in healthy subjects, but also the anti-DNA autoantibodies characteristic of patients with SLE [56, 57].

To analyze the contribution of the somatically generated CDR3s and that of other different Ig V regions to polyreactivity, as well as to assess the impact of class switch to IgG on the ability of an originally polyreactive IgM antibody to bind multiple antigens, we performed recombinatorial experiments, involving a human polyreactive IgM, mAb55 [20], and a human monoreactive antigen-induced anti-insulin IgG, mAb13 [58]. These two mAbs were chosen because they use the same V_H, J_H, $V\kappa$, and $J\kappa$ gene segments in a highly similar configuration and with highly conserved FR structures [19, 47], but differ significantly in the length and composition of the H chain CDR3. mAb13 was previously characterized in experiments designed to analyze the structural correlates underlying the insulin-dependent emergence of a specific anti-insulin producing cell clone. By constructing the germline revertants for this somatically mutated anti-insulin IgG monoclonal antibody, and analyzing the antigen binding activity of the gene products, we determined that the full germline revertant bound specifically to insulin, although with lower affinity than that of the wildtype mAb13 [59]. Utilization of the same germline V_H, J_H, $V\kappa$ and $J\kappa$ gene segments of the "insulin-specific" full germline revertant mAb13 by a variety of other antibodies with different antigen binding activities suggests a primary role of the H chain CDR3 in antigen binding. The analysis of the chimeric molecules generated by replacing different portions of the polyreactive mAb55 H and L chain V segments with the corresponding portions of the monoreactive mAb13 and by expressing the "wild-type" or recombinant H and L chain V gene segments juxtaposed with the same $C\gamma 1$ and $C\kappa$ chains, respectively, demonstrated that antibody polyreactivity was not affected by class switch from IgM to IgG and was primarily dependent on the structure of the H chain CDR3. The unmutated $V\kappa$ FR1-FR3 segment facilitated the inherent multiple antigen binding activity of the H chain CDR3 [60]. These findings suggest that polyreactivity can be primarily a function of somatically generated structures. In addition, they show that such structures may also play a crucial role in antigen binding by monoreactive antigen-induced antibodies.

Natural Antibody-Producing B-1 Cells in Autoimmune Diseases

Due to their broad self-reactivity, natural antibodies found in healthy individuals may provide the templates for autoantibodies in many autoimmune diseases. Recognition of self is an early and possibly crucial step in the development of the immune system. Such self-recognition is initiated and mediated by natural antibodies, mainly IgM expressed on the surface of $CD5^+$ B cells occurring at high frequency in the fetus and neonate [61-63]. The random processes of V_H-D-J_H and V_L-J_L recombination as well as V_H and V_L gene pairing ensure the potential for the emergence of B clonotypes able to recognize self antigens. Such potential is frequently found among B-1 cells. Once generated, these cells may escape normal regulatory mechanisms; elimination of self-reactive B cells takes place in the periphery and may be a relatively inefficient process. Since B-1 cells are self-replenishing [26, 27, 64] they would provide a source of autoantibody-producing cell precursors throughout adult life.

In several autoimmune diseases B-1a cells are greatly increased in number, including rheumatoid arthritis [12-14], Sjogren's syndrome [65], and primary antiphospholipid syndrome [66]. In rheumatoid arthritis patients, B-1a cells can account for up to 60% of circulating B cells and produce rheumatoid factor autoantibodies that are monoreactive, high affinity, and somatically mutated [50, 67]. In contrast, in SLE patients, B-1a cells are generally not increased in number and do not constitute the main source of autoantibodies; a high proportion of anti-DNA autoantibodies are produced by lymphocytes that exhibit a surface $CD5^-$ phenotype [37, 68]. Our recent analysis of the segregation of anti-DNA autoantibody-producing cell precursors in SLE patients demonstrated that B-1b cells can account for most of the surface $CD5^-$ B cells that have been shown to produce anti-DNA autoantibodies [51]. These autoantibodies are IgG, IgA, and to a lesser extent, IgM, directed to single-stranded and/or double-stranded DNA; many of them cross-react with nucleic acids, phospholipids, and other antigens. As in the case of RFs isolated from patients with rheumatoid arthritis, the genes encoding the V regions of these antibodies are not dissimilar to those encoding the V regions of natural antibodies, and they bear the imprints of an antigen-driven selection process, i.e. extensive somatic mutations yielding high R:S mutation ratios in the CDRs but not the FRs [69-72]. These findings suggest that B-1 cells provide most of the autoantibody producing cell precursors in at least two important autoimmune diseases. They also suggest that they can somatically diversify, questioning the established dogma that B-1 lymphocytes are primordial cellular elements incapable of undergoing somatic hypermutation. Rather they indicate that these lymphocytes can participate in affinity maturation processes in response to self antigens.

Summary and Conclusions

Natural antibodies arise independently of known antigenic stimulation, are mostly IgM, polyreactive, and are generally encoded by V genes in germline configuration. Polyreactive IgM natural antibodies are produced by mainly B-1 cells which account for most of the B cell repertoire in the fetus and neonate, and possibly play a major role in the development and physiology of the human B cell repertoire. Although endowed with self-reactivity, natural antibodies also bind exogenous antigens [73, 74]. Exposure to environmental antigens is not necessary for the emergence of natural antibody-producing cell precursor clones to exogenous antigens, as suggested by the significant population of B cells capable of producing antibodies to a variety of bacterial antigens in germ-free animals. Because of their ability to bind a variety of exogenous antigens, including those on bacteria and viruses, natural antibodies play a major role in the primary line of defense against infections.

A central issue related to the understanding of the physiopathologic roles of natural antibodies is whether precursors of cells producing natural antibodies, B-1a and B-1b lymphocytes, are capable of undergoing an antigen-driven clonal selection process, thereby producing autoantibodies with a high affinity for the selecting antigen. In this respect, we have clearly established that B-1 cells can express a hypermutation mechanism similar to that of conventional (B-2) cells. Furthermore, we have shown by gene shuffling, site-directed mutagenesis, and *in vitro* human Ig gene expression, that the main structural correlate for antibody polyreactivity is provided by the somatically generated H chain CDR3. We have also shown that this Ig V region provides the main structural correlate for antigen-binding in monoreactive antigen-induced autoantibodies. These findings in the human are at the basis of our proposed structure-function model in which the antigen binding features of the germline template antibody are dictated by the somatically generated H chain CDR3, and perhaps, but at a lower degree, L chain CDR3; the point-mutation changes underlying the antigen-driven affinity maturation process would impact mainly the Ig V gene encoded segments. This structure-function model is being tested in our laboratory by analyzing the antigen binding activity of somatically mutated polyreactive autoantibodies that have been structurally reverted to their original putative unmutated configuration. Precise identification of the Ig gene and/or somatic recombination products mediating recruitment of unmutated B cell clonotypes, as well as those that are preferentially modified by an antigen-dependent selection process, should further our understanding of the mechanisms that shape the B cell repertoire in development and disease.

Acknowledgments

The experimental work discussed here was performed with funds from the United States Public Health Service grants AR-40908 and CA-68541. No funds were received from Dow Corning or from any other commercial sources. This is publication 10 from the Division of Molecular Immunology.

References

1. Boyden S (1965) Natural antibodies and the immune response. Adv Immunol 5:1-28
2. Michael JG (1969) Natural antibodies. Curr Top Microbiol Immunol 48:43-62
3. Casali P, Notkins AL (1989) CD5$^+$ B lymphocytes, polyreactive antibodies and the human B-cell repertoire. Immunol Today 10:364-368
4. Avrameas S (1991) Natural autoantibodies: from "horror autotoxicus" to "gnothi seauton." Immunol Today 12:154-159
5. Riboldi P, Kasaian MT, Mantovani L, Ikematsu H, Casali P (1993) Natural antibodies. In: Bona CA, Siminovitch K, Zanetti M, Theophilopoulos AN (ed) Molecular Pathology of Autoimmunity. The Harwood Academic Publisher, New York, pp 45-64
6. Turman MA, Casali P, Notkins AL, Bach FH, Platt JL (1991) Polyreactive antibodies from CD5$^+$ B cells: antigen specificity and relationship to xenoreactive natural antibodies. Transplantation 52:710-717

7. Kasaian MT, Ikematsu H, Casali P (1992) Identification and analysis of a novel human surface CD5⁻ B lymphocyte subset producing natural antibodies. J Immunol 148:2690-2702
8. Kasaian MT, Casali P (1992) Analysis of the human $CD5^-CD45RA^{lo}$ B cell subset. Ann NY Acad Sci 651:59-69
9. Nakamura M, Burastero SE, Notkins AL, Casali P (1988) Human monoclonal rheumatoid factor-like antibodies from CD5 (Leu-1 $^+$) B cells are polyreactive. J Immunol 140:4180-4186
10. Durandy A, Thuillier L, Forveille M, Fischer A (1990) Phenotypic and functional characteristics of human newborns' B lymphocytes. J Immunol 144:60-65
11. Gadol N, Ault KA (1986) Phenotypic and functional characterization of human Leu 1 (CD5) B cells. Immunol Rev 95:23-34
12. Burastero SE, Casali P (1989) Characterization of human CD5 (Leu-1 OKT1)$^+$ B lymphocytes and the antibodies they produce. Contrib Microbiol Immunol 11:231-262
13. Casali P, Notkins AL (1989) Probing the human B-cell repertoire with EBV: Polyreactive antibodies and $CD5^+$ B lymphocytes. Ann Rev Immunol 7:513-535
14. Burastero SE, Casali P, Wilder RL, Notkins AL (1988) Monoreactive high affinity and polyreactive low affinity rheumatoid factors are produced by $CD5^+$ B cells from patients with rheumatoid arthritis. J Exp Med 168:1979-1992
15. Casali P, Kasaian MT, Haughton G (1994) B-1 (CD5 B) cells. In: Coutinho A, Kazatchkine MD (ed) Autoimmunity: Physiology and Disease. John Wiley and Sons, Inc., New York, pp 57-88
16. Kasaian MT, Casali P (1993) Autoimmunity-prone B-1 (CD5 B) cells, natural antibodies and self recognition. Autoimmunity 15:315-329
17. Van Voorhis WC, Schlekewy L, Trong HL (1991) Molecular mimicry by *Trypanosmoa cruzi*: the F1-160 epitope that mimics mammalian nerve can be mapped to a 12-amino acid peptide. Proc Natl Acad Sci USA 88:5993-5997
18. Lafer EM, Rauch J, Andrzejewski JR, Mudd D, Furie B, Schwartz RS, Stollar DB (1981) Polyspecific monoclonal lupus autoantibodies reactive with both polynucleotides and phospholipids. J Exp Med 153:897-909
19. Ikematsu H, Harindranath N, Notkins AL, Ueki Y, Casali P (1993) Clonal analysis of a human antibody response. II. Sequences of the V_H genes of human monoclonal IgM, IgG and IgA to rabies virus reveal preferential utilization of the V_HIII segments and somatic hypermutation. J Immunol 150:1325-1337
20. Ueki Y, Goldfarb I, Harindranath N, Gore M, Koprowski H, Notkins AL, Casali P (1990) Clonal analysis of a human antibody response: Quantitation of precursors of antibody-producing cells and generation and characterization of monoclonal IgM, IgG, and IgA to rabies virus. J Exp Med 171:19-34
21. Foote J, Milstein C (1991) Kinetic maturation of an immune response. Nature 352:530-532
22. Hayakawa K, Hardy RR, Honda M, Herzenberg LA, Steinberg AD, Herzenberg LA (1984) Ly-1 B cells: Functionally distinct lymphocytes that secrete IgM autoantibodies. Proc Natl Acad Sci USA 81:2494-2498
23. Engleman EG, Warnke R, Fox RI, Dilley J, Benike C, Levy R (1981) Studies of a human T lymphocyte antigen recognized by a monoclonal antibody. Proc Natl Acad Sci USA 78:1791-1795
24. Huang HJ, Jones NH, Strominger JL, Herzenberg LA (1987) Molecular cloning of Ly-1, a membrane gycoprotein of mouse T lymphocytes and a subset of B cells: Molecular homology to its human counterpart Leu-1/T1 (CD5). Proc Natl Acad Sci USA 84:204-208
25. Jones NH, Clabby ML, Dialynas DP, Huang, HJ, Herzenberg LA, Strominger JL (1986) Isolation of complementary DNA clones encoding the human lymphocyte glycoprotein T1/Leu-1. Nature 323:346-349
26. Herzenberg LA, Stall AM, Lalor PA, Sidman C, Moore WA, Parks DR, Herzenberg LA (1986) The Ly-1 B cell lineage. Immunol Rev 93:81-102
27. Lalor PA, Herzenberg LA, Adams S, Stall AM (1989) Feedback regulation of murine Ly-1 B cell development. Eur J Immunol 19:507-513
28. Hayakawa K, Hardy RR (1988) Normal, autoimmune, and malignant $CD5^+$ B cells: The Ly-1 B lineage? Ann Rev Immunol 6:197-218

29. Boumsell L, Bernard A, Lepage V, Degos L, Lemerle J, Dausset J (1978) Some chronic lymphocytic leukemia cells bearing surface immunoglobulins share determinants with T cells. Eur J Immunol 8:900-904
30. Boumsell L, Coppin H, Pham D, Raynal B, Lemerle J, Dausset J, Bernard A (1988) An antigen shared by human T cell subsets and B cell chronic lymphocytic leukemia cells: Distribution on normal and malignant cells. J Exp Med 152:229-234
31. Royston I, Majoa JA, Baird SM, Meserve GL, Griffiths JC (1980) Human T-cell antigens defined by monoclonal antibodies: The 65,000-dalton antigen of T cells (T65) is also found on chronic lymphocytic leukemia cells bearing surface immunoglobulin. J Immunol 125:725-731
32. Caligaris-Cappio F, Gobbi M, Bofill M, Janossy G (1982) Infrequent normal B lymphocytes express features of B-chronic lymphocytic leukemia. J Exp Med 155:623-628
33. Gobbi M, Caligaris-Cappio F, Janossy G (1983) Normal equivalent of cells of B cell malignancies: Analysis with monoclonal antibodies. Brit J Haematol 54:393-403
34. Antin JH, Emerson SG, Martin P, Gadol N, Ault KA (1986) Leu-1+ (CD5+) B cells: A major lymphoid subpopulation in human fetal spleen: phenotypic and functional studies. J Immunol 136:505-510
35. Hayakawa K, Hardy RR, Herzenberg LA (1986) Peritoneal Ly-1 B cells: Genetic control, autoantibody production, increased lambda light chain expression. Eur J Immunol 16:450-465
36. Kipps TJ, Fong S, Tomhave E, Chen PP, Goldfien RD, Carson DA (1987) High frequency expression of a conserved kappa variable region gene in chronic lymphocytic leukemia. Proc Natl Acad Sci USA 84:2916-2920
37. Casali P, Burastero SE, Nakamura M, Inghirami G, Notkins AK (1987) Human lymphocytes making rheumatoid factor and antibody to ssDNA belong to the Leu-1+ B-cell subset. Science 236:77-81
38. Hayakawa K, Hardy RR, Parks DR, Herzenberg LA (1983) The "Ly-1 B" cell subpopulation in normal, immunodefective, and autoimmune mice. J Exp Med 157:202-218
39. Hasegawa K, Nishimura H, Ogawa S, Hirose S, Sato H, Shirai T (1990) Monoclonal antibodies to epitope of CD45R(B220) inhibit interleukin 4-mediated B cell proliferation and differentiation. Internat Immunol 2:367-375
40. Mittler RS, Greenfield RS, Schacter BZ, Richard NF, Hoffmann MK (1987) Antibodies to the leukocyte antigen (T200) inhibit an early phase in the activation of resting human B cells. J Immunol 138:3159-3166
41. Yakura H, Kawabata I, Ashida T, Katagiri M (1988) Differential regulation by Ly-5 and Lyb-2 of IgG production induced by lipopolysaccharide and B cell stimulatory factor-1 (IL-4). J Immunol 141:875-880
42. Yakura H, Kawabata I, Shen FW, Katagiri M (1986) Selective inhibition of lipopolysaccharide-induced polyclonal IgG response by monoclonal Ly-5 antibody. J Immunol 136:2729-2733
43. Yakura H, Shen FW, Bourcet E, Boyse EA (1983) On the function of Ly-5 in the generation of antigen-driven B cell differentiation. Comparison and contrast with Lyb-2. J Exp Med 157:1077-1088
44. Kantor AB (1991) The development and repertoire of B-1 cells (CD5 B cells). Immunol Today 12:389-391
45. Matsuda F, Shin EK, Nagaoka H, Matsumura R, Haino M, Fukita Y, Taka-ishi S, Imai T, Riley JH, Anand R, Soeda E, Honjo T (1993) Structure and physical map of 64 variable segments in the 3' 0.8-megabase region of the human immunoglobulin heavy-chain locus. Nature Genet 3:88-94
46. Cook GP, Tomlinson IM, Walter G, Riethman H, Carter NP, Buluwela L, Winter G, Rabbitts TH (1994) A map of the human immunoglobulin V_H locus completed by analysis of the telomeric region of chromosome 14q. Nature Genet 8:162-168
47. Ikematsu H, Ichiyoshi Y, Schettino EW, Nakamura M, Casali P (1994) V_H and $V\kappa$ segment structure of anti-insulin IgG autoantibodies in patients with insulin-dependent diabetes mellitus. Evidence for somatic selection. J Immunol 152:1430-1441

48. Ikematsu H, Kasaian MT, Schettino EW, and Casali P (1993) Structural analysis of the V_H-D-J_H segments of human polyreactive IgG mAb. Evidence for somatic selection. J Immunol 151:3604-3616
49. Kasaian MT, Ikematsu H, Balow JE, Casali P (1994) Structure of the V_H and V_L segments of monoreactive and polyreactive IgA autoantibodies to DNA in patients with systemic lupus erythematosus. J Immunol 152:3137-3151
50. Mantovani L, Wilder RL, Casali P (1993) Human rheumatoid B-1a ($CD5^+$ B) cells make somatically hypermutated high affinity IgM rheumatoid factors. J Immunol 151:473-488
51. Kasaian MT, Casali P (1995) B-1 cellular origin and V_H segment strucutre of IgG, IgA, and IgM anti-DNA autoantibodies in patients with systemic lupus erythematosus. Ann NY Acad Sci In press
52. Colman PM (1988) Structure of antibody-antigen complexes: Implications for immune recognition. Adv Immunol 43:99-132
53. Kabat EA (1988) Antibody complementarity and antibody structure. J Immunol (suppl) 141:S25-S36
54. Amit AG, Mariuzza RA, Phillips SE, Poliak RJ (1986) Three-dimensional structure of an antigen-antibody complex at 2.8 A resolution. Science 233:747-753
55. Stanfield RL, Fieser TM, Lerner RA, Wilson IA (1990) Crystal structure of an antibody to a peptide and its complex with peptide antigen at 2.8 A. Science 248:712-719
56. Eilat D, Webster DM, Rees AR (1988) V region sequences of anti-DNA and anti-RNA autoantibodies from NZB/NZW F1 mice. J Immunol 141:1745-1753
57. Shlomchik M, Mascelli M, Shan H, Radic MZ, Pisetsky D, Marshak-Rothstein A, Weigert MG (1990) Anti-DNA antibodies from autoimmune mice arise by clonal expansion and somatic point mutation. J Exp Med 171:265-292
58. Casali P, Nakamura M, Ginsberg-Fellner F, Notkins AL (1990) Frequency of B cells committed to the production of antibodies to insulin in newly diagnosed patients with insulin-dependent diabetes mellitus and generation of high affinity monoclonal IgG to insulin. J Immunol 144:3741-3747
59. Ichiyoshi Y, Zhou M, Casali P (1995) A human anti-insulin IgG autoantibody apparently arises through clonal selection from an insulin-specific "germ-line" natural antibody template. J Immunol 154:226-238
60. Ichiyoshi Y, Casali P (1994) Analysis of the structural correlates for antibody polyreactivity by multiple reassortments of chimeric human immunoglobulin heavy and light chain V segments. J Exp Med 180:885-895
61. Kipps TJ, Robbins BA, Carson DA (1990) Uniform high frequency expression of autoantibody-associated crossreactive idiotypes in the primary B cell follicles of human fetal spleen. J Exp Med 171:189-196
62. Pisetsky DS, Jelinek DF, McAnally LM, Reich CF, Lipsky PE (1990) In vitro autoantibody production by normal adult and cord blood B cells. J Clin Invest 85:899-903
63. Lydyard PM, Quartey-Papafio R, Broker B, Mackenzie L, Jouquan J, Blaschek MA, Steele J, Petrou M, Collins P, Isenberg D, Youinou PY (1990) The antibody repertoire of early human B cells: I. High frequency of autoreactivity and polyreactivity. Scand J Immunol 31:33-43
64. Herzenberg LA, Herzenberg LA (1989) Toward a layered immune system. Cell 59:953-954
65. Dauphinee M, Tovar Z, Talal N (1988) B cells expressing CD5 are increased in Sjogren's syndrome. Arthritis Rheum 31:642-647
66. Velasquillo MC, Alcocer-Varela J, Alarcon-Segovia D, Cabiedes J, Sanchez-Guerrero J (1991) Some patients with primary antiphopholipid syndrome have increased circulating $CD5^+$ B cells that correlate with levels of IgM antiphospholipid. Clin Exp Rheum 9:1-5
67. Harindranath N, Goldfarb IS, Ikematsu H, Burastero SE, Wilder RL, Notkins AL, Casali P (1991) Complete sequence of the genes encoding the V_H and V_L regions of low- and high-affinity monoclonal IgM and IgA1 rheumatoid factors produced by $CD5^+$ B cells from a rheumatoid arthritis patient. Int Immunol 3:865-875
68. Suzuki N, Sakane T, Engleman EG (1990) Anti-DNA antibody production by $CD5^+$ and $CD5^-$ B cells of patients with systemic lupus erythematosus. J Clin Invest 85:238-247

69. Mannheimer-Lory A, Katz JB, Pillinger M, Ghossein C, Smith A, Diamond B (1991) Molecular characteristics of antibodies bearing an anti-DNA-associated idiotype. J Exp Med 174:1639-1652
70. Dersimonian H, Schwartz RS, Barrett KJ, Stollar DB (1987) Relationship of human variable region heavy chain germ-line genes to genes encoding anti-DNA autoantibodies. J Immunol 139:2496-2501
71. Van Es JH, Gmelig-Meyling FHJ, Van De Akker WRM, Aanstoot H, Derksen RHWM, Logtenberg T (1991) Somatic mutations in the variable regions of a human IgG anti-double-stranded DNA autoantibody suggest a role for antigen in the induction of systemic lupus erythematosus. J Exp Med 173:461-470
72. Diamond B, Katz JB, Paul E, Aranow C, Lustgarten D, Scharff MD (1992) The role of somatic mutation in the pathogenic anti-DNA response. Ann Rev Immunol 10:731-757
73. Bos, NA, Kimura H, Meewsen CG, De Visser H, Hazenberg MP, Wostmann BS, Pleasants JR, Benner R, Marcus DM (1989) Serum immunoglobulin levels and naturally occurring antibodies against carbohydrate antigens in germ-free BALB/c mice fed chemically defined ultrafiltered diet. Eur J Immunol 19:2335-2339
74. Underwood JR, Pederson JS, Chalmers PJ, Toh BH (1985) Hybrids from normal, germ-free, nude and neonatal mice produce monoclonal autoantibodies to eight different intracellular structures. Clin Exp Immunol 60:417-426

Antibodies to Cholesterol: Biological Implications of Antibodies to Lipids

Carl R. Alving[1], Nabila M. Wassef[1], and Michael Potter[2]
[1]Department of Membrane Biochemistry, Walter Reed Army Institute of Research, Washington, DC 20307-5100 USA, and [2]Michael Potter, Laboratory of Genetics, DCBDC, NCI, NIH, Bethesda, MD 20892 USA.

Summary

Injection of silicone gel or silicone oil intraperitoneally into BALB/c mice induced the formation of antibodies that reacted by ELISA with highly purified crystalline cholesterol and, to a much lesser extent, antibodies that reacted with a phospholipid (dimyristoyl phosphatidylglycerol). Although IgM and IgG antibodies to cholesterol were detected, the titers of IgG antibodies were low when compared with IgM. The titers of IgM antibodies to cholesterol in certain sera exhibited activities that reached baseline values at dilutions as high as 1:5000, thus making them equivalent to titers that have been previously published for ascites fluid containing murine monoclonal antibodies to cholesterol. The antibodies to cholesterol induced by silicone compounds are indistinguishable in their binding to crystalline cholesterol from naturally-occurring antibodies to cholesterol in normal human serum. They are also indistiguishable from antibodies induced by a proposed vaccine to cholesterol that is currently in late preclinical development for prevention of hypercholesterolemia in humans. The anti-cholesterol vaccine, which consists of liposomes heavily laden with cholesterol as an antigen and lipid A as an adjuvant, induces antibodies that react with low density lipoproteins (LDL) and opsonize them for removal by liver macrophages. It appears that silicone gel or silicone oil causes recruitment and adsorption of cholesterol at the injection site, and also serves as an adjuvant that may have immunostimulant properties similar to lipid A for inducing antibodies to lipids. Antibodies to lipids such as cholesterol or phospholipids are not harmful to intact cell membranes because of steric hindrance from surrounding lipids and larger macromolecules that block binding of the antibodies.

Introduction

Antibodies to many lipids, including phospholipids and cholesterol, can be readily induced in rabbits and mice by injection of liposomes containing lipid A, the lipid moiety of Gram-negative bacterial lipopolysaccharide (Schuster et al., 1979; Alving, 1986; Alving and Swartz, 1991). Lipid A serves as a potent adjuvant that induces "anti-liposome" antibodies that recognize individual lipid constituents in the liposomal lipid bilayer. Highly specific murine monoclonal antibodies (mAbs) to phospholipids have been produced by injection of appropriate liposomes (Banerji et al., 1982; Wassef et al., 1984; Alving, 1986). Monoclonal antibodies to cholesterol have also been produced in mice by injection of liposomes containing both lipid A and a high concentration of highly purified cholesterol (cholesterol/phospholipid ratio of 2.5/1, or 71%) (Swartz et al., 1988). The mAbs to cholesterol recognized purified crystalline cholesterol both by immunogold electron microscopy and by ELISA. Injection of mice with 71% cholesterol liposomes lacking lipid A did not induce antibodies to cholesterol.

Naturally-occurring Antibodies to Cholesterol in Human Sera

Upon screening human sera by ELISA, the interesting discovery was made that naturally-occurring antibodies to highly purified crystalline cholesterol are present in varying titers in virtually all normal human sera (Alving et al., 1989). Recent analysis of 742 normal human sera revealed that all of the sera contained antibodies to cholesterol, often in very high levels (Alving et al., 1995a). Although the exact origin of natural antibodies to cholesterol is still unknown, it has been proposed that the ubiquitous appearance of such antibodies might have effects on the regulation of cholesterol metabolism (Alving et al., 1995a).

Anti-cholesterol vaccine

Rabbits that had been injected with cholesterol-rich liposomes containing lipid A to induce antibodies to cholesterol were fed a high cholesterol diet to cause hypercholesterolemia and atherosclerosis. When compared with nonimmunized animals, the immunized animals developed significantly reduced levels of serum cholesterol, reduced aortic sudanophilia in certain areas, and smaller plaque lesions in certain regions of the aorta (Alving et al., 1995a, b). Antibodies to cholesterol also bound to low, intermediate, and very low density lipoprotein isolated from nonimmunized cholesterol-fed rabbits (Alving et al., submitted for publication). Based on these results it has been proposed that naturally-occurring antibodies to cholesterol might play a role in cholesterol metabolism that could result in protective effects against hypercholesterolemia associated with elevated low density lipoproteins (Alving et al., 1995a, b). The unique possibility that antibodies to cholesterol might have beneficial effects has led to the proposal that active immunization of humans with an anti-cholesterol "vaccine" might provide beneficial prophylactic effects against hypercholesterolemia and atherosclerosis (Alving, 1995b). Phase I trials in human volunteers for initial testing of an anti-cholesterol vaccine are anticipated in the near future.

Induction of Antibodies to Cholesterol and Phospholipids by Injection of Silicone Oil or Gel

BALB/c mice that were injected only a single time intraperitoneally with silicone oil (dimethylpolysiloxane, also known as DMPS) or silicone gel (Potter et al., 1994) developed substantial levels of IgM antibodies to highly purified crystalline cholesterol by ELISA (Fig. 1A). IgG antibodies were also observed, but in much lower amounts (not shown). As noted earlier, mice that are injected with 71% cholesterol liposomes lacking lipid A do not develop antibodies.

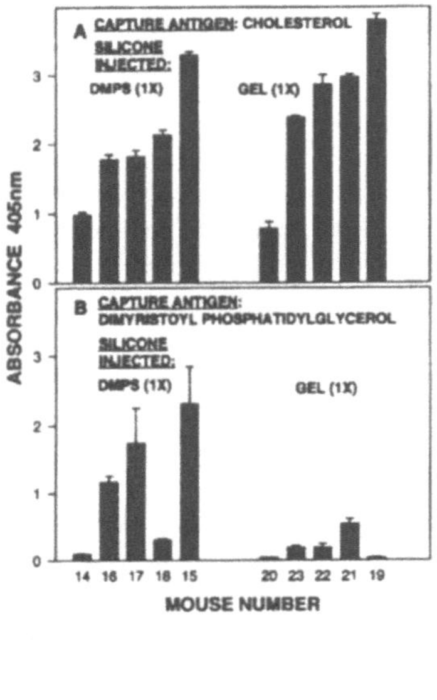

Fig. 1. Induction of antibodies to lipids by injection of silicone compounds. BALB/cAnPt mice were injected once i.p. with either silicone oil (1000- centistoke DMPS) or gel. Sera (50 µl of 1:100 dilution) were analyzed by solid phase ELISA for antibodies to purified cholesterol (A) or phosphatidylglycerol (B).

The same process that caused the induction of antibodies to cholesterol also resulted in the appearance of lower amounts of antibodies to certain phospholipids. As shown in Fig. 1B, DMPS and, to a much lower extent, gel induced IgM antibodies that reacted with dimyristoyl phosphatidylglycerol by ELISA. This is compatible with previous observations that have suggested that, under conditions where it is immunogenic, cholesterol is a potent antigen that induces a stronger antibody response than that observed against phospholipids.

Upon dilution of serum from mice injected twice with DMPS, the anti-cholesterol activity diminishes rapidly at 1:1000, and reaches baseline at 1:5000 (Fig. 2). For purposes of comparison, two out of four ascites fluids containing murine mAbs to cholesterol were still detectable by ELISA at dilutions of 1:31250, but one other reached baseline at a dilution of 1:2500 (Swartz et al., 1988).

The results of Figs. 1 and 2 therefore suggest that injection of silicone oil or gel, each of which is known to cause a substantial granuloma at the site of injection (Potter et al., 1994), might promote recruitment of tissue cholesterol or phospholipid, perhaps on the surface of silicone-containing particles. The silicone compound then might serve as a potent adjuvant for inducing antibodies to cholesterol or phospholipid. If this hypothesis is true it would imply that silicone oil and gel each has adjuvant activity that is equivalent to that of lipid A. This would be compatible with the adjuvant activities that have been reported to be associated with these materials (Naim et al., 1993).

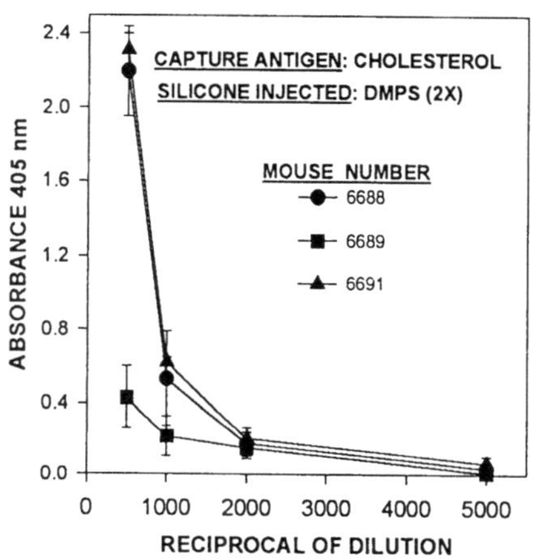

Fig. 2. Titration of antibodies to cholesterol. The mice were injected twice (0, 60 days) and sera were analyzed at day 83

Biological Implications of Antibodies to Cholesterol and Other Lipids

A frequently asked question relating to antibodies to cholesterol is whether such antibodies can bind to cholesterol that is present in cell membranes. Obviously, any antibodies that are circulating have not bound to membrane cholesterol. If any such binding does take place the available binding sites presumably have already been filled when circulating antibodies are detected in the serum The most likely place for antibody binding to take place would be on the surface of circulating very low, low, or intermediate density lipoproteins. Normal human plasma contains immunoglobulins (mainly IgM and IgA) that bind to low density human lipoprotein (Bauer et al., 1982) and rabbit antibodies to cholesterol bind to low and very low density lapine lipoproteins. The binding of antibodies to certain lipoproteins may occur because of the very high concentration of cholesterol in the lipoprotein surface that may permit exposure of cholesterol epitopes for binding of antibodies. As discussed earlier, antibodies to cholesterol may provide beneficial prophylactic effects against elevated cholesterol in low density lipoproteins.

It is highly unlikely that the cholesterol that is present in any cell membranes exposed to circulating antibodies would be easily accessible to the binding of the antibodies. This is because the presumed major binding site, the C3-OH group, which represents the only polar group on the cholesterol molecule, is exceedingly small when compared with the size of the other adjacent polar groups on the surface of the lipid bilayer of the cell membrane. As illustrated in Fig. 3, the polar region of cholesterol (arrow) is very small when compared with the zwitterionic polar headgroup of

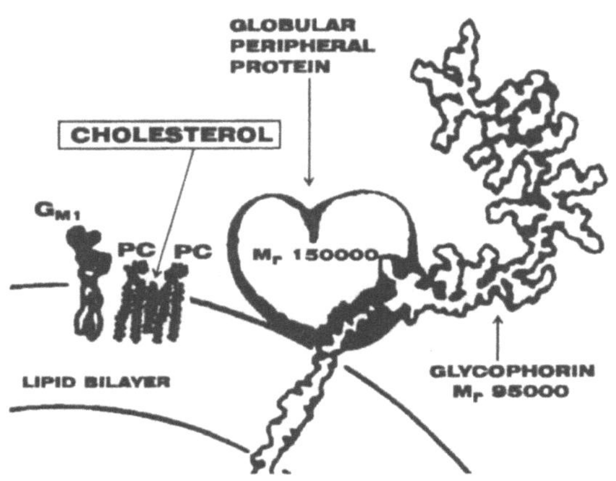

Fig. 3. Comparative sizes of cholesterol, phosphatidylcholine, ganglioside G_{MI}, glycophorin, and a peripheral globular protein. Proportions of molecules are derived as a composite of proportions described by Grant (1986) and Alving and Swartz (1991).

phosphatidylcholine (PC), and this latter moiety is small when compared with the anionic polar headgroup of ganglioside G_{MI}. Overlaying all of these molecules at the surface of the lipid bilayer are other large macromolecules, such as glycophorin, that might cause interference with antibody binding to underlying molecules. The antigen-binding group of an immunoglobulin molecule would be expected to be too bulky to gain easy access to the polar group of cholesterol at the normal concentration of cholesterol in the cell membrane. However, at higher cholesterol/phospholipid ratios, self-association of cholesterol might provide a "landing zone" for the anti-cholesterol molecule. Evidence for this mechanism is further derived from the observation that accessibility of liposomal cholesterol or viral cholesterol to cholesterol oxidase is greatly facilitated by increased cholesterol/phospholipid ratios (Pal et al., 1980).

Previous work with monoclonal antibodies to phospholipids has demonstrated that the presence of relatively simple glycolipids, such as globoside (ceramide tetrahexoside), can cause steric interference that blocks the binding of antibodies to liposomal phospholipids (Shichijo et al.,

1985). Liposomal gangliosides can also cause steric interference with binding of a mAb to liposomal Forsmann glycolipid (ceramide pentahexoside) (Shichijo et al. 1986). Binding of an anti-phospholipid mAb did not occur with suspended macrophages, but did occur when the macrophages were treated lightly with trypsin (Fogler et al., 1987). This latter observation is compatible with early studies that demonstrated that the ability of polyclonal antibodies to globoside to agglutinate human erythrocytes is increased 1000-fold when the cells are trypsinized (Koscielak et al., 1968). The above studies demonstrate that polar antigenic moieties of cell membrane lipids normally are either too small to allow efficient binding of antibodies or are blocked from binding by steric hindrance from adjacent lipids or proteins. From a practical standpoint, the inaccessibility of cell membrane lipids to binding by antibodies provides a strong logical basis for confidence that antibodies to lipids will not produce deliterious effects against normal cell membranes. In fact it has been proposed that naturally-occurring antibodies to lipids could serve a useful normal function for removing debris derived from damaged or dead cells (Alving, 1990).

Acknowledgements and Note

The authors acknowledge the excellent technical assistance of SGT Keith Ellis and SPC Anthony Schmidt. Dr. Alving is a coinventor of the anti-cholesterol vaccine and has a financial interest in EntreMed, Inc.

References

Alving CR (1986) Antibodies to liposomes, phospholipids, and phosphate esters. Chem Phys Lipids 40:303-314

Alving, CR, (1990) Antibodies to liposomes, phospholipids, and cholesterol: Implications for autoimmunity, atherosclerosis, and aging. In: Nicholau C, Chapman D (eds) Horizons in Membrane Biotechnology A R Liss, New York 41-51

Alving CR, Swartz Jr GM (1991) Antibodies to cholesterol, cholesterol conjugates, and liposomes: Implications for atherosclerosis and autoimmunity. CRC Crit Rev Immunol 10:441-453

Alving CR, Swartz Jr GM, Wassef NM (1989) Naturally-occurring autoantibodies to cholesterol in humans. Biochem Soc Trans 17:637-639

Alving CR, Swartz Jr GM, Wassef NM, Herderick EE, Virmani R, Kolodgie FD, Matyas GR, Ribas JL, Kenner JR, Cornhill JF (1995a) Vaccination against cholesterol: immunologic modulation of diet-induced hypercholesterolemia and atherosclerosis. In: Woodford P, Davignon J, Sniderman A (eds) Atherosclerosis X Elsevier Science BV, Amsterdam 944-948

Alving CR, Swartz Jr GM, Wassef NM, Herderick EE, Virmani R, Kolodgie FD, Matyas GR, Ribas JL, Kenner JR, Cornhill JF (1995b) Prospects for an anti-cholesterol vaccine. Clin Immunother 3:409-414

Banerji B, Lyon JA, Alving CR (1982) Membrane lipid composition modulates the binding specificity of a monoclonal antibody against liposomes. Biochim Biophys Acta 689:319-326

Bauer BJ, Blashfield K, Norris R, Buthala DA, Ginsberg LC (1982) Immunoglobulin as the major low density lipoprotein binding protein in plasma. Atherosclerosis 44:153-160

Fogler WE, Swartz Jr GM, Alving CR (1987) Antibodies to phospholipids and liposomes: Binding of antibodies to cells. Biochim Biophys Acta 903:265-272

Grant CWM (1986) Model membranes bearing glycolipids and glycoproteins. Chem Phys Lipids 40:285-302

Koscielak J. Hakomori S, Jeanloz RW (1968) Glycolipid antigen and its antibody. Immunochemistry 5:441-445

Naim JO, Lanzafame RJ (1993) The adjuvant effect of silicone-gel on antibody formation in rats. Immunol Invest 22:151-161

Pal R, Barenholz Y, Wagner RR (1980) Effect of cholesterol concentration on organization of viral and vesicle membranes. J Biol Chem 225:5802-5806

Potter M, Morrison S, Wiener F, Xiaokui KZ, Miller FW (1994) Induction of plasmacytomas with silicone gel in genetically susceptible strains of mice. J Cancer Natl Inst 86:1058-1065

Schuster B, Neidig M, Alving BM, Alving CR (1979) Production of antibodies against phosphocholine, phosphatidylcholine, sphingomyelin, and lipid A by injection of liposomes containing lipid A. J. Immunol 122:900-905

Shichijo S, Alving CR (1985) Influence of glycolipids on immune reactions of phospholipid antigens in liposomes. Biochim Biophys Acta 820:289-294

Shichijo S, Alving CR (1986) Inhibitory effects of gangliosides on immune reactions of antibodies to neutral glycolipids in liposomes. Biochim Biophys Acta 858:18-124

Swartz Jr GM, Gentry MK, Amende LM, Blanchette-Mackie, EJ, Alving CR (1988) Antibodies to cholesterol. Proc Natl Acad Sci USA 85:1902-1906

Wassef NM, Roerdink F, Swartz Jr GM, Lyon JA, Berson, B.J., Alving, C.R. (1984) Phosphate binding specificities of monoclonal antibodies against phosphoinositides in liposomes. Mol Immunol 21:863-868

T Cell, NK Cell Responses to Silicones

Silicone-Induced T Cell Proliferation in Mice

A. H. McDonald*, K.Weir* and J. R. Sanger†.
*Department of Pathology, Medical College of Wisconsin and †Department of Plastic and Reconstructive Surgery, Medical College of Wisconsin, Milwaukee, Wisconsin.

Introduction

The silicone polymers used in mammary implants have been linked anecdotally to the development of autoimmune connective tissue diseases in women (1-7). Although, retrospective studies do not indicate an increased risk of developing autoimmune disease in women with silicone gel breast implants (8-10), there remains a legitimate concern among physicians and plastic surgeons alike regarding whether silicone gel breast augmentation induces and/or enhances the development of autoimmune diseases in the 1% of the population who are estimated to be genetically-susceptible. Recent studies by other labs indicate that silicone gel can enhance the production of anti-BSA antibodies in Sprague-Dawley rats and, therefore, function in an adjuvant-like manner to stimulate B cell responses (11). In this study, we demonstrate that silicone gel induces an *in vitro* T cell proliferative response in certain inbred strains of mice, i.e., BALB/cAnPt, (BALB/cAnPt x DBA/2N)F1 and C57BL/6, but not in DBA/2N and BALB/cJax. This response is mediated by silicone-induced peritoneal cells, which stimulate spleen, lymph and mesenteric lymph nodes cells from syngeneic mice injected subcutaneously with silicone gel, pristane or thioglycollate but not with Hank's balanced salt solution (HBSS). In contrast, pristane, thioglycollate or HBSS-generated peritoneal cells do not induce T-cell proliferation. In BALB/c mice, this response is dose dependent, enhanced by enrichment of CD4+ cells (stimulation index > 9.0) and inhibited with antibodies to either IL-2 or IL-4. Environmental factors play a critical role in the development of a T cell response, since neither specific pathogen-free (SPF)-BALB/c mice nor conventionally-housed (CON) BALB/c mice maintained on a low-fat diet respond well to silicone. These results demonstrate that silicone-induced T cell proliferation in mice is mediated nonspecifically by CD4+ Th cells and is influenced by both genetic and environmental factors.

Results and Discussion

Silicone-induced peritoneal cells stimulate a proliferative response in BALB/cAnPt mice. To address the question whether silicone gel induces an antigen-specific lymphoproliferative response that can be measured *in vitro* and to circumvent the difficulty of adding small, accurately measured quantities of silicone

Support for this work was provided by clinical funds from the Medical College of Wisconsin, Milwaukee, Wisconsin.

Table I. Silicone-induced presenting cells stimulate spleen cells to proliferate in silicone, thioglycollate and pristane challenged BALB/c mice, but not in HBSS-injected BALB/c mice.

Presenting Cells[a]	Responding Cells[b]	Spleen Cells CPM[c] ± 1 SEM	SI[d]
Silicone	Silicone	**6199 ± 182**	**4.04**
"	Thioglycollate	**3534 ± 197**	**2.94**
"	Pristane	**2127 ± 408**	**2.25**
"	HBSS	1412 ± 225	1.37
Thioglycollate	Silicone	2008 ± 169	1.03
"	Thioglycollate	1357 ± 196	1.24
"	Pristane	1253 ± 107	1.31
"	HBSS	1281 ± 171	1.12
Pristane	Silicone	1790 ± 279	1.40
"	Thioglycollate	1891 ± 168	1.88
"	Pristane	828 ± 109	1.10
"	HBSS	836 ± 57	1.00
Saline	Silicone	710 ± 184	0.57
"	Thioglycollate	1086 ± 171	0.64
"	Pristane	998 ± 38	0.70
"	HBSS	1058 ± 336	0.70

[a]Presenting cells are whole populations of peritoneal cells induced by the intraperitoneal injection of either 0.2ml silicone gel, 0.5ml pristane, 2ml thioglycollate or 0.5ml HBSS 3-10 days previously and irradiated with 1000 rads prior to cell co-culture. Presenting cells were added at a concentration of $1x10^5$ cells/well.

[b]Responder cells are whole spleen cell (SpC) suspensions made from female mice injected sc with either 0.2ml silicone gel, pristane, saline or 2ml thioglycollate 3-10 days previously. Responder cells were cultured at a concentration of $4x10^5$ cells/well. Co-cultures were incubated for 5 days at 37°C/5% CO_2 and pulsed with 1 uCi ^{3}H-thymidine overnight on the final day. Cultures were harvested onto glass fiber filter strips (Cambridge Technology, Inc, Watertown, MA).

[c]CPM = experimental counts per minute of co-cultures containing both presenting and responding cells ± 1 standard error of the mean (SEM) as measured on a Tri-Carb 2000CA liquid scintillation counter.

[d]Stimulation index (SI) = Experimental CPM/(Presenting cell background CPM + Responder cell background CPM) Results in bold lettering highlight results statistically higher ($p < .001$) than controls (backround cpm) as determined by the student *t* test. These results are representative of more than 3 separate experiments.

gel *in vitro* the following assay system was developed. Ten to twelve-week-old female BALB/cAnPt (BALB/c) mice (generously provided by Dr. Michael Potter, NCI contract N01-CP-21075, Perimmune Corp, Rockville, MD) were given two subcutaneous (sc) 0.1ml injections of silicone gel from a sterile breast implant (Lot Number HH4077, Dow Corning, Midland, MI) in the abdominal area. Ten days later, the mice were sacrificed and the spleens, lymph nodes and mesenteric lymph nodes were prepared as single cell suspensions (12) and used as reponding cells. Silicone-containing 'presenting cells'/peritoneal cells were obtained from the peritoneal cavity of male or female BALB/c mice injected intraperitoneally (ip) with 0.2ml silicone gel 3 - 10 days previously and irradiated with 1000 rads from a cesium irradiator (J.L. Shepard and Associates, San Fernando, CA). Intraperitoneal injection of silicone gel has been shown to induce an influx of

Table II. Cellular composition of peritoneal exudate cells after ip injection with HBSS, silicone gel, pristane and thioglycollate.

	Percent Positive			
	Silicone	*Pristane*	*Thioglycolate*	*Saline*
Mac-1+	69	61	75	15
CD45/B220	11	18	11	72
CD4+	8	6	3	8
CD8+	NT	2	2	3

Male and female BALB/c mice were injected ip with either 0.2ml silicone gel, 0.5ml pristane, 0.5ml HBSS or 2.0ml thioglycollate. Ten days later, mice were sacrificed and peritoneal cells collected by peritoneal lavage as previously described (12). Thioglycollate injected mice were sacrificed three days after injection. Peritoneal cells were stained with immunofluorescently labeled monoclonal antibodies against murine CD4, CD8, CD45/B220 (PharMingen, San Diego, CA) and Mac-1 (Boerhinger Mannheim Biochemicals, Indianapolis, IN) as previously described (12) and analyzed by an Epics-Profile II Flow Cytometer (Coulter Electronics).

macrophages that ingest droplets of silicone gel (13). BALB/c mice injected ip with either Hank's balanced salt solution (HBSS) (Gibco Life Technologies, Grand Island, NY), pristane (Sigma Chemical CO., St. Louis, MO) or thioglycollate (Becton Dickinson and Company, Cockeysville, MD) served as normal and specificity controls. As seen in Table 1, when responding and presenting cells were co-cultured for 5 days *in vitro*, silicone-induced presenting cells were able to produce a statistically significant proliferative response (SI > 2) in the spleen cells (SpC) of mice previously injected with either silicone, thioglycollate or pristane, but not with HBSS. In contrast, neither HBSS, thioglycollate nor pristane-induced peritoneal cells were capable of stimulating a proliferative response in any of the responding cell populations (SI < 2) (Table 1). Identical results were obtained using mesenteric lymph node cells (MLNC) or lymph node cells (LNC) from silicone-injected BALB/c mice (data not shown). These results indicate that silicone-containing peritoneal cells are capable of inducing a lymphoproliferative response in silicone-injected mice. However, because silicone-containing peritoneal cells were seen to stimulate lymphocytes from pristane and thioglycollate-injected mice, as well as silicone-injected mice, it is unlikely that the observed proliferation is antigen-specific. The lack of a response to either HBSS, pristane or thioglycollate-induced presenting cells suggests that the lymphoproliferation induced by silicone-containing presenting cells is due to silicone and not to an autologous mixed leukocyte response (AMLR) (14). Therefore, these results suggest that silicone-induced lymphoproliferation while not antigen-specific, is unique to silicone when compared to pristane, thioglycollate and HBSS.

Mac-1+ cells predominate in the peritoneal exudate from silicone, pristane and thioglycollate-injected BALB/c mice. The cellular composition of peritoneal cells from silicone, HBSS, pristane and thioglycollate injected mice were compared by flow cytometry (Table 2). Intraperitoneal injection of silicone gel, pristane and thioglycollate produced an inflammatory infiltration composed predominantly of macrophages and neutrophils (61-75% Mac-1+ cells). T and B cells were present in small percentages (T + B cells ≤ 26%) (Table 2). In contrast, presenting cell preparations from mice injected with HBSS were composed predominantly of B cells, a pattern similar if not identical to that of the resting peritoneum in uninjected mice (12) (Table 2). These results demonstrate that the

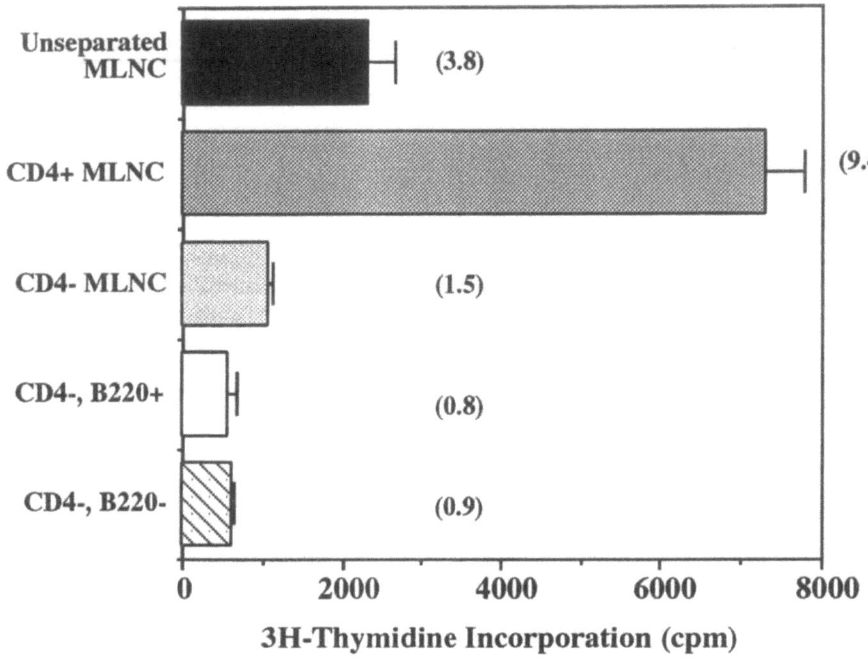

Figure 1. Silicone-containing peritoneal cells stimulate CD4+ T cells to proliferate in BALB/c mice. Mesenteric lymph node cells (MLNC) from 3-4 sc injected female mice were pooled and separated into CD4+, CD4-, CD4-/B220+ and CD4-/B220- fractions by magnetic activated cell separation using anti-CD4 and anti-CD45/B220 beads (15). Fractions were cultured with irradiated silicone-containing peritoneal cells and proliferation determined 5 days later. Numbers in parentheses represent the stimulation index (SI).

cellular composition of the peritoneal exudate after injection with either silicone gel, pristane or thioglycollate is not significantly different and, therefore, unlikely to be responsible for the inability of pristane and thioglycollate to induce a lymphoproliferative response.

CD4+ T cells from silicone-injected BALB/c mice proliferate when cultured with silicone-containing peritoneal cells and are inhibited by monoclonal antibodies against IL-2 and IL-4. Mesenteric lymph node cells (MLNC) from BALB/c mice sc injected with silicone gel were separated into CD4+ and CD4- fractions by anti-L3T4 (CD4) beads (Miltenyi Biotec Inc, Sunnyvale, CA) and magnetic column fractionation (15). CD4- cells were further separated into CD45/B220+ (B cell) and CD45/B220- (CD8+) fractions using anti-CD45/B220 beads (Miltenyi). When fractionated and unfractionated MLNC were cultured with irradiated silicone-containing peritoneal cells, only unfractionated MLNC (SI = 3.8) and CD4+ MLNC (SI = 9.4) incorporated ^{3}H-thymidine greater than background (Fig.1). Thus, only those populations containing CD4+ T cells proliferated in response to silicone-containing peritoneal cells. These results were confirmed by the demonstration that monoclonal antibodies against murine IL-2 and IL-4, but not NK1.1 when added at the beginning of culture inhibit the proliferation

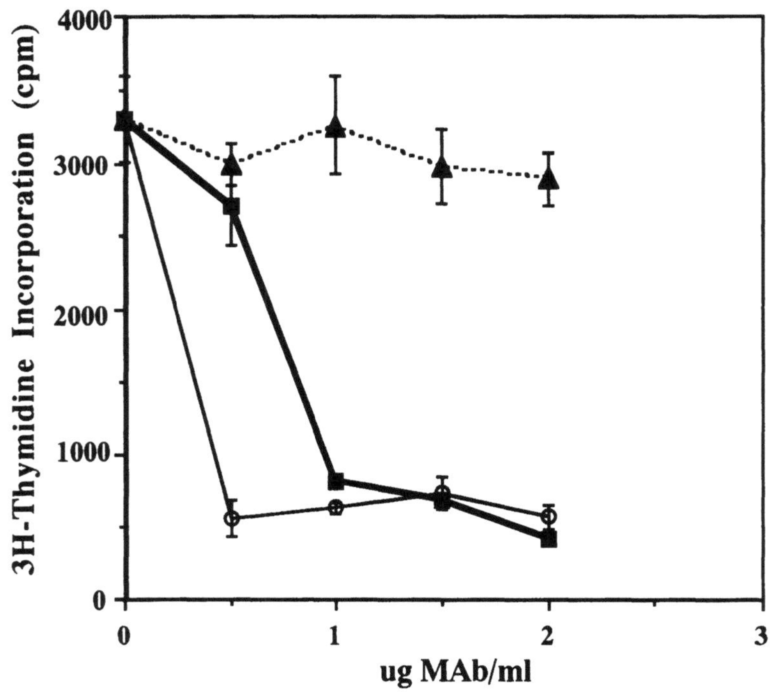

Figure 2. Monoclonal antibodies against IL-2 and IL-4 inhibit silicone gel-induced T cell proliferation in BALB/c mice. Mesenteric lymph nodes cells from silicone-injected female BALB/c mice were incubated with irradiated silicone-containing peritoneal cells and either rat anti-murine IL-2 (O) (Endogen, Cambridge, MA), rat anti-mouse IL-4 (■) (PharMingen) or rat anti-mouse NK1.1 (▲) (PharMingen). Incorporation of 3H-thymidine was determined 5 days later. Results listed are the average of two or more separate experiments ± 1 SEM.

of responding cells to silicone-laden peritoneal cells (Fig. 2). Interestingly, a less than two-fold enrichment of CD4+ cells (data not shown) resulted in lymphoproliferation greater than the degree of enrichment (Fig.1), suggesting the presence of a regulatory cell(s) in the CD4- fraction.

Silicone gel-induced T cell proliferation is dependent on the concentration of silicone-containing peritoneal cells *in vitro* and silicone gel *in vivo*. To a constant concentration ($4x10^5$ cells/well) of responding SpC, LNC and MLNC from silicone-injected BALB/c mice, increasing concentrations of silicone-gel containing peritoneal cells was added. As controls, increasing concentrations of peritoneal cells from HBSS-injected mice were cultured with the same responding cells. As depicted in Fig.3A, responding cells cultured with increasing concentrations of silicone-containing peritoneal cells showed a significant increase in proliferation at the maximum concentration of $1x10^5$ peritoneal cells/well. At this concentration, stimulation indexes for SpC, LNC and MLNC were 2.3, 3.9 and 4.7, respectively. In contrast, responding cell preparations cultured with peritoneal cells from HBSS-injected BALB/c mice did not proliferate significantly (SI = 0.67 - 1.33)(Fig 3A). These results suggest that in BALB/c mice, silicone gel-induced CD4+ proliferation is dependent upon the

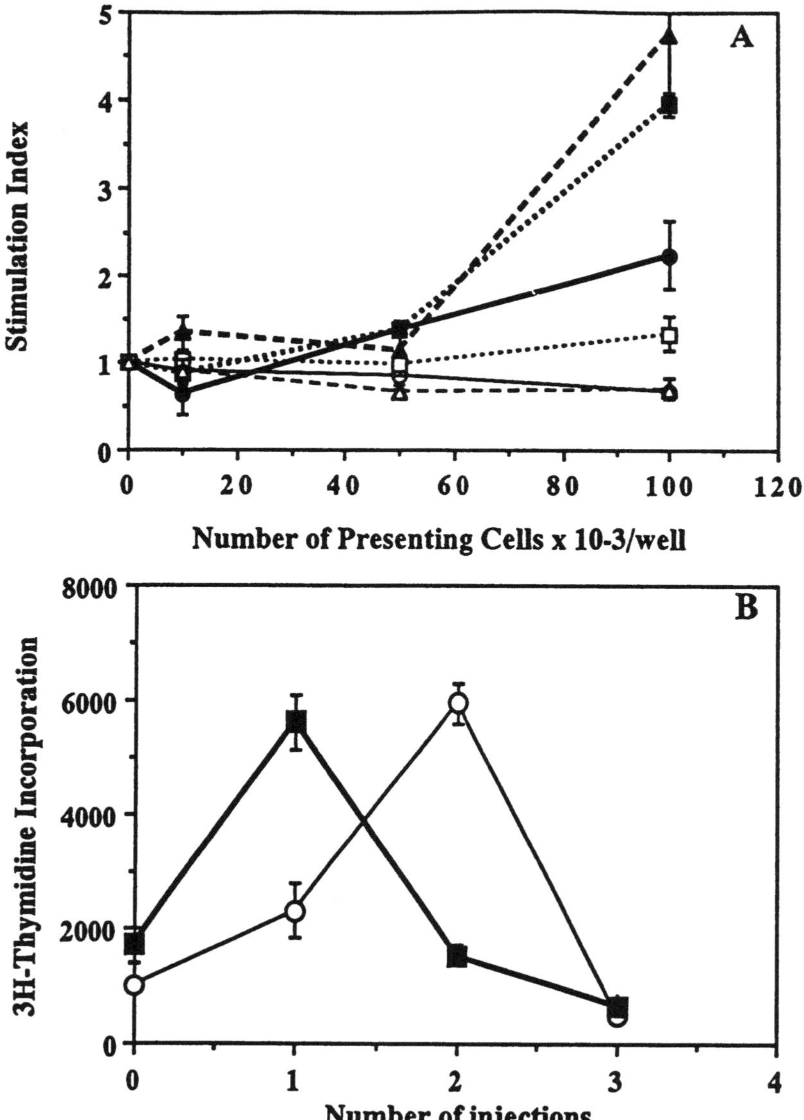

Figure 3. Silicone-induced CD4+ proliferation is dependent on the concentration of silicone gel *in vivo* and *in vitro*. Panel A: Female BALB/c mice were sc injected with 0.2ml silicone gel. SpC, LNC and MLNC were cultured with either $1x10^4$, $5x10^4$ and $1x10^5$ irradiated, silicone-containing peritoneal cells or similar concentrations of irradiated peritoneal cells from HBSS-injected mice. Proliferation was determined by the incorporation of 3H-thymidine and the calculation of the stimulation index (SI). SpC, MLNC and LNC cultured with silicone-containing peritoneal cells are represented as filled circles, squares and triangles, respectively. SpC, MLNC and LNC cultured with HBSS peritoneal cells are represented by open circles, squares and triangles, repectively. Panel B: Female BALB/c mice were given 1, 2 or 3 0.1ml sc injections of silicone gel abdominally. Ten days later, $4x10^5$ SpC (■) and MLNC (O)were cultured with $1x10^5$ irradiated silicone peritoneal cells and proliferation measured. Panel A and B show representative results from one of three separate experiments. All results are the mean of triplicate samples ± 1 SEM.

concentration of silicone-containing peritoneal cells. To determine whether the *in vitro* proliferative response was directly dependent on the concentration of silicone gel injected *in vivo*, female BALB/c mice were given 1 to 3 sc injections of 0.1ml of silicone gel. SpC and MLNC from these mice were co-cultured with silicone-containing peritoneal cells and the proliferative responses recorded in Fig.3B. SpC from mice given a single injection of silicone gel proliferated significantly above background. Additional injections of silicone appeared inhibitory. Similarly, the maximum silicone-induced proliferation in MLNC was observed in mice that had received 2 injections of silicone-gel, while 3 injections appeared inhibitory (Fig 3B). These results indicate that the *in vitro* T cell response to silicone gel is dependent on the concentration of silicone gel injected *in vivo* and that larger doses may inhibit the development of T cell responses in both spleen and mesenteric lymph nodes.

Silicone stimulates a proliferative response in BALB/c, (BALB/c x DBA/2N)F1 and C57BL/6 mice, but not in DBA/2N and BALB/cJax mice. Female BALB/c, DBA/2N, BALB/cJax, C57BL/6 and (BALB/cAnPt x DBA/2N)F1 (CDF1) mice (generously provided by Dr. Michael Potter, NCI, NIH) were injected sc with 0.2ml silicone gel. SpC, LNC and MLNC were collected from the female mice and used as responding cells. Male mice received either 0.2ml of silicone gel, 0.5ml pristane or 0.5ml HBSS ip. Peritoneal cells were collected from the male mice by peritoneal lavage and the cells irradiated as 'presenting cells.' After a 5 day co-culture of responding and presenting cells, proliferation was measured and the stimulation index calculated as previously described (Table I). As previously shown, responding cells from BALB/c mice cultured with silicone-laden peritoneal cells proliferate significantly (Fig.4). No proliferation was observed when responding cells were cultured with peritoneal cells from BALB/c mice injected with either pristane or HBSS (data not shown). Statistically significant proliferative responses were also observed in the spleens and lymph nodes of CDF1 mice and the spleens of C57BL/6 mice. Interestingly, neither DBA/2N nor BALB/cJax cells were stimulated by silicone-containing, syngeneic presenting cells (Fig.4). Indeed, the stimulation indexes actually seemed to be depressed in these mice. This was surprising since BALB/c, DBA/2N and BALB/cJax all have the same MHC (H-2^d) haplotype, and if silicone gel is being processed and presented in association with MHC, then MHC haplotype and expression could significantly affect the ability of each strain to respond (16). However, since BALB/c CD4+ cells proliferate when cultured with silicone-containing peritoneal cells and DBA/2N and BALB/cJax do not, one must conclude that MHC does not play a role in determining silicone responsiveness in these mice. Moreover, in those strains that did proliferate, i.e., BALB/c, CDF1 and C57BL/6 mice, responses varied between strain and lymphoid tissue (Fig.4), suggesting the possibility of different mechanisms of activation. These results, then, demonstrate that silicone-induced T cell proliferation is genetically determined, but do not indicate what or how many genes may be involved.

Diet and environment can modulate silicone-induced T cell proliferation. While performing these studies, it quickly became apparent that both environment and diet could have major effects on the extent of lymphoproliferation generated by the injection of silicone gel. BALB/c mice maintained in a nonbarrier, conventional colony were the mice used for all of the studies reported above. These conventional (CON) BALB/c mice are kept in open-air cages, have circulating antibody titers to common murine viruses and normal microbial colonization of the gastrointestinal tract (17). Specific pathogen-free

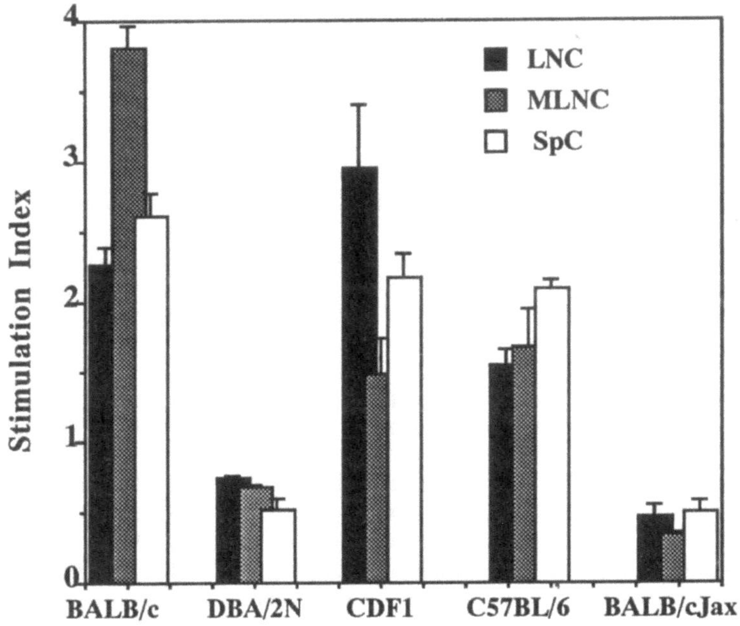

Figure 4. Silicone stimulates a proliferative response in BALB/c, (BALB/c x DBA/2N)F1 and C57BL/6 mice, but not in DBA/2N and BALB/cJax mice. Co-cultures of silicone responding and silicone presenting cells were established and incubated as described in Table 1. Proliferation was determined by the incorporation of 3H-thymidine (cpm) and the calculation of the stimulation index (Table I). Results are the mean of triplicate samples ± 1 SEM. Only those responses with a stimulation index (SI) > 2.0 with a $p < .05$ (student t test) were considered statistically significant.

(SPF) BALB/c mice (generously provided by Dr. Sandra J. Smith-Gill, NCI, NIH) are maintained in a barrier facility where all food, water and caging materials are autoclaved. Personnel are required to wear gowns, gloves, masks, shoe covers and bonnets before entering the facility. SPF mice do not have circulating antibody titers to murine viruses, but do have normal microbial colonization of the gastrointestinal tract (17). SPF- and CON-BALB/c mice maintained on a standard, low fat, autoclavable rodent chow (rodent laboratory chow 5010, Purina Mills, Inc, Richmond, IN) were sc injected with silicone gel and the SpC and MLNC checked for lymphoproliferation against silicone-containing peritoneal cells. As seen in Fig.5, SPF SpC and MLNC did not proliferate significantly above background (SI < 2.0), while CON SpC and MLNC did (SI = 2.0 and 2.8, respectively), although, the responses for CON mice were relatively weak. However, if at the time of silicone injection, the diet was changed to a high fat, high energy diet (rodent chow 5015, Purina Mills), lymphoproliferation was increased in both SPF and CON mice (Fig.5). For example, proliferation in SPF SpC and MLNC (SI = 2.3 and 2.2, respectively) was small but statistically greater than the responses observed in SPF mice fed a low fat diet. Diet had no significant effect on SPF responses

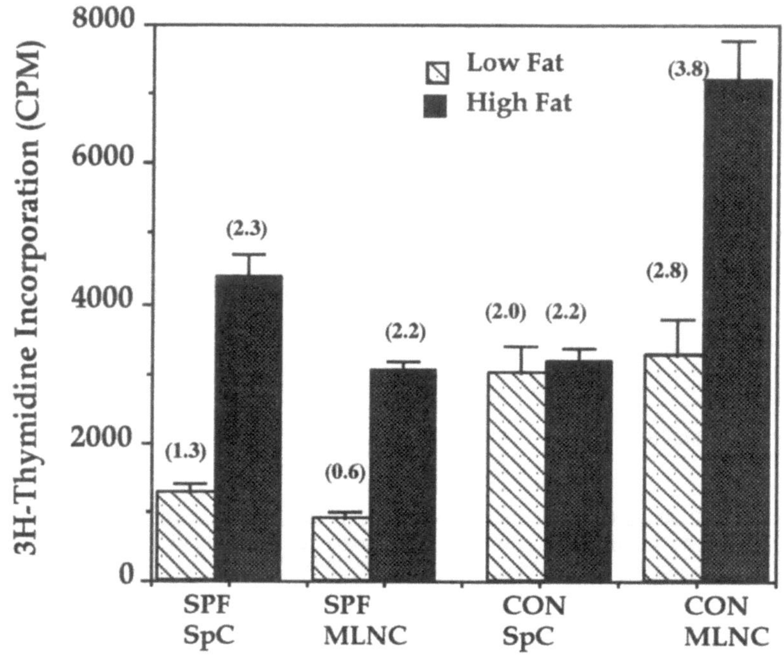

Figure 5. In BALB/c mice, diet and environment can effect the proliferative response to silicone gel. Conventionally-housed (CON) and specific pathogen-free (SPF) BALB/c mice were injected sc or ip with silicone gel and co-cultures of responding cells and silicone-containing peritoneal cells established as previously described in Table 1. The results represent the mean cpm ± 1 SEM. The stimulation index is in parentheses. These results are representative of more than three separate experiments.

in CON mice, but enhanced the response of MLNC to levels greater than that of SPF mice. Therefore, diet alone cannot totally restore the SPF silicone response to that of CON mice, but it can enhance the silicone response in both groups. These results suggest that dietary and environmental exposure to antigens can influence the extent of silicone-induced lymphoproliferation. Moreover, these environmental effects may account for the lack of reports documenting lymphoproliferation to silicone gel in other experimental animal models.This study demonstrates that in certain inbred strains of mice, i.e., BALB/c, CDF1 and C57BL/6, the subcutaneous injection of silicone gel *in vivo* can produce a statistically significant CD4+ lymphoproliferative response *in vitro*. Although this response is small compared to secondary proliferative responses to protein antigens like hen egg lysozyme (16), it is dose dependent and greatly enhanced by enrichment of CD4+ cells. Moreover, proliferation was inhibited by the addition of neutralizing antibodies against IL-2 and IL-4, confirming the role of CD4+ T cells in silicone-induced lymphoproliferation. However, it seems unlikely that this response is antigen-specific, since silicone-containing peritoneal cells stimulated lymphocytes from silicone, pristane and thioglycollate-injected mice. Silicone-containing peritoneal cells, therefore, may stimulate pre-activated and/or memory cells, regardless of the initial stimulus. A change of diet or a conventional housing environment may simply provide an increase in antigenic exposure leading to an increase in pre-activated/memory cells and an increased response to silicone. The small lymphoproliferative response may reflect the low numbers of T cells initially activated by the compounds injected in this study or a limited subset of CD4+ cells that can actually be activated by silicone. Regardless of the precise mechanism of lymphocyte activation, these studies demonstrate that silicone gel can stimulate T cells in genetically-susceptible strains of mice and that this stimulation is unique to silicone when compared to pristane, HBSS and thioglycollate. Studies investigating the effect of longterm stimulation by silicone gel in BALB/c mice may provide valuable information concerning a possible role for silicone in the induction of autoimmune disease.

References

1. Myoshi K, Miyoaka T, Kobayoshi U, Itakura T, Nishijo K, Higashibara M, Shiragami H and Ohno F (1964) Hypergammaglobulinemia by prolonged adjuvanticity in man: disorders developed after augmentation mammoplasty. Ijishimpo 2122:9.
2. Kumagai Y, Shiokawa Y, Medsger TA and Rednan GP. (1984) Clinical spectrum of connective tissue disease after cosmetic surgery. Observations on eighteen patients and a review of the Japanese Literature. Arth and Rheum 27:1.
3. Travis WD, Balegh K and Abraham JL (1985) Silicone granulomas: Report of three cases and review of the literature. Human Path 16:19.
4. Weisman, MH, Vecchione TR, Albert D, Moore, LT and Mueller, MR. (1988) Connective tissue disease following breast augmentation: A preliminary test of the human adjuvant disease hypothesis. Plast and Reconst Surg 82:626.
5. Varga J, Schumacher R and Jimenez SA (1989) Systemic sclerosis after augmentation mammoplasty with silicone implants. Annal Int Med 111:377.
6. Endo LP, Edwards L, Longley S, Corman LC and Panush RS (1987) Silicone and rheumatic diseases. Sem Arth Rheum 17:112.
7. Lin, RP, DiLeonardo M and Jacoby RA (1993) Silicone lymphadenopathy: A case report and review of the literature. Am J Dermatopath 15:1.
8. Gabriel SE, O'Fallon WM, Kurland LT, Beard CM, Woods JE, and Melton LF (1994) Risk of connective tissue diseases and other disorders after breast implantation. New Engl J Med 330:1697.
9. Duffy, MJ and Woods JE (1994) Health risks of failed silicone breast implants: A 30year clinical experience. Plast and Reconstr Surg 94:295.
10. Pidutti, R and Morales A (1993) Silicone gel filled testicular prosthesis and systemic disease. Urology 42:155.
11. Naim JO and Lanzafame RJ (1993) The adjuvant effect of silicone gel on antibody formation in rats. Immunol Invest 22:151.
12. McDonald AH and DeGrassi A (1993) Pristane induces an indomethacin inhibitable inflammatory influx of CD4+ T cells and IFN-γ production in plasmacytoma-suseptible BALB/cAnPt mice. Cell Immunol 146:157.
13. Picha GJ and Goldstein JA (1991) Analysis of the soft-tissue response to components used in the manufacture of breast implants: Rat animal model. Plast and Reconst Surg 87:490.
14. Wolos JA and Smith JB (1982) Helper cells in the autologous mixed lymphocyte reaction III. Production of helper factors(s) distinct from interleukin-2. J Exp Med 156:1807.
15. Miltenyi S, Mueller W, Werchel W and Radbruch A (1990) High gradient magnetic cell separation with MACS. Cytometry 11:231.
16. Hill SW and Sercarz EE (1975) Fine specificity of the H-2 linked immune response gene for the gallinaceous lysozymes. Eur J Immunol 5:317.
17. Byrd LG, McDonald AH, Gold LG and Potter M (1991) Specific pathogen-free BALB/cAn mice are refractory to plasmacytoma production by pristane. J Immunol 147:3632.

Silicone-induced Modulation of Natural Killer Cell Activity

S.D. Wilson and A.E. Munson

Department of Pharmacology/Toxicology, Medical College of Virginia/Virginia Commonwealth University, Richmond, VA

Abstract

Current controversy regarding the effects of silicone gel mammary implants on the immune system has led to increased focus on the potential biological activity of silicone materials. Studies were undertaken in the B6C3F1 mouse to evaluate the immunotoxicological effects of the following components of a mammary gel prosthesis: polydimethylsiloxane fluid, silicone gel, elastomer shell and a polyurethane implant cover. Material was implanted subcutaneously (s.c.) for either 10 or 180 days. The only toxicological or immunological parameter which differed from control values was the natural killer (NK) cell activity in gel implanted mice. In these animals, basal NK activity was decreased. NK activity was comparably inhibited in female Fischer 344 rats implanted with silicone gel following short term (14 or 30 days) as well as chronic (1 year) exposure. The response was variable in both the rat and mouse. Host resistance to B16F10 melanoma in the mouse is known to be related to NK activity. Despite suppression of NK activity following gel implantation, host resistance was unaltered. Inhibition of NK activity by the administration of anti-asialo GM1 indicated that resistance was not adversely affected until NK activity was decreased by 40 to 50%. As with basal NK activity, augmented NK activity was inhibited in gel implanted rats when compared to controls. Administration of polyinosinic:polycytidylic acid to gel implanted rats resulted in an increase of approximately 65% in NK activity compared to gel implanted controls. This level of augmented NK activity was significantly less than the level of augmented NK activity in vehicle implanted animals where 100% enhancement in NK activity was noted. The results of these studies indicate that (1) NK cytolytic activity is altered in two animal models, the mouse and rat, although the results were variable, that (2) the level of suppression noted in the mouse is ineffective when compared to the level of suppression required to alter host resistance to B16F10 melanoma and that (3) the gel implanted animals exhibit a suppressed response to NK augmentation.

Introduction

For a number of years, the use of silicone materials has been widespread in both consumer products and medical devices. Medical uses include non-implantable applications in tubing, catheters, dialysis pump inserts and lubricants in syringes. Implantable uses include drug release capsules, hydrocephalus shunts as well as prosthetic devices for the breast, chin, ear, testicle and joint. Until recently, the general consensus regarding silicone materials has been that not only are they chemically stable but they are biologically compatible as well. Now, however, there is considerable controversy regarding the biocompatibility of these compounds with most of the recent interest focusing on silicone gel mammary implants.

Estimates of the number of women who have received breast implants in the United States is variable but range from a low of 300,000 [1] up to two million [2,3]. Beginning in the early 1980's, increasing numbers of case reports and case studies began to appear in the literature purporting a causal relationship between silicone gel mammary augmentation and autoimmune, immune mediated and connective tissue disease [for review see 1,4]. However, there are also a number of studies suggesting that there is no link [1,5,6]. This inconsistency is also apparent in the experimental data evaluating the effects of silicone gel on various components of the immune system [7-9]. Epidemiological studies have indicated that there does not appear to be a correlation between breast augmentation and the development of connective tissue disease [10,11]. Therefore, an unambiguous correlation between silicone implantation and disease conditions in humans has not been established.

The data delineating the immunotoxic effects of silicone materials is minimal. Therefore, studies were undertaken to ascertain the potential immunotoxic effects of silicone implants using the B6C3F1 mouse as the animal model. The principle components of a breast implant were evaluated. It should be noted that the studies were designed to evaluate immunotoxicity not immunogenicity. The caveat remains that if the silicone implant materials are capable of eliciting chronic antigenic stimulation, the results of the assays may be altered. Evaluation of toxicological and immunological parameters indicated that natural killer (NK) cell cytolytic activity was the only functional assay which was adversely affected (8,9).

Natural killer cells are large granular lymphocytes which exhibit a heterogeneity of function, phenotype and morphology. They exert pleiotropic effects within the immune system. They were first described based on their innate ability to lyse certain tumor cells and cells infected with intracellular pathogens without prior exposure. They have subsequently been found to play an equally important regulatory role. These functions include elaboration of cytokines (i.e. interferon γ and tumor necrosis factor α), regulation of antibody production and hematopoiesis as well as self regulation [12-14]. It has also been suggested that they may play a role in the expression of various autoimmune syndromes [15,16].

The potential consequences of perturbations of NK activity are significant. Therefore, these studies were designed to further elucidate the alterations of NK activity following gel implantation.

Materials and Methods

Animals

Either female B6C3F1 mice or female Fischer 344 rats were used.

Test Materials

The silicone test materials were provided by Dow Corning Corporation, Midland, MI. The gel and elastomer were obtained from Silastic II mammary implants. The polydimethylsiloxane (PDMS) fluid used in these studies was 1000 cs medical grade fluid. The polyurethane implant material, which is an alternative implant cover, was purchased from Natural Surgical Specialties Incorporated, Paso Robies, CA. As a comparative control in one study, altered high molecular weight polyethylene 2 cm spheres (Crown Plastic Company, Harrison, OH) were obtained courtesy of Dow Corning. Anti-asialo GM1 (AAGM1) was obtained from WAKO BioProducts, Richmond, VA. Polyinosinic-polycytidylic acid (poly I:C) was obtained from Sigma Chemical Co., St. Louis, MO.

Administration and implantation

The two matrices below delineate the test materials and the volumes utilized in the studies for mice (Table 1) and rats (Table 2).

Table 1: Materials implanted into mice

Material	Implant Volume
Phosphate Buffered Saline	1 cc
Dow Corning PDMS fluid, 1000 cs	1 cc
Dow Corning Gel	0.5 to 3 cc
Dow Corning Elastomer Shell	0.6 cm diameter
Polyurethane prosthesis cover	0.6 cm diameter
Positive control	Assay dependent

Table 2: Materials implanted into rats

Material	Implant Volume and Duration of Implantation		
	14 Days	30 Days	1 Year
Phosphate Buffered Saline	20 cc	15 cc	15 cc
Dow Corning Gel	1, 2.5, 5, 7.5,10, 12.5, 15 or 20 cc	5, 10 or 15 cc	5, 10, or 15 cc
Comparative control - polystyrene implants	None	3 implants each - 2 cm in diameter	None

Materials in both the mouse and rat were implanted with the animal anesthetized using pentobarbital (55 mg/kg intravenously [i.v.]) for the mouse and 40 mg/kg i.v. for the rat). Material was implanted s.c. on the ventral surface of the animal following surgical preparation of the skin. A maximum volume of 1 cc for the mouse and 5 cc for the rat was implanted per site. Incisions were closed with Flexible Collodion USP in the mouse and with surgical staples in the rat.

Toxicological, Immunological and Host Resistance Studies

Choice of studies conducted in mice was based on the National Toxicology Program Tier I and Tier II tests [17]. These tests are outlined in Table 3. Methods for each of these tests have been previously described by Bradley et. al. [8,9]. Time points for all studies were either 10 or 180 days of exposure unless otherwise indicated. No dose response study was performed in the first protocol. Each parameter that showed statistical significance at $p \leq 0.05$ was repeated as a dose response study.

Table 3: Parameters assessed in implanted mice

Toxicology	Immunology	Host Resistance
Body weights	Spleen IgM and IgG response to sRBC	*Streptococcus pneumoniae*
Gross pathology	Mixed leukocyte response	*Listeria monocytogenes*
Hematology including RBC and WBC counts and differentials	Spleen cell proliferation (PHA, CON A, LPS and anti-Fab'2)	Metastatic pulmonary B16F10 melanoma
Selected serum chemistries including glucose, albumin, urea nitrogen, alanine aminotransferase	Macrophage studies including peritoneal exudate number and differential, gamma interferon activation, phagocytic activity (sRBC, covaspheres), function reticuloendothelial system function	
	Cytotoxic T lymphocyte response	
	Serum complement	
	Spleen cell phenotyping (B cells and T cells and subsets)	
	Natural killer cell response	
	Bone marrow CFU-GM and CFU-M	

Studies Evaluating NK Activity vs B16F10 Melanoma Resistance

These studies were performed in nonimplanted female B6C3F1 mice. Mice were administered dilutions of AAGM1 i.v. ranging from 1:40 to 1:260 on day 1. AAGM1 is an antibody to the asialo GM1 surface marker found on NK cells. Administration of this antibody results in suppression of NK activity [13]. On day 2, the mice were challenged i.v. with 1.5, 2 or 3 X 10^5 B16F10 melanoma cells. After 10 to 14 days, mice were pulsed with radiolabeled iododeoxyuridine for 4 hours. Animals were sacrificed, the lungs excised and placed into Bouin's solution. Nodules per lung and cpm per lung were enumerated.

Augmentation Studies

Female Fischer 344 rats were implanted s.c. with either 10 ml of phosphate buffered saline (PBS) or 10 ml of silicone gel on day 1. On day 27, either PBS or poly I:C was administered i.v. at 2 mg/kg. On day 28, the rats were sacrificed and a standard 4-hour ^{51}Cr release assay was performed.

Statistical Analysis

Statistical analysis was performed as described by Bradley et. al. [8,9] and included a one-way analysis of variance for evaluation of homogeneous data analysis and the Dunnett's t Test to define experimental and control group differences. Non-homogenous data was examined using a non-parametric analysis of variance. For significant differences, experimental and control groups were compared by the Wilcoxon Rank Test. Trends towards dose dependency were determined by the Jonckheere's Test. Statistical significance for mortality data was determined using the Fisher's Exact Test.

Results

Toxicology

No effects were seen after ten days or six months of exposure to any of the test articles used. Data shown elsewhere [8,9].

Immune Assays

No alterations were observed in the functional studies in mice implanted for 10 days or 6 months except for the natural killer (NK) cell activity. Data shown elsewhere [8,9].

Host Resistance Studies

No effect on host resistance models was seen with any of the test materials. The following host resistance models were used in the mouse: *Listeria monocytogenes, Streptococcus pneumoniae* or B16F10 melanoma. Data not shown.

Natural Killer Cell Activity

A. Mice - A series of seven experiments assessing NK activity was performed. Data is expressed as percent of control cytotoxicity to normalize for the decrease in NK function associated with aging [9]. Table 4 outlines the NK activity in gel implanted mice. Values were obtained by averaging the percent decrease in NK activity from control for all three effector-to-target ratios (100:1, 50:1, 25:1). No inhibition was seen after a 10 day exposure period. A significant decrease in NK activity was observed in mice implanted with silicone gel in the initial 180 day study.

In the 180 day dose response study, the dose that had produced a significant effect in the first study did not produce a statistically significant suppression in the repeat study. NK activity, however, did decrease in a dose dependent fashion with significance at the highest dose level.

A time course utilizing 1, 2 and 3 ml of gel was performed. The decrease in NK activity was dose dependent at 30 and 90 days but not at 180 days. At 60 days there was essentially no change from the vehicle treated animals.

B. Rats - Additional studies were performed in a second animal model, female Fischer 344 rats. The results indicate that suppression of NK cell activity after exposure to silicone gel is not a species specific response. NK activity inhibition (38% to 61%) was observed as early as 14 days after implantation of silicone gel. The dose response at both the 14 and 30 day time points, as illustrated in Figure 1, was biphasic with the peak response between 10 to 15 ml of implanted material. This corresponds to a dose of 50 to 100 ml/kg of silicone gel. After exposure to 5, 10 or 15 ml of silicone gel for 30 days, there was a 57.8, 65.1 and 51.9% decrease in NK activity respectively. Animals implanted with the comparative control, polystyrene spheres, did not tolerate the implants well exhibiting wound dehiscence, seroma formation and pressure necrosis. Despite these problems, there was no significant change in their NK activity compared to control. Data not shown.

Table 4. Effect of silicone gel implantation on natural killer cell activity in B6C3F1 mice

Dose	PERCENT CHANGE						
	10 Days	180 Days	180 Days	30 Days	60 Days	90 Days	180 Days
0.5 ml	ND	ND	-2.5	ND	ND	ND	ND
1.0 ml	NE	-43	-9.5	-7.0	+9.2	-11.2	-23.9
2.0 ml	ND	ND	-57.9	-9.3	+19.8	-11.6	-11.9
3.0 ml	ND	ND	ND	-25.4	+10.7	-19.8	-23.4

ND = not determined, NE = no effect
(-) denotes suppression and (+) indicates enhancement

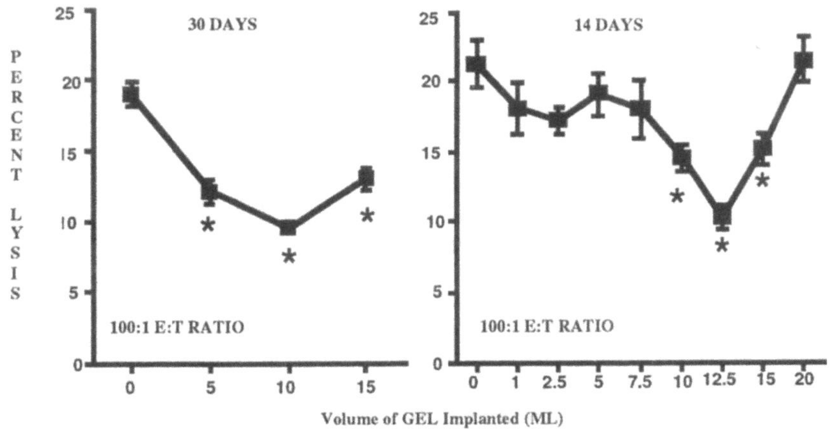

Fig. 1. Natural killer cell activity in female Fischer 344 rats implanted with gel. Rats were implanted with the volumes indicated for either 14 or 30 days. Following exposure, a standard 4-hr chromium release NK assay was performed. Spontaneous lysis was <10%. Effector to target ratios were 200:1, 100:1, 50:1, 25:1, 12.5:1 and 6.25:1. The 100:1 E:T ratio is representative of the results. For the 30 day study N = 8 for both vehicle and gel implanted rats. For the 14 day study N =8 for vehicles and N=4 for implanted animals. * $p < 0.05$.

After chronic exposure (one year) to silicone gel, a dose-dependent decrease in NK activity was observed (Fig 2). There was a significant decrease (51.8%) in NK cytolysis at the 15 ml dose level. Three animals developed solid state tumors and were eliminated from the study. Two of these animals, one implanted with 10 and one implanted with 15 ml of gel, had fibrosarcomas associated with the capsule surrounding the gel material. The fibrosarcoma in one rat implanted with 10 ml of

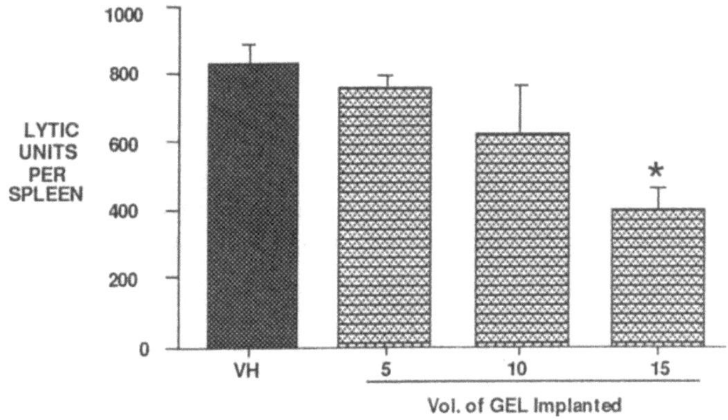

Fig. 2. Natural killer cell activity in Fischer 344 rats following chronic implantation of silicone gel. Rats were implanted with the volume of gel indicated above for 398 days. Following exposure an NK assay was performed. Spontaneous lysis was <10%. E:T ratios ranged from 200:1 to 6.25:1 Data is expressed in lytic units per spleen which is based on the number of cells required to lyse 10% of the target cells as well as the total lymphocyte count per spleen. N=5 for 5 ml, N=6 for 10 and 15 ml and N=7 for vehicle rats. *$p < 0.05$.

gel was associated with the uterine wall. However, a study by Klykken et. al. [18] indicated that silicone gel is subject to solid state tumorigenesis but has no potential chemical carcinogenicity. The capsule surrounding the gel material in the other rats was thin and transparent with minimal vascularization. There was no gross migration of the gel material evident at any time point. An additional five rats, one vehicle animal, three implanted with 5 ml and 1 implanted with 15 ml of gel, were eliminated from the study due complications secondary to blood collection under anesthesia.

As noted in the mouse model, there was also variability in the response in the rat model. No inhibition in NK activity was observed in 3 of 9 studies. Data not shown.

B16F10 Melanoma Studies

As mentioned earlier, NK activity correlates with resistance to the development of metastatic disease [13]. Although implanted mice exhibited decreased NK activity *in vitro*, there was no change in resistance to B16F10 melanoma. These studies were designed, therefore, to clarify the degree of NK inhibition that translates into altered host resistance in a tumor model, specifically B16F10 melanoma. NK activity in nonimplanted B6C3F1 mice was suppressed to various levels by the i.v. administration of AAGM1 on day 1. The dilutions used were based on preliminary studies. Data not shown. Dilutions ranged from 1:40 which resulted in >95% suppression to 1:260 which resulted in <15% suppression. The 1:120 dilution resulted in approximately a 50% suppression. Mice were challenged with B16F10 melanoma on day 2. These studies indicate that a 50 to 60% decrease in NK activity is required before changes in host resistance to B16F10 melanoma becomes apparent (Fig 3). Therefore, the level of suppression noted in the initial studies in mice is ineffective when compared to the level of suppression that is required to observably alter resistance in this model.

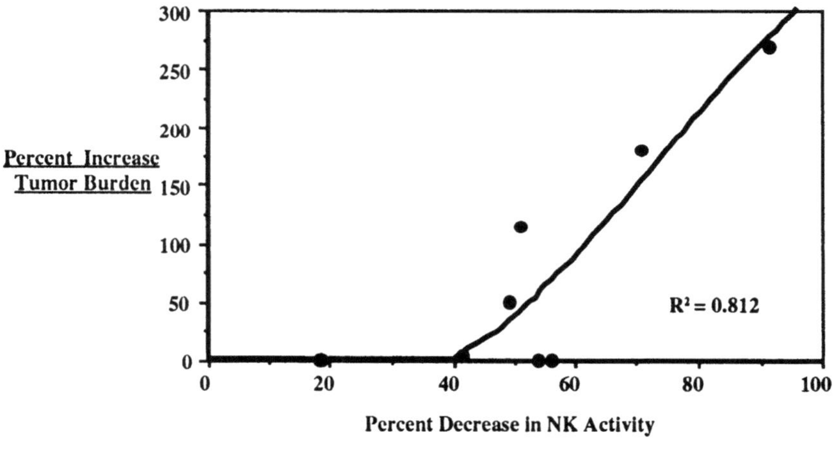

Fig. 3. Relationship between NK activity and B16F10 Tumor Burden. This is a composite graph representing the results from 3 studies. Mice were administered dilutions of AAGM-1 i.v. on day 1 to incrementally decrease NK activity. On day 2, they were challenged i.v. with B16F10 melanoma. The level of tumor burden was assessed between 10 to 14 days. The data is expressed as percent increase in tumor burden based on cpm per lung. N = 12

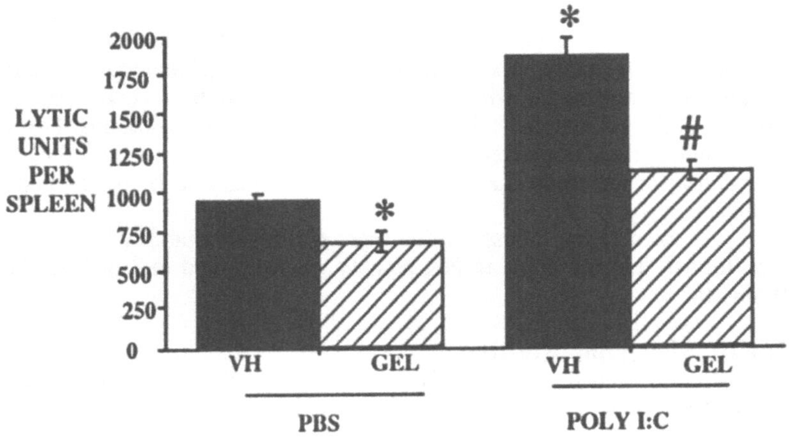

Fig. 4. Effects on augmented NK cell activity in rats implanted with silicone gel. On day 27 after rats were implanted with silicone gel (10 ml), either PBS or poly I:C was administered i.v. On day 28, an NK assay was performed. Spontaneous lysis was <10%. E:T ratios ranged from 200:1 to 6.25:1 Data is expressed in lytic units per spleen which is based on the number of cells required to lyse 10% of the target cells as well as the total lymphocyte count per spleen. N = 6. *$p < 0.05$ compared to VH:PBS animals. #$p < 0.05$ compared to VH:POLY I:C animals. This represents a single study.

Augmentation Studies

Results describing effects on augmented NK activity in rats implanted with silicone gel are shown in Fig. 4. NK activity was suppressed by approximately 28% in rats implanted with 10 ml of silicone gel for 28 days compared to control animals. In PBS implanted rats administered poly I:C, NK activity was enhanced approximately 100%. Gel implanted rats partially responded to the poly I:C with a 65% increase in NK activity. This level of activity was comparable to control animals but was significantly less than that in the augmented PBS implanted mice.

Discussion

Assuming a specific density of 1 gm/ml for the gel, a dose of 1 to 3 ml of gel in the mouse constitutes approximately 5 to 15% of the body weight. In the rat, the volume of gel implanted ranging from 1 to 20 ml represents approximately 0.6 to 13% of the body weight. In women, implantation of two 300 ml mammary implants is not unusual. In a 50 kg woman, this volume of implanted material would correspond to 1.2% of her body weight. Compared to a 1 ml implant in the mouse or a 5 ml implant in the rat, this would be approximately a 4 or 3 fold factor difference respectively

The suppression in the level of NK activity in both the rat and mouse was repeatable although there was variability in the response. For example, following gel implantation in the mouse at 180 days, the decrease in NK activity from controls ranged from 9.5% to 43%. The source of the variability was not determined. However, Potter et. al. [19] observed a 50% difference in the ability of one lot of the gel material versus another to induce plasmacytomas when injected intraperitoneally.

The natural killer cell has been shown to play a critical role in the control of metastasis of many tumor cells [13, 20, 21] . This role was further supported by these studies. As indicated earlier, no perturbation in host resistance in the B16F10 metastatic melanoma was observed in mice implanted with gel for 180 days. This can be explained by the fact that in this system a 40 to 50% decrease in NK activity is required before changes would be seen. The level of inhibition in the implanted mice was less than 50% in the majority of the studies.

Augmentation of NK activity by poly I:C was impaired in the rats implanted with gel. Poly I:C is a synthetic double stranded RNA. The body responds to administration of this compound in much the same manner as it would a viral infection. There is a rapid increase in the serum level of interferons and a subsequent increase in NK activity [22-24]. The decrease in the response observed in the above studies raises the question of the ability of these animals to adequately respond to a pathogenic challenge. Furthermore, a study by Levy et al [25] concluded that individuals exhibiting a persistently low level of spontaneous NK activity are at greater risk of developing infectious problems.

Vodjani, Campbell and Brautbar [26] suggested that there is a correlation between silicone gel mammary augmentation in women and low NK activity. The NK activity in symptomatic implanted women when compared to healthy age matched women was significantly lower. Proper internal controls, however, were lacking in this study so that two questions remain. First, what is the NK activity in healthy implanted vs healthy nonimplanted women. Second, what is the NK activity in nonimplanted women exhibiting the same symptomatology as the unhealthy implanted women. It is of interest that many autoimmune diseases and most rheumatic diseases are associated with a decreased NK function. In several of these disorders, i.e. Systemic Lupus Erythematosus and Rheumatoid Arthritis, the level of NK activity is inversely proportional to the severity of signs [15]. In addition, NK lytic dysfunction may indicate alterations in the immunoregulatory role of these cells. Inhibition of the regulation of antibody production and polyclonal B cell proliferation by the NK cell could potentially result in hypergammaglobulinemia [15,16]. This could contribute to the development of autoimmune or immune mediated disorders. However, at this time it is unclear whether this alteration in NK activity as it relates to autoimmunity is cause or effect.

Acknowledgments

This manuscript is supported in part by grants from the National Institute of Environmental Health Sciences Contract ES 0522, Immunotoxicology Training Grant ES 07087, and Dow Corning.

References

1. Gott, DM, Tinkler, JJB (1994) Silicone implants and connective tissue disease: Evaluation of evidence for an association between the implantation of silicones and connective tissue disease. Medical Devices Agency. London.
2. Department of Health and Human Services (1991) Background information on the possible risks of silicone breast implants. Rockville, MD.
3. Shons, AR, Schubert, W (1992) Silicone breast implants and immune disease. Ann Plast Surg 28:491-501
4. Sergent, JS, Fuchs, H. Johnson, JS (1993) Silicone implants and rheumatic diseases. In: Kelley, Harris, Ruddy, Sledge (ed) Textbook of rheumatology update series. WB Saunders Co. Philadelphia, pp 1-79.

5. Schusterman, MA, et al (1993) Incidence of autoimmune disease in patients after breast reconstruction with silicone gel implants versus autogenous tissue: A preliminary report. Ann Plast Surg 31(1):1-6.
6. Peters, W, Keystone, E, Snow, K, Rubin, L, Smith, D (1994) Is there a relationship between autoantibodies and silicone-gel implants? Ann Plast Surg 32(1):1-7.
7. Brantley, SK (1990) Assessment of the lymphocyte response to silicone. Plast Recon Surg 86(6):1131-1137.
8. Bradley, SG et al (1994) Subchronic 10 day immunotoxicity of polydimethylsiloxane (silicone) fluid, gel and elastomer and polyurethane disks in female B6C3F1 mice Drug Chem Tox 17(3):175-220.
9. Bradley, SG et al (1994) Immunotoxicity of 180 day exposure to polydimethylsiloxane (silicone) fluid, gel and elastomer and polyurethane disks in female B6C3F1 mice. Drug Chem Tox 17(3):221-269.
10. Gabriel, SE, O'Fallon, WM, Kurland, LT, Beard, CM Woods, JE and Melton, LJ (1994) Risk of connective tissue diseases and other disorders after breast augmentation. N Engl J Med 330:1697.
11. Engler, HJ and Brooks, P (1994) Scleroderma and augmentation mammoplasty - A causal relationship? Aust NZ J Med 24:74.
12. Whiteside, TL and Herberman, RB (1990) The biology of human natural killer cells. Ann. 1st Super. Sanita. 26(3-4):335-348.
13. Trinchieri, G. (1989) Biology of natural killer cells. Adv Immun 47:187-376.
14. Abruzzo, LV, Mullen, CA, Rowley, DA (1986) Immunoregulation by natural killer cells. Cell Immun 98:226-278.
15. Grunenbaum, E, Maltzky-Goshen, E and Schoenfeld, Y (1989) Natural killer cells and autoimmunity. Immunol Res 8:292-304.
16. Bassan, R, et al (1989) Autoimmunity and B-cell dysfunction in chronic proliferative disorders of large granular lymphocyte/natural killer cells. Cancer 63:90-95.
17. Luster, MI et al (1992) Risk Assessment in Immunotoxicity: I. Sensitivity and predictability of immune tests. Fundam Appl Toxicol 18:200-210.
18. Klykken, PA, Woolhiser, MR, Nelson, SA, Goodman, DG, Mast, RW (1995) A life-time implant study of silicone mammary gel in female Sprague Dawley rats. Abstract. Fund and Appl Toxicol 15(1):199.
19. Potter, M, Morrison, S, Wiemer, F, Zhang XK, Miller, FW (1994) Induction of plasmacytomas with silicone gel in genetically susceptible strains of mice. JNCI 86(14):1058-1065.
20. Gorelik,C et al (1982) Role of NK cells in the control of metastatic spread and growth of tumor cells in mice. Int J Cancer 30:107-112.
21. Wiltrout, RH et al (1985) Role of organ-associated NK cells in decreased formation of experimental metastases in lung and liver. J Immunol. 134(6):4267-75.
22. Wiltrout, RH, Salub, RR, Twilley, TA and Talmadge, JE (1985) Immunomodulation of natural killer activity by polyribonucleotides. J Bio Response Mod 4:512-517.
23. Vaage. KT, Reynolds, CW, Reynolds, D, Fossum, S. and Rolstad, B (1989) The proliferation and life-span of rat large granular lymphocytes: Effects of cytokines. Eur J Immunol 19:1895-1902.
24. Ishikawa, R, Biron, CA (1993) IFN induction and associated changes in splenic leukocyte distribution. J Immunol 150(9):3713-3727.
25. Levy, SM et al (1991) Persistently low natural killer cell activity, age, and environmental stress as predictors of infectious morbidity. Nat Immun Cell Growth Regul. 10:289-307.
26. Vojdani, A, Campbell,A and Brautbar, N (1992) Immune functional impairment in patients with clinical abnormalities and silicone breast implants. Tox and Ind Health 8(6):415-429.

HLA Typing in Women With and Without Silicone Gel-filled Breast Implants

V.L. Young, MD,[1] J.R. Nemecek, MD,[2] B.D. Schwartz, MD, PhD,[3] D.L. Phelan, MT (HEW), CHS (ABHI),[4] and M.W. Schorr, MA[1]

[1] Division of Plastic and Reconstructive Surgery, Washington University School of Medicine, St. Louis, Missouri; [2] Park Nicollet Medical Center, Minneapolis Minnesota; [3] Division of Rheumatology, Dept. of Medicine, Washington University School of Medicine; and [4] HLA Laboratory, Barnes Hospital, St. Louis, Missouri

During the past 10 years or so, numerous anecdotal reports have appeared in the literature describing a small percentage of women who underwent breast augmentation or reconstruction with silicone gel-filled implants and later developed unexplained symptoms of weakness, chronic fatigue, myalgias/arthralgias, fever of unknown origin, burning breast pain and, in some instances, recognized rheumatologic disease. Many good investigations have been conducted recently to look for an explanation of what is happening with implant patients who seem to have symptoms suggestive of a connective tissue disease. Unfortunately, central questions remain unanswered. We do not know whether silicone gel-filled implants are causally related to the symptoms some patients are experiencing. To date, research has not shown that breast implants can cause disease, but if they do, we need to determine whether it is an already-defined disease or a new one. Alternatively, implants could be causing some women to experience a delayed hypersensitivity reaction that may or may not have an immune-mediated basis. If they are, we don't know whether patients are responding to silicone gel, elastomer, or some component used in or resulting from the implant manufacturing process.

After being convinced that a small percentage of our patients with silicone breast implants suffer from real physical complaints, we undertook a collaborative study involving the Divisions of Plastic Surgery and Rheumatology at Washington University School of Medicine and the HLA Laboratory at Barnes Hospital in St. Louis. If an immune-mediated process were responsible for causing some women with breast implants to develop the complaints reported by symptomatic patients, we wondered whether an association with certain HLA antigens might be involved. This study was designed to conduct human leukocyte antigen (HLA) typing on different groups of subjects in an effort to determine whether symptomatic patients with silicone gel-filled implants have a specific HLA antigen which differentiates them from asymptomatic women with implants, healthy controls, and symptomatic patients without breast implants.

This research project received no funding from any company or organization. Dr. Young is a co-inventor of the Trilucent™ triglyceride-filled breast implant manufactured by LipoMatrix, and he serves as a medical and research consultant for that company. He has also received implant research funding from McGhan Medical Corp., LipoMatrix, and the Plastic Surgery Research Fund for studies unrelated to silicone gel-filled implants.

This prospective study began with the hypothesis that no correlation would be found between specific HLA molecules and the presence of symptoms in implant patients. This null hypothesis was proven false as increased frequencies of HLA antigens (most importantly DR53 and DQ2) were found in symptomatic women with implants. The study additionally determined that asymptomatic women with implants had a significantly increased frequency of a different antigen (DR1).

Study Subjects and Methods

In this study, 199 women were divided into four groups based on the presence of symptoms and breast implants. We observed that the majority of our implant patients presenting with musculoskeletal complaints had symptoms which are more vague than those seen with well-defined rheumatologic diseases. We therefore decided to study a group of patients with ill-defined, connective tissue disease-like problems. Strict criteria were defined to discriminate between symptomatic and asymptomatic implant patients. To be considered symptomatic, a woman had to experience one or more of the following symptoms: burning breast pain, chronic fatigue, vague generalized upper torso pain, or myalgias and/or arthralgias. In an attempt to separate chronic problems from general complaints everyone occasionally suffers, women in the symptomatic implant group had to experience persistent symptoms for at least four months that were debilitating in nature and interfered with activities of daily living.

Seventy-seven women with silicone gel-filled breast implants were judged to be symptomatic by these criteria and were categorized into Group I. For Group II, 37 women who closely approximated Group I members in terms of age and duration of implantation but did not meet the symptomatic criteria were recruited from patients reporting for routine appointments. A healthy control group (Group III) of 54 asymptomatic women without implants and no history of autoimmune diseases was made up of office or hospital staff plus all healthy Caucasian women whose HLA typing records were part of the internal controls used by the HLA Laboratory at Barnes Hospital. Group IV consisted of 31 women without breast implants who have received a diagnosis of primary fibromyalgia; their symptoms have several similarities with Group I subjects, but fibromyalgia is not known to have an immune-mediated basis. The age- and race-matched fibromyalgia patients were recruited from nearby rheumatology practices for HLA typing.

All implant patients and approximately three-quarters of the healthy controls were interviewed for demographic data and a general medical history by a surgeon from the Division of Plastic and Reconstructive Surgery at Washington University School of Medicine. For the majority of fibromyalgia patients, we reviewed patient histories from their rheumatologists' records. Data regarding personal and family history of rheumatologic or connective tissue disorders were recorded. Subjects were then asked an open-ended question pertaining to chronic fatigue, fevers, and generalized aches and pains. They were also questioned about keratoconjunctivitis sicca, dry mouth, and dermatitis. Women considered symptomatic were asked in more detail about their medical history and given a musculoskeletal examination that included inspection for swelling, erythema, tenderness, and range of motion.

When appropriate, patients were referred for consultation with an ophthalmologist, rheumatologist, or dermatologist.

All women with breast implants were asked about the date and reason for the initial implantation surgery and any subsequent breast surgery, postoperative complications, or history of closed capsulotomy. All women with implants underwent a physical examination of the breasts while in sitting and supine positions. Data regarding masses, axillary or supraclavicular lymphadenopathy, and capsular contracture were recorded, and patients were examined for possible implant rupture and questioned about ruptures in the past. In addition, all Group I members had diagnostic mammography regardless of age; those with a possible ruptured implant received further studies with ultrasound, CT, or magnetic resonance imaging. Asymptomatic women with breast implants (Group II) who were 35 years or older underwent diagnostic mammography.

Despite our care in assigning patients to the symptomatic and asymptomatic implant groups, this study design has several sources of possible bias that could not be avoided. Because patients assigned to Groups I or II referred themselves for consultation, our study subjects should not be considered a community sample. In addition, HLA typing began in March of 1992, after media reports questioning the safety of implants had begun appearing. Group II asymptomatic implant patients were easy to identify; they came to the office to ask if they should be concerned about silicone, but they did not report any symptoms. Identifying Group I members was more challenging. Even though the symptoms used to categorize the groups are largely subjective, we had no doubt about the symptomatic status of subjects selected for Group I. We excluded a few women because they had sustained an injury that might account for their symptoms. Some potential subjects were also rejected because of doubts about their symptomatic status: either their reports of symptoms were inconsistent, or we had concerns about their emotional stability. In addition, anyone who seemed more interested in possible litigation than in the symptoms they reported was excluded from the study.

Serological Testing

This project received no outside funding, and patients were not asked to pay for HLA typing or T and B cell auto crossmatch tests, which would have cost nearly $1,300 per study subject. Since the costs of this testing were absorbed by the HLA Laboratory, we asked patients (or their insurance carriers) to pay for the more routine serological studies, which included a CBC, SMA-6, SMA-12, rheumatoid factor (RF), antinuclear antibody (ANA), and erythrocyte sedimentation rate (ESR). These tests were therefore made voluntary. Not surprisingly, all subjects did not volunteer, though cooperation was greater among women with symptoms.

For all 199 study participants, the HLA Laboratory at Barnes Hospital in St. Louis used complement-dependent microlymphocytotoxicity (CDC) assays to test peripheral blood and determine the antigens carried by class I HLA molecules (A, B, and C) and class II HLA molecules (DR$\alpha\beta$1, DR$\alpha\beta$3, DR$\alpha\beta$4, and DQ).

Serum from all 199 subjects was also tested for the presence of autoantibodies to B cells and T cells by lymphocytotoxicity crossmatch assays, which were done at the same time and in the same lab as the HLA typing. As is standard testing protocol, two lymphocytotoxicity crossmatch assays were used: Three Wash Amos and Antiglobulin-augmented, the latter of which is considered more sensitive and accurate for assessing the complete specificity of antibodies in sera (particularly antibodies against cross-reactive, public epitopes). The Antiglobulin-augmented lymphocytotoxicity assay is a complement-dependent assay that detects both non-complement fixing antibodies as well as serum antibody to cell surface antigens. Both tests are performed similarly. After the B and T cells are harvested from the blood, the B cells are labeled (dyed) with fluorescein conjugated antibody so they can be differentiated from T cells. The lymphocytes are co-incubated with serum for a period of time, after which a pre-titered antiglobulin reagent is added, followed by the addition of complement and a second incubation. Any antibody in the sera that is reactive to T or B cells will bind to these cells respectively and activate a complement cascade, which kills T or B lymphocytes. The dead cells are visualized by a vital stain, counted to obtain a percentage of lysis and scored numerically (8-6-4-2-1). A higher score means more antibodies to T or B cells are present.

Rheumatoid factor was assessed with the latex human IgG slide agglutination technique, wherein a titer level of ≥1:20 is considered positive. To detect circulating antibodies to nuclear antigens, the indirect immunofluorescence technique with a HEp-2 substrate was used. An ANA titer level of ≥1:40 is considered positive for this method.

Statistical Analysis

Statistical analysis of data is complicated when multiple variables are involved. Analysis of HLA typing data is even more complex; if the HLA-A, B, C and D antigens are thoroughly screened, as they were in this study, scores of variables are possible. Results from the screening of A, B, and C antigens were tabulated and compared, but no pattern or increased frequency of specific antigens was observed in any of the four subject groups. When data were analyzed for the 20 DR antigens screened, identifiable patterns became apparent in the molecules determined by DR β1 (DR1–18) and DRβ4 (DR53), but not by DRβ3 (DR52). Patterns of increased frequencies were also found in the 8 DQ antigens screened (DQ1–DQ8). The HLA antigens that appeared with the greatest frequency, other lab test results, and data collected in interviews were tabulated and analyzed for statistical significance using chi-square to test the hypothesis that no differences exist between the four groups. When the number of cell entries was too small for chi-square to be valid, Fisher's Exact test was used.

Our biostatistician recommended that for an exploratory study of this nature, pairwise comparisons, which look at differences between two groups, would provide no more useful information than the standard chi-square tests, which analyzed the four groups together. The large number of variables examined, as well as the presence of four groups, would have required a substantial number of pairwise comparisons. The more comparisons that are performed, the more likely you are to see a significant difference simply by chance. If the study had been based on a more specific hypothesis—e.g., "women with silicone breast implants are more apt to develop systemic symptoms if they have a certain HLA antigen"—then pairwise comparisons of differences might be a more appropriate method of statistical analysis. With the analysis method used, a statistically significant P value (≤0.05) means there is very strong evidence *against* the null hypothesis ("no differences exist between the four groups").

Traditionally, the most conservative way of statistically analyzing studies with multiple variables is to apply the Bonferroni adjustment, which adjusts probabilities by multiplying the achieved P value and the number of variables in the study. In an investigation of HLA antigens, however, data analysis must consider the phenomenon of linkage disequilibrium, which means that many variables are interdependent.

Although a Bonferroni correction can be applied with dependent data, it is nearly impossible to decide on the correct number of variables to use when multiplying the initial P value. For this exploratory study, unadjusted probabilities were used. Even if a Bonferroni adjustment had been made, the Group I women would still be statistically different from their asymptomatic counterparts in terms of the presence of DR53 and B cell autoantibodies.

Results

The 199 women who underwent HLA typing were divided into four groups according to their symptomatology and the presence of breast implants **(Table 1)**. Unfortunately, Group II is less than half the size of Group I since implant patients without any symptoms tend not to make appointments with their surgeons. Group IV, which consists of women who have received a diagnosis of primary fibromyalgia, is the smallest group, in part because it was difficult to get these patients to participate in a study with no obvious relevance to their disease. Readers are referred to a more detailed report on this study's findings published elsewhere [1].

Table 1. HLA testing population groups

Study Groups Total n=199	Classification	Mean Age (Range)	Mean Duration of Implantation (Range)
Group I (n=77)	symptoms with implants	46.2 (26-68)	12.1 yrs. (4-24)
Group II (n=37)	no symptoms with implants	46.0 (27-68)	10.3 yrs. (2-24)
Group III (n=54)	no symptoms/no implants	36.9 (14-65)	NA
Group IV (n=31)	symptoms/no implants	46.8 (29-76)	NA

For Groups I, II, and IV, the mean age is in the 46th year. Group III is approximately 10 years younger than the other three groups, but an individual's HLA genotype is independent of age. Duration of implantation is more pertinent than age, especially since Group I women reported a mean of nine years between implantation and symptom onset. As shown in Table 1, the mean duration of exposure to gel-filled breast implants among symptomatic women is nearly two years longer than it is for the asymptomatic women.

Complete information on the types of implants and their manufacturers could not be obtained because relevant medical records were unavailable for the many patients who had undergone breast augmentation or reconstruction years ago by other surgeons, sometimes in other parts of the country. All but one Group II subject knew they had silicone gel-filled implants, and we assume most had smooth elastomer shells based on dates of implantation. So many manufacturers and implant types were unknown that we could not draw any meaningful conclusions from these variables. From what could be determined, however, the distribution of implant manufacturers and shell designs seemed similar in the asymptomatic and symptomatic groups.

Of the 199 women included in this study, all but one were Caucasian; one Group II member was African-American. Among the 77 Group I members, 53 initially received implants for breast augmentation, while 24 underwent reconstruction after mastectomy for carcinoma or subcutaneous mastectomy for prophylactic reasons. Among the 37 Group II subjects, 30 received implants for augmentation and 7 for reconstruction. The reason for implant surgery had no influence on any of the variables examined in this study.

Reported symptoms and physical examination findings are tabulated in **Table 2**. Small numbers of women considered to be asymptomatic (Groups II and III) by the strict criteria of this study experienced occasional burning breast pain, myalgias and arthralgias, or fatigue. Curiously, some symptoms were more frequent among the healthy controls without implants than in asymptomatic women with implants. The few women in Group II who experienced breast pain, myalgia/arthralgia, or fatigue did not meet the symptomatic criteria because their complaints were of insufficient duration and severity. Those judged to be symptomatic (Groups I and IV) had multiple complaints, which explains why the numbers of reported symptoms greatly exceed the number of subjects in the groups. The highly significant ($P<0.0001$) difference found when the four groups are compared according to symptoms is expected since the presence of symptoms was the primary criteria used for categorizing the study subjects.

Table 2. Frequencies of symptoms and physical exam findings for the four study groups

	Group I (n=77)	Group II (n=37)	Group III (n=43)‡	Group IV (n=20)§	P value (chi-square)
PHYSICAL SYMPTOMS					
Breast pain	70%	5%	7%	10%	<0.0001
Myalgia/Arthralgia	83%	3%	14%	100%	<0.0001
Fatigue	83%	11%	7%	60%	<0.0001
General upper torso pain	36%	0	0	90%	<0.0001
BREAST EXAM FINDINGS					
Capsular contracture	74%	68%			0.509
Breast mass	5%	5%			1.000
Implant rupture (at least 1)	42%	32%			0.414
Lymphadenopathy	3%	0			1.000

‡ We did not interview 11 normal controls typed for HLA Laboratory purposes.

§ We had access to charts for only 20 out of 31 fibromyalgia patients.

Positive findings on physical breast examination of implant patients (Table 2) included capsular contracture (Baker grades III and IV), palpable breast masses, lymphadenopathy, and a history of ruptured implants, but none of these findings was statistically significant when Groups I and II were compared. The palpable masses found in four Group I members and two Group II members were judged to be silicone granulomas. Two Group I patients had adenopathy of the supraclavicular or axillary lymph nodes. The high frequencies of capsular contracture and implant rupture probably relate to the mean duration of implantation greater than 10 years: most subjects received implants with smooth shells, and many of the implants had aged, making them more prone to failure. The fact that capsular contracture and a history of implant rupture are similar in the two groups suggests these two variables do not account for the symptoms seen in Group I patients.

Table 3. Serological tests [columns show percent of group (# of patients)]

	Group I (n=58) symptoms with implants	Group II (n=5) no symptoms with implants	Group IV (n=11) symptoms/ no implants	P Value (chi-square)
Rheumatoid factor positive	11% (6)	0	0	0.728
Antinuclear antibodies ≥ 80	24% (14)	0	18% (2)	0.762
Sed rate > 20 mm/hr	5% (3)	20% (1)	17% (2)	0.134

Table 3 presents results of the voluntary screening for rheumatoid factor, antinuclear antibodies (ANA), and erythrocyte sedimentation rate (ESR). None of the healthy controls (Group III) volunteered for serological screening. Regarding the autoantibodies examined in these screenings, no statistically significant differences were found between the groups, but so few Group II and III subjects were tested, and so few tested positive, that only vast differences in the groups would yield significant results. It is nevertheless interesting that 24% of symptomatic women with implants had elevated ANA titer levels. By the indirect immunofluorescence method used for ANA testing, a titer level of 1:40 is considered positive. In Group I, titer levels (and number of patients) were as follows: 1:80 (6), 1:160 (4), 1:640 (2), 1:1280 (1), and 1:5120 (1).

When the frequencies of HLA antigens were tabulated and compared for the four groups, no differences were found in the distribution of HLA-A, B, and C antigens. **Table 4** compares the groups according to the presence of autoantibodies to B cells and the HLA-D antigens which appeared with greater frequency. Determination of antigens carried by the DRβ1 molecule revealed an increased frequency of DR4 and DR7 in both of our symptomatic groups (I and IV). This difference reached statistical significance for DR7. Asymptomatic patients with implants (Group II) had a statistically significant increased frequency of DR1.

Table 4. Frequency of HLA-DR and DQ antigens and autoantibodies to B cells [columns show percent of group (# of patients)]

	Group I symptoms with implants (n=77)	Group II no symptoms with implants (n=37)	Group III no symptoms/ no implants (n=54)*	Group IV symptoms/ no implants (n=31)	P value (chi-square)
DR1	18% (14)	38% (14)	16% (8)	26% (8)	0.048
DR4	44% (34)	27% (10)	31% (17)	45% (14)	0.188
DR7	34% (26)	11% (4)	20% (11)	29% (9)	0.046
DR53	68% (52)	35% (13)	52% (28)	65% (20)	0.007
DR4,7,53	10% (8)	3% (1)	2% (1)	10% (3)	0.143
DQ1	65% (50)	81% (30)	57% (29)	58% (18)	0.097
DQ2	57% (44)	27% (10)	35% (18)	45% (14)	0.010
DQ3	42% (32)	32% (12)	41% (21)	23% (7)	0.240
B cell auto-antibodies	42% (32)	14% (5)	2% (1)	19% (6)	<0.0001

* Three women in Group III were not tested for DQ antigens.

The determination of antigens carried by the DRβ4 molecule revealed a highly statistically significant increase (P=0.007) in the presence of DR53 in both symptomatic groups. The 52% frequency of DR53 in the healthy controls without implants (Group III) is similar to the 49.1% frequency expected in a large group of Caucasian women according to published frequency tables; the expected frequency of DR53 is 36.1% for Blacks and 69% for Orientals [2].

Table 4 reveals a striking similarity between symptomatic patients with and without implants (Groups I and IV) in terms of an HLA haplotype bearing DR53 and DR4 or DR7. In all populations studied to date, DR53 is found in strong linkage disequilibrium with DR4 and DR7. Thus, an increased frequency of DR53 in a group predicts that DR4 and/or DR7 will also be increased. Eight subjects in the symptomatic implant group are DR4/DR7 heterozygotes and DR53 positive. Due to the strong linkage disequilibrium of DR53 with DR4 and 7, these eight women are presumed to be DR53 homozygotes. There is one DR53 homozygous individual in the asymptomatic Group II, one in Group III, and three in Group IV. None of the study subjects is a DR4 or DR7 homozygote; in other words, no one has DR4/4 or DR7/7 but is DR53 negative.

The strong similarity seen in Groups I and IV with respect to HLA-DR antigens is less impressive with DQ antigens (Table 4). DQ1 and DQ3 are considered *broad parent molecules*. DQ5 and 6 are two specific epitopes, or *splits*, of DQ1, and DQ7 and 8 are splits of DQ3. Thus, everyone with DQ5 and/or DQ6 will have DQ1, and everyone with DQ7 and/or DQ8 will have DQ3. These four splits are not shown on Table 4 because we were more interested in the parent molecules. DQ4 also is not shown because only 10 of the 199 study subjects had this antigen.

As with the DR antigens, the DQ typing results reveal that the symptomatic and asymptomatic women with implants are different. The frequency of DQ2 in symptomatic women with implants (Group I) was significantly increased. DQ2 is closely associated with DR7, and this may partially explain the increased frequency of DQ2 in Group I. However, the significance of the DQ2 frequency is much greater than for DR7. The frequency of DQ1 is increased in asymptomatic patients with breast implants (Group II), but it did not reach statistical significance. Since DQ1 is often found in haplotypes bearing DR1 and DR2, we assume the increase of DQ1 in Group II is at least partly related to the fact that this group had a statistically significant increased frequency of DR1.

The most highly statistically significant finding of this study is that 42% of symptomatic Group I women have produced autoantibodies directed against their own B cells, which are indicative of an immune response directed against host tissues. Although the frequency of autoantibody production gradually increases with age, the variable of age does not account for the magnitude of difference in B cell autoantibodies found in our symptomatic implant patients. Of the Group I members who have formed autoantibodies to B cells, 22 of the 32 are younger than 50, compared to one of five Group II women and four of six Group IV patients.

Table 5 illustrates the association between DR53 and autoantibodies to B lymphocytes in the two symptomatic groups. Of the patients with implants who produced autoantibodies to their own B cells, 81% are DR53 positive. This compares to the 33% of fibromyalgia patients who are positive for autoantibodies and DR53. Only one of the five Group II women with autoantibodies to B cells is positive for DR53 (data not shown). The formation of B cell autoantibodies seems to be associated with DR53 in Group I (statistically significant at P=0.047 by Fisher's Exact test), but this is not true for Group IV (P=0.156).

Table 5. Frequency of autoantibodies to B cells associated with HLA-DR53 in Groups I and IV

	Group I (symptoms with implants)		Group IV (fibromyalgia patients)	
	B cell Positive % (# of Pts.)	B cell Negative % (# of Pts.)	B cell Positive % (# of Pts.)	B cell Negative % (# of Pts.)
DR53 Positive	81% (26)	58% (26)	33% (2)	71% (17)
DR53 Negative	19% (6)	42% (19)	67% (4)	29% (7)

Since we found such a striking association between DR53 and the formation of autoantibodies to B cells in patients with symptoms and implants, we also compared these autoantibodies, DQ1, and DQ2. Though the number of DQ2 positive subjects was significantly increased in Group I, **Table 6** reveals no association between this antigen and B cell autoantibodies. Formation of these autoantibodies therefore seems related to DR53 positivity, not to DQ2. When the presence of DQ1 was considered, we found that Group I patients positive for this antigen had a *decreased* frequency of B cell autoantibodies that approached statistical significance. It may be that DQ1 offers some protection against the formation of these autoantibodies.

Table 6. Frequency of autoantibodies to B cells associated with DQ1 and DQ2 in symptomatic patients with implants (Group I)

	B cell Positive (n=32) % (# of Pts.)	B cell Negative (n=45) % (# of Pts.)	P value (chi-square test)
DQ1 Positive	53% (17)	73% (33)	0.067
DQ1 Negative	47% (15)	27% (12)	
DQ2 Positive	59% (19)	56% (25)	0.739
DQ2 Negative	41% (13)	44% (20)	

The high frequencies of ruptured implants and capsular contractures in both implanted groups prompted us to compare these variables to the presence of DR53 and autoantibodies to B cells (data not shown). The frequency of patients with contractures who are positive for DR53 is nearly twice as high in Group I as in Group II (P=0.0079). The frequency of autoantibodies to B cells in women with capsular contractures is three times as high in Group I as in Group II (P=0.034). When comparing the variable of implant rupture with DR53 and B cell autoantibodies, the difference between Groups I and II is not significant when women with and without DR53 are compared (P=0.088 with Fisher's Exact test). However, we did find a statistically significant association between ruptured implants and autoantibodies to B cells, with 47% of Group I being both autoantibody and rupture positive, compared to 8% of Group II (P=0.032). This suggests some connection between exposure to silicone and production of these autoantibodies. There was no similar association between ruptured implants and elevated ANA titer levels.

These data should be viewed with some caution. It may be that the higher frequencies of DR53 and autoantibodies to B cells seen in Group I women with capsular contracture or ruptured implants arise from the fact that Group I patients as a whole have a highly significant increased frequency of both DR53 and B cell autoantibodies. We believe the variables of capsular contracture and implant rupture are much less important in the context of patients' symptoms, especially since these variables were not significantly different in symptomatic and asymptomatic women with implants.

Several investigators have found positive titer levels of antinuclear antibodies in symptomatic women with breast implants. Because 24% of our symptomatic patients with implants were ANA positive, we looked for an association between ANA and HLA-DR53 but, as **Table** 7 shows, no association was evident.

Table 7. Frequency of antinuclear antibodies (ANA) associated with HLA-DR53 in Group I

	ANA Positive (n=14) % (# of Pts.)	ANA Negative (n=44) % (# of Pts.)	P Value (chi-square)
DR53 Positive	71% (10)	70% (31)	0.944
DR53 Negative	29% (4)	30% (13)	

Discussion

Associations between specific HLA antigens and a variety of autoimmune, allergic, and metabolic diseases have been found during the last few decades. At the same time, researchers have learned that three different types of pathogenic mechanisms are known to be responsible for diseases associated with HLA antigens [3]. In one type, autoimmune disease, the pathogenic mechanism results from the direct effects of a specific immune response (either an autoantibody or an autoreactive T-cell response) directed against host tissues. Examples of autoimmune diseases fitting this description include rheumatoid arthritis (associated with DR4 and DR1), ankylosing spondylitis (B27), and insulin-dependent diabetes mellitus (DR3, DR4, and DQ7/8). A second type of pathogenicity causes immune complex-mediated disease, which is characterized by the formation of autoantibodies and insoluble immune complexes, such as those seen in systemic lupus erythematosus (SLE), which is associated with DR2 and two antigens—DR3 and B8—found in strong linkage disequilibrium [4]. The third type of HLA-associated disease has no known pathogenic immune component. One example is narcolepsy, associated with DR15.

In addition to rheumatoid arthritis and SLE, other connective tissue diseases with HLA associations have been reported in patients with silicone breast implants. Sjögren's syndrome [5], CREST syndrome [6], and inflammatory myositis [7] have all been linked with DR3. Scleroderma patients also have increased frequencies of DR3 [8] as well as DR5 [9,10]. Unfortunately, anecdotal reports of these diseases in implant patients do not help definitively answer a central question: were these patients fated to develop a rheumatologic disease regardless of their breast surgery, or are their implants causally related to development of the disease? While some believe that scleroderma is overrepresented among women with breast implants [11-13], recently published epidemiological studies have found that when the number of reported rheumatologic disease cases in women who also have silicone gel implants is compared to incidence and prevalence figures for the general population, no increased incidence of any disease can be found [14-18].

Since previous studies have revealed HLA associations with several defined connective tissue diseases, we tried to exclude patients with such diseases from our study groups so our data would not be biased and we could determine which HLA antigens might not be random. However, one Group I member did have diagnosed SLE. Her HLA typing was consistent with the antigens associated with lupus; she had both DR2 and DR3 but not DR53. She also had an ANA titer of 1:5120 and was negative for B cell autoantibodies. Although our symptomatic patients with implants have significantly increased frequencies of specific class II molecules, the ones significant in the group (DR53, DR7, and DQ2) are different from those associated with known rheumatologic diseases. This suggests that if symptomatic implant patients have mounted an immune-mediated response, it differs somewhat from that which occurs in patients with defined connective tissue diseases and is governed by different class II HLA molecules.

We considered the possibility that our symptomatic implant patients are suffering from fibromyalgia, and this became more intriguing when the HLA typing revealed striking similarities between Groups I and IV in terms of the DR4, DR7, and DR53 antigens (see Table 4). Two other HLA typing studies of fibromyalgia patients have been conducted, but only the DR1–DR8 antigens were tested. One study found that 67% of 18 fibromyalgia patients were DR4 positive, compared to 30% of 23 normal controls [19]. In a larger study, this DR4 association was not confirmed [20]. In the fibromyalgia group we tested, the frequency of DR4 was not increased to a statistically significant degree, although DR7 and DR53 were.

We don't believe any of our symptomatic patients with implants fit the 1990 American College of Rheumatology (ACR) diagnostic criteria for fibromyalgia. According to the ACR, a fibromyalgia diagnosis requires that patients have pain in at least 11 of 28 tender point sites on digital palpation plus a history of widespread pain [21]. Pain is considered widespread when all of the following are present: pain in left and right sides of the body, pain above and below the waist, and axial skeletal pain. Our symptomatic implant patients had nowhere near 11 tender points and did not report axial pain; the majority did not have pain below the waist. Group I women also did not report the kinds of non-musculoskeletal complaints common among fibromyalgia patients, such as GI problems, frequent respiratory infections, numbness in the extremities, or headaches.

Although both class I and II HLA molecules seem to be involved in a variety of functions related to an individual's ability to mount an immune response, the class II molecules are considered the most important in terms of predisposing individuals to develop autoimmune diseases and immunopathologic disorders. When the HLA molecules expressed on the surface of antigen-presenting phagocytic cells bind foreign antigenic peptide, they form an HLA–peptide complex. This complex is then recognized by T lymphocytes, which determine whether, and how great, an immune response will be mounted against that antigen [22,23].

Not all HLA antigens are expressed on all cell types. Class I antigens (HLA-A, B and C) are the most widely distributed and are found on almost all nucleated cells; they regulate the ability of lymphocytes to recognize foreign antigens on the surfaces of cells. Class II antigens (HLA-DR, DQ, and DP) are critical in immunoregulation. Because they control the interactions between regulatory T cells, B cells, and antigen-presenting cells, they govern the ability of lymphocytes to mount an immune response. Class II HLA molecules have a more restricted distribution than do class I molecules. Thus far, DQ antigens have been found only on B cells, while DP antigens are expressed on B cells and some macrophages and activated T cells. DR antigens are more widely expressed; they are found on B cells, antigen-presenting cells, some macrophages, and some activated T cells, as well as on the endothelial and epithelial cells of the thymus, intestine, breast, bladder, and bronchi

[24]. It is interesting that breast tissue contains more DR antigen expression (more DR positive cells) than do other frequent sites of silicone implantation. Although the full implications of this are unknown, it may partially explain why the development of systemic symptoms is not seen in patients receiving implanted silicone devices in other parts of the body.

Our study results lead us to speculate that a combination of factors underlies the symptoms seen in some patients with silicone breast implants. While we cannot say whether an autoimmune process is involved, multiple interacting factors are known to contribute to the development of autoimmune diseases: 1) immunologic abnormalities, 2) genetic backgrounds that predispose to autoimmunity, 3) local tissue alterations, and 4) microbial infections [25]. A genetic characteristic which predisposes an individual to respond immunologically as a consequence of silicone exposure is strongly implicated by the fact that a relatively small percentage of women with implants develop symptoms suggestive of rheumatologic disease. A report by Vasey et al. of identical twins who developed symptoms after a similar duration of implantation provides further evidence for this possibility [26]. In addition, the composition and perhaps location of breast implants may play a role in the body's response to silicone exposure. The literature contains virtually no reports of systemic symptoms or possible autoimmune problems in the millions of people who have received implanted silicone elastomer for bone, joint, genitourinary, vascular, cardiac, or other applications in which silicone devices are widely used. It is possible that silicone gel may be capable of stimulating an autoimmune or hypersensitivity response, but elastomer is not. Alternatively, perhaps breast tissue, or soft tissue in general, has distinct immunological characteristics that cause it to react to silicone in a way which bones and blood vessels do not [27].

Two investigator groups have recently performed HLA typing in women with breast implants, but their findings have thus far been presented only in abstract form, so we do not know the details of their methodologies or controls. However, both groups seem to have conducted molecular typing of tissue samples by polymerase chain reactions, whereas we used lymphocytes from peripheral blood to perform standard two-stage microcytotoxicity assays. In an investigation by Love et al., 9 of 12 (75%) patients who developed myositis after receiving silicone implants were found to have the DQα1*0102 allele, compared to a 16% frequency of this allele in studies of patients with idiopathic inflammatory myopathy [28]. In our study, 65% of symptomatic patients had DQ1, but the frequency of this antigen was even higher in asymptomatic implant patients, at 81%.

In a study by Morse et al., 60 women with silicone breast implants and musculoskeletal complaints were typed for HLA-DRβ1,3,4,5 and DQβ1 [29]. The 16 who had a defined connective tissue disease had increased frequencies of DR1, DR5 and DQ5, as well as decreased DR7 and DR3. When all 60 subjects with defined diseases and vague complaints were considered as a group, they had statistically significant decreased DR3 and DQ2 and increased DR5 when compared to more than 2,500 historical controls. Whereas Morse's symptomatic group had a decreased frequency of DQ2 compared to historical controls, our symptomatic implant patients had a statistically significant increased frequency of this antigen when compared to asymptomatic women with implants.

The investigations by Love and Morse point to important issues related to HLA typing study design. Neither of their studies seem to have used an asymptomatic control group with implants. We were primarily interested in determining whether differences exist between symptomatic and asymptomatic women with breast implants in terms of their HLA genotype. Based on our screening of class II HLA molecules, we must conclude that our two groups of patients with implants are indeed different from one another with respect to important genetic characteristics which govern immunological responses.

Autoantibodies

The most statistically significant finding of this study relates to the formation of autoantibodies to B lymphocytes by 42% of Group I symptomatic patients with implants (see Table 4). Remarkably, 81% of autoantibody-positive Group I women are also positive for HLA-DR53 (Table 5). This finding was a complete surprise to us. The B and T cell autoantibody tests were run routinely as part of the HLA typing, not because we expected any noteworthy results to emerge with respect to these autoantibodies. Such a highly significant frequency of B cell autoantibodies is clearly abnormal. Production of autoantibodies to B cells was the greatest point of difference between Groups I and IV, which were nearly identical in terms of the HLA-DR antigens significant in this study. While more than four times as many Group I women with these autoantibodies are DR53 positive than DR53 negative, only one-third of Group IV members with B cell autoantibodies are DR53 positive. The fibromyalgia patients are more like the asymptomatic Group II women with respect to this variable; of the five subjects in Group II with autoantibodies to B cells, four are DR53 negative.

If autoantibodies to B cells are formed in response to silicone gel or one of its components, then the asymptomatic implant group might also be expected to have high frequencies. On the other hand, if the autoantibodies are somehow related to the presence of HLA-DR53, then the fibromyalgia patients might be expected to have higher frequencies of B cell autoantibodies. Although we cannot fully explain the highly statistically significant formation of autoantibodies to B cells by Group I members, their presence may suggest the activation of an immune-mediated process that is related to both DR53 positivity and breast implant exposure. However, there is no proof that silicone breast implants, nor an HLA antigen, resulted in the production of these B cell autoantibodies. We also cannot be certain these autoantibodies are related to symptoms.

The close association between B cell autoantibodies, a specific class II HLA molecule (DR53), and the presence of symptoms in Group I subjects is difficult to interpret because the clinical significance of these autoantibodies is unknown. B lymphocytes always have the potential to produce autoantibodies, but this function is normally held in check by sufficient numbers of suppressor T cells (CD8+), a lack of helper T cells (CD4+), or a combination of the two [30]. T cell populations have received the most attention in studies of autoimmunity and HLA associations because it is HLA molecules which present peptide fragments derived from protein antigens to T cells. When an autoimmune process is activated, an imbalance in the ratio between helper and suppressor T cells occurs, disrupts the immunoregulatory network and activates autoreactive B cell clones. Autoreactive clones are cells that react to *self* as if foreign.

Even though our symptomatic implant patients did not form autoantibodies to T cells, their B cell autoantibodies might be due to abnormalities of T cell populations. Some have speculated that B cell autoantibody production may be stimulated by an antigen that contains foreign epitopes recognized by specific helper T cells [25]. Another possibility is that Group I subjects have experienced a loss of helper T lymphocytes. It has also been suggested that helper T cells may stimulate autoreactive B cells following exposure to a multideterminant antigen in which one epitope binds to autoreactive B cells but another linked epitope is foreign [25]. In a study that looked for T-cell proliferation after exposure to silicon, silicone gel, and silica, Ojo-Amaize determined that 25% of women exposed to silicone gel breast implants had an abnormal T-cell proliferative response [31]. All of the T cells that reacted to silicon(e) were CD4+. They hypothesize that the production of autoantibodies often seen in implant patients may be due to amplification of T-cell help for autoreactive B cells, and our findings may support this hypothesis.

Other studies have determined that polyclonal B cell activation may be induced by microbial products, and polyclonal T cell activation can be initiated by local inflammation or bacterial superantigens [25]. It may be that the presence of an implant predisposes some people to subacute infection or an ongoing inflammatory response, which could play a role in the formation of the autoantibodies to B cells found in our study. The inflammation that often accompanies capsular contracture plus the bacterial colonization that can occur in an implant capsule could lead to chronic inflammatory stimulation of the immune system and polyclonal B cell or T cell activation. This possibility is supported by recent work done at the National Cancer Institute in which mice grew plasmacytomas in response to intraperitoneal injections of silicone gel [Michael Potter, personal communication].

The B cell autoantibodies we found might also be left over from the body's attempt to eliminate autoreactive B cell clones, which is usually accomplished by suppressor T cells (CD8+). Perhaps Group I patients with these autoantibodies lack sufficient numbers of suppressor T cells to eliminate the autoreactive B cell clones. Analyzing the ratio of CD4:CD8 T cells in symptomatic patients with implants may provide insight into the question of whether the ratio of T cell subsets is out of balance.

To our knowledge, no other studies have looked for autoantibodies to B and T cells in implant patients, although other antibodies are receiving attention. Most serological investigations have focused on antinuclear antibodies and, to a lesser extent, rheumatoid factor, which are frequently found in patients with connective tissue diseases. In several large studies of symptomatic women with silicone breast implants, 26% of 655 symptomatic patients were ANA positive, and 10% of 503 patients were RF positive [13,26,32-36]. This closely compares to our symptomatic implant patients, 24% of whom are ANA positive and 11% of whom are RF positive. Among our 32 symptomatic patients who have produced autoantibodies to B cells, only six are also ANA positive.

A few points about ANA results are worth noting. Our finding of no association between implant rupture and elevated ANA titer levels has been observed by others. For example, Claman and Robertson found that among 82 patients with ill-defined symptoms, 23 had ruptured implants; of these, 22% were ANA positive [13]. In our symptomatic implant group, 27 patients had a known history of rupture, and 26% were ANA positive. A recent investigation by Peters et al. of 200 patients with intact implants, 29 with ruptured implants, and 100 age-matched controls found that 27% of implant patients were ANA positive, as were 17% of those with ruptures and 28% of the controls [16]. (Not all implant patients in Peters' study were symptomatic.) Peters' finding of a nearly identical frequency of positive ANAs in patients with implants and controls without implants greatly obscures the meaning of these antibodies.

With respect to positive ANA titers, there seems to be a difference between implant patients who have a diagnosed connective tissue disease and those with more ill-defined symptoms that do not meet the diagnostic criteria for a known disease. Claman found that 26% of 82 implant patients with symptoms of fatigue, arthralgias, and myalgias were ANA positive [13]. However, 64% of a group of 11 women with implants who have a defined autoimmune disease were ANA positive. Bridges et al. tested 156 women with breast implants and rheumatologic disease complaints (29 of whom had received a connective tissue disease diagnosis) [37]. Among all their symptomatic implant patients, 22% were ANA positive and 9% were RF positive. Of the 29 women who had a defined rheumatologic disease, the frequency of elevated titer levels was much higher: 45% were ANA positive and 17% were RF positive. The greater frequency of elevated ANA titers in implant patients with defined connective tissue diseases suggests they differ from those patients with more vague symptoms. Thus, the immunological processes at work in these two populations of implanted women may not be identical.

Conclusion

Due to the phenomenon of gel bleed, we can assume that everyone with silicone breast implants is exposed to silicone gel and its byproducts. Yet a relatively small percentage develop musculoskeletal complaints, and most do so only after an extended period of time. This clinical picture suggests that some factor related to an individual's genetic characteristics may predispose certain women to develop the symptoms seen in some implant patients. The study reported here examined whether there is any association between the symptoms seen in implant patients and HLA antigens. We performed HLA typing on 199 subjects categorized into four groups: symptomatic patients with implants (Group I), asymptomatic women with implants (Group II), healthy female volunteers without implants (Group III), and fibromyalgia patients without implants (Group IV).

A statistically significant 68% of Group I are positive for HLA-DR53, compared to 35% of Group II and 52% of Group III. The fibromyalgia patients were strikingly similar to Group I women in terms of HLA-DR antigens, with 65% of Group IV being positive for DR53. Group I also had a statistically significant increased frequency of HLA-DQ2. The most statistically significant study finding is that 42% of symptomatic women with implants have formed B cell autoantibodies. In these symptomatic patients, the DR53 antigen seems to be strongly associated with the production of these autoantibodies since 81% of Group I members with autoantibodies to B cells are DR53 positive. Though similar to Group I with respect to DR53, only a few fibromyalgia patients produced these autoantibodies. Thus, the autoantibody production seems related to both the presence of silicone and the DR53 antigen, especially since no association was found between B cell autoantibodies and the significantly increased frequency of DQ2 in Group I.

In contrast to both groups with symptoms, the asymptomatic women with implants (Group II) had increased frequencies of DR1 and DQ1. Our data suggest that symptomatic patients with implants share important genetic characteristics (primarily HLA-DR53 positivity) which differentiate them from their asymptomatic counterparts. DR53 may be a marker of women who are genetically predisposed by their HLA genotype to develop an immune-mediated reaction following exposure to some component of silicone gel breast implants.

References

1. Young VL, Nemecek JR, Schwartz BD, Phelan DL, Schorr MW (1995) HLA typing in women with breast implants. Plast Reconstr Surg (in press)
2. Terasaki PI (ed) (1980) Histocompatibility testing. UCLA Tissue Typing Laboratory, Los Angeles, pp 567-69
3. Lechler R (1994) Mechanisms of HLA and disease associations. In: Lechler R (ed) HLA and disease. Academic Press, London, pp 83-91
4. Hamilton RG, Harley JB, Bias WB, Roebber M, Reichlin M, Hochberg MC, Arnett FC (1988) Two Ro (SS-A) autoantibody responses in systemic lupus erythematosus: correlation of HLA-DR/DQ specificities with quantitative expression of Ro (SS-A) autoantibody. Arthritis Rheum 31:496-505
5. Campbell RD, Milner CM (1993) MHC genes in autoimmunity. Curr Opin Immunol 5:887-893
6. Germain BF, Espinoza LR, Bergen LL, Vagesh M, Vasey FB (1981) Increased prevalence of DRw3 in the CREST syndrome. Arthritis Rheum 24:857-859
7. Goldstein R, Duvic M, Targoff IN, et al. (1990) HLA-D region genes associated with autoantibody responses to histidyl-transfer RNA syntetase (Jo-1) and other translation-related factors in myositis. Arthritis Rheum 33:1240-1248
8. Kallenberg CGM, Van der Voort-Beelen JM, D'Amaro J, The TH (1981) Increased frequency of B8/DR3 in scleroderma and association of the haplotype with impaired cellular immune response. Clin Exp Immunol 43:478-485
9. Black CM, Welsh KI, Maddison PJ, Jayson MIV, Bernstein RM (1984) HLA antigens, autoantibodies and clinical subsets in scleroderma. Br J Rheumatol 23:267-271
10. Gladman DD, Keystone EC, Baron M, Lee P, Cane D, Mervert H (1981) Increased frequency of HLA-DR5 in scleroderma. Arthritis Rheum 24:854-856
11. Bridges AJ, Vasey FB (1993) Silicone breast implants: history, safety, and potential complications. Arch Intern Med 153:2638-2644
12. Spiera H, Kerr LD (1993) Scleroderma following silicone implantation: a cumulative experience of 11 cases. J Rheumatol 20:258-261
13. Claman HN, Robertson AD (1994) Antinuclear antibodies and breast implants. West J Med 160:225-228
14. Sánchez-Guerrero J, Schur PH, Sergent JS, Liang MH (1994) Silicone breast implants and rheumatic disease: clinical, immunologic, and epidemiologic studies. Arthritis Rheum 37: 158-168
15. Wigley FM, Miller R, Hochberg MC, et al. (1992) Augmentation mammoplasty in patients with systemic sclerosis: data from the Baltimore scleroderma research center and Pittsburgh data bank. Arthritis Rheum 35:Suppl., S46
16. Peters W, Keystone E, Snow K, Rubin L, Smith D (1994) Is there a relationship between autoantibodies and silicone-gel implants? Ann Plast Surg 32:1-7
17. Gabriel SE, O'Fallon WM, Kurland LT, Beard CM, Woods JE, Melton LJ (1994) Risk of connective-tissue diseases and other disorders after breast implantation. N Engl J Med 330: 1697-1702
18. Giltay EJ, Moens HJB, Riley AH, Tan RG (1994) Silicone breast prostheses and rheumatic symptoms: a retrospective follow up study. Ann Rheum Dis 53:194-196
19. Burda CD, Cox FR, Osborne P (1986) Histocompatability antigens in the fibrositis (fibromyalgia) syndrome. Clin Exp Rheumatol 4:355-357
20. Horven S, Stiles TC, Holst A, Moen T (1992) HLA antigens in primary fibromyalgia syndrome. J Rheumatol 19:1269-1270
21. Wolfe F (1990) Fibromyalgia. Epidemiol Rheum Dis 16:681-698
22. Segall M, Bach FH (1990) HLA and disease: the perils of simplification. N Engl J Med 322: 1879-1881
23. Hong R (1991) Autoimmunity: present-day concepts and future prospects. Curr Probl Pediatr 21:253-258

24. Tizard IR (1988) Immunology: an introduction. Saunders College Publishing, Philadelphia
25. Abbas AK, Lichtman AH, Pober JS (1994) Cellular and molecular immunology, 2nd ed. W.B. Saunders Company, Philadelphia
26. Vasey FB, Havice DL, Bocanegra TS, Seleznick MJ, Bridgeford PH, Martinez-Osuna P, Espinoza LR (1994) Clinical findings in symptomatic women with silicone breast implants. Semin Arthritis Rheum 24 (Suppl.) 1:22-28
27. Brautbar N, Vojdani A, Campbell AW (1992) Silicone implants and systemic immunological disease: review of the literature and preliminary results [Editorial]. Toxicol Ind Health 8: 231-237
28. Love LA, Weiner SR, Vasey FB, et al. (1992) Clinical and immunogenetic features of women who develop myositis after silicone implants. Arthritis Rheum 35: Suppl. S46
29. Morse JH, Spiera H, Zhang Y, Fotino M (1992) Autoimmune diseases and HLA typing in 60 females with silicone breast implants. Arthritis Rheum 35:Suppl. S132
30. Shoenfeld Y, Schwartz RS (1984) Immunologic and genetic factors in autoimmune diseases. N Eng J Med 311:1019-1027
31. Ojo-Amaize EA, Conte V, Lin H-C, Brucker RF, Agopian MS, Peter JB. (1994) Silicone-specific blood lymphocyte response in women with silicone breast implants. Clin Diagn Lab Immunol 1:689-695
32. Freundlich B, Altman C, Sandorfi N, Greenberg M, Tomaszewski J (1994) A profile of symptomatic patients with silicone breast implants: a Sjögren's-like syndrome. Semin Arthritis Rheum 24 (Suppl.) 1:44-53
33. Teuber SS, Rowley MJ, Yoshida SH, Ansari AA, Gershwin ME (1993) Anti-collagen autoantibodies are found in women with silicone breast implants. J Autoimmun 6:367-377
34. Bridges AJ (1994) Autoantibodies in patients with silicone implants. Semin Arthritis Rheum 24 (Suppl.) 1:54-60
35. Borenstein D (1994) Siliconosis. Semin Arthritis Rheum 24 (Suppl.) 1: 1-7
36. Solomon G (1994) A clinical and laboratory profile of symptomatic women with silicone breast implants. Semin Arthritis Rheum 24 (Suppl.) 1:29-37
37. Bridges AJ, Conley C, Wang G, Burns DE, Vasey FB (1993) A clinical and immunologic evaluation of women with silicone breast implants and symptoms of rheumatic disease. Ann Int Med 118:929-936

T Cell-Mediated Immune Response to Silica in Silicone Breast Implant Patients

D. R. Shanklin, M.D., FRSM[1,2], D. L. Smalley, Ph.D.[1,3], M. F. Hall[3], and M. V. Stevens, Ph.D.[3]

University of Tennessee, Departments of [1]Pathology and [2]Obstetrics and Gynecology, Memphis, Tennessee 38163 and Baptist Memorial Health Care System, [3]Baptist Regional Laboratories, Memphis, Tennessee 38105

During the last 25 or more years, silicone has been used as a filler in breast implants and is the major constituent of the outer elastomer. It was once thought to be biologically and metabolically inert; however, studies strongly suggested that silicone can be metabolized to lower molecular weight structures and that it deteriorates to silica [1-3]. Biologically, silicone has been shown to produce reactions by macrophages *in vivo* to promote the release of interleukin 1 [4], and to be antigenic with the production of antibodies to silicone [5] and to the native proteins that adhere to the silicone [6]. Recently, it has been shown that breast implant patients can develop T cell response to silicon dioxide [7,8], and to silicone [9]. In the studies with silicon dioxide, the primary form of silica used was a crystalline form, yet the form used in the outer elastomer was an amorphous silica. The present study undertook to further define the cell-mediated immune response to silica by evaluating the potential of blocking the reactions with an antibody directed against interleukin 2 (IL2). In addition, various forms of silica were tested in parallel with the crystalline form to determine if the silica form varied the immune recognition, and two elements not involved with silicone breast implants were tested to evaluate the specificity of T cell reactions in implant recipients.

Drs. Shanklin and Smalley have served as expert witnesses in the past, mainly for claimants and have one active case in mediation Funding of this and related work has been entirely internal. Dr. Stevens and Ms. Hall have not served as expert witnesses.

T Cell Response to Crystalline Silica

The first phase of the study was a retrospective evaluation of 106 breast implant recipients who were tested in the laboratory for clinical purposes to determine if the level of positivity was similar to that reported previously [7]. These patients' records were examined under the following criteria: they were requested by a physician for clinical purposes; the medical records clearly documented that the patient had silicone implants and manufacturer was not considered; the patient had at least two or more symptoms as described by Bridges et al. [10]. The results of the stimulation studies were recorded so as to avoid patient identification and to maintain patient anonymity. The data were examined in the same manner as previously reported in groups of less than a stimulation index (SI) of 25, SI of 25 to 50, SI of 50 to 100, and SI of >100 [7]. No further statistical studies were done on this group of patients since the objective was to verify that the distribution of immune responses were similar to previous studies [7].

Two levels of silica were used as antigen in the *in vitro* system (0.335 g/ml diluted in RPMI was the standard dose; 0.167g/ml in RPMI was also used). A total of 20 normal adult females without symptoms or silicone implants were tested and 40 breast implant patients were also tested. Distribution of responses were defined by establishing the mean SI and a cutoff of 2.5 times the mean representing a positive response. In addition, each response to the lower concentration was compared to that of the higher silica level to determine the potential of false positive and false negative responses.

Immune Blocking by Antibody to Interleukin 2

In this series of experiments, the blood of three randomly selected patients submitted to the laboratory for lymphocyte stimulation studies to silicon dioxide were tested with the addition of antibody to IL2. Briefly, each patient had lymphocyte stimulation studies performed by the criteria previously described [8] using triplicate wells for each patient for unstimulated cells for background, concanavalin A (Con A) stimulated cells to confirm immune stimulatory response by the T cells, and crystalline silicon dioxide stimulated cells to determine specific immune response to the antigen. In addition, each series described above had triplicate wells set up with the following: unstimulated wells with an additional 2.5 ug/ml of antibody to IL2, Con A wells with addition of 2.5 ug/ml of antibody to IL2, silicon dioxide wells set up in triplicate with 2.5 ug/ml, 5.0 ug/ml and 10.0 ug/ml of antibody to IL2.

The lymphocyte stimulation studies used a standard tritiated thymidine incorporation method as described previously [8]. However, in the wells containing antibody to IL2, the counts per minute (cpm) were determined in duplicate wells and the third well for each patient and with each agent was used to verify the percent viability after harvest of lymphocytes. The percent of decline in cpm was determined for each patient and for each agent or concentration of antibody.

Lymphocyte Stimulation with Various Forms of Silica

Amorphous silica (Sigma Chemical Co., St. Louis, MO) was used to stimulate lymphocytes. The same concentration of amorphous silica as was used before with crystalline silicon dioxide (0.335 g/ml in RPMI) [8]. The stimulation studies were performed as previously reported and used in the anti-IL2 studies described above. A total of 50 randomly selected implant patients were tested along with ten normal adult controls. The patients and controls were selected blindly to avoid identification and to maintain anonymity. The average of triplicate cpm for each patient was determined as well as SI for the amorphous silica for each patient and control. Two-tailed, Fisher's exact test was performed in comparing the response to amorphous silica with the crystalline silica in both groups.

Fumed amorphous silica (Sigma) was used in identical fashion as that described with amorphous silica with the exception that 51 different randomly selected implant patients were tested along with ten normal controls. Statistics were determined on data as described with the amorphous silica. These same 51 patients and ten normal controls were also tested against beryllium dioxide (Sigma) and titanium dioxide (Sigma) using the same protocol and statistical evaluation for patients and controls.

Results

The results of the stimulation studies of the 106 patients is shown in Fig. 1. The distribution of positive and negative response are quite similar to that previously reported [7]. The level of negative response to crystalline silica was 6.6% compared to 9.1% in previous studies. However, the positive response was nearly 93% compared to 91% previously.

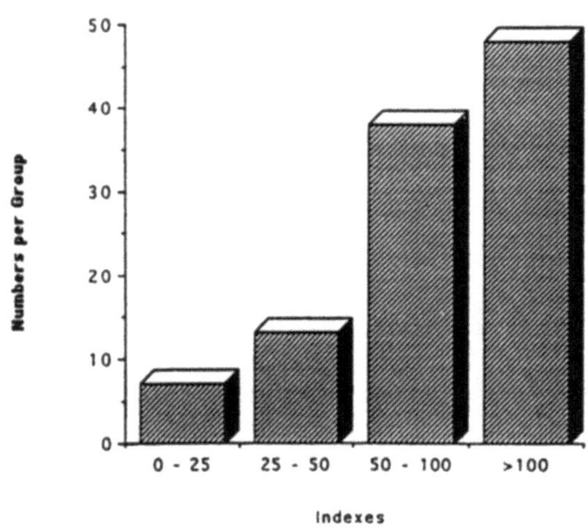

Fig 1. Distribution stimulation indexes found in 106 symptomatic breast implant recipients

In evaluating the dose response, the lower concentration of crystalline silica had a mean SI for the normal controls as 6 with a cutoff of positivity established as 15. Based on this format, 19 of the 20 normal controls would have been considered negative. The one control exceeding this level had a SI of 17. Among the implant patients, 35 patients exceeded the SI of 15. In comparing the 40 implant patients with high level silica, the mean SI was 9 which was nearly identical to our previous studies where the mean SI in 220 normal controls was 10. All 20 normal controls were below a cutoff of 23 based on 9 being the mean for this study group. Thirty-six implant patients exceeded the cutoff of 23. In comparing these two levels, five patients had levels below 15 on low silica concentrations but two of these had SI's exceeding 23 in the higher silica tests which would yield a sensitivity of 94.4% for the lower concentration of silica. In addition, one false positive would have been seen among the normal controls in the lower silica stimulations but was not seen in the higher silica stimulations. This would have yielded a specificity of 91.7% for the lower silica level. These findings validate prior results [7,8].

The three patients that had antibody to IL2 added to each of the components tested are shown in Table 1. The viability of all wells was not affected by the presence or absence of the antibody to IL2. The cpm for the unstimulated wells showed essentially no significant changes in the presence of antibody to IL2. The wells with Con A showed a significant decrease (approximately 98%) in cpm in the presence of antibody to IL2. The silica stimulated cpm also showed a significant decrease in the presence of the antibody to IL2 as shown in Table 1. In Fig. 2., the individual percentage of decreased cpm is shown per patient at each level of antibody used. The level of decline in cpm was 97 to 98% in all three patients at all three levels tested.

Table 1. Inhibition of lymphocyte proliferation responses by antibody to IL2

Activator	Anti-IL2	[^{3}H] Thymidine incorporation mean cpm	Viability (%)
None	-	30 ± 6.1	94 ± 1
	+	54 ± 16 3	91 ± 2
Con A	-	3160 ± 1631	89 ± 4
	+ (2 5 ug)	46 ± 13.5	92 ± 2
SiO_2	-	3389 ± 1424	89 ± 4
	+ (10 ug)	68 ± 9.7	88 ± 2
	+ (5 ug)	116 ± 43 2	87 ± 2
	+ (2 5 ug)	56 ± 11.6	84 ± 2

Counts were based on three silicone breast implant recipients tested independently but during the same days.

The cpm of implant patients' T cells with amorphous silica are shown in Fig. 3. The comparison of SI data with the crystalline silica are shown in Table 2. Among the 50 implant patients, 39 exceeded the standard SI of 25 established for this laboratory. Eleven patients stimulated above the SI of 25 with amorphous silica but not crystalline silica. No statistical evaluation was done since all patients were stimulated by one or both of the forms of silica. The normal controls stimulated with amorphous and crystalline silica are shown in Table 3. No normal controls were stimulated above the SI of 25 by either form of silica.

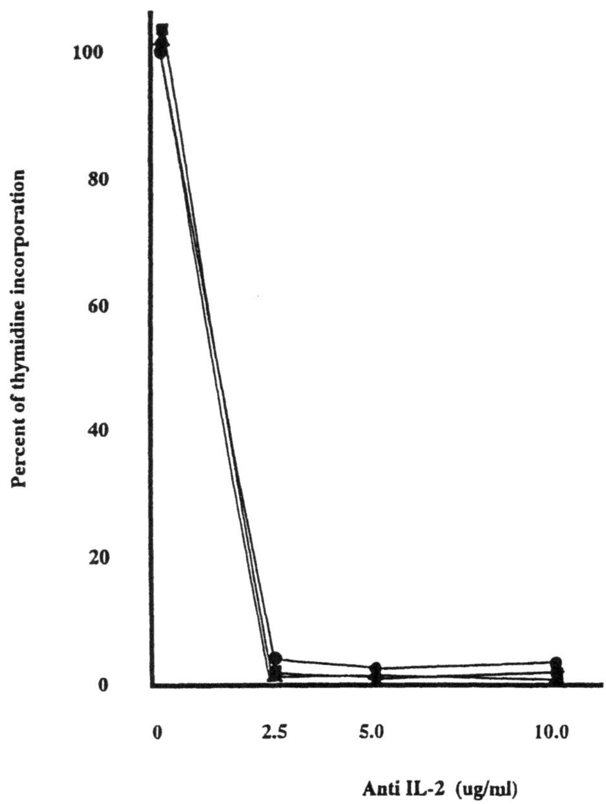

Fig 2. Percentage of decrease in thymidine uptake in the presence of various concentrations of anti-IL2

Table 2. Comparison of stimulation indexes between colloidal silicon dioxide and amorphous silica in 50 random breast implant patients

Amorphous Silica	Colloidal Silicon Dioxide	
	Positive *	Negative
Positive	39	11
Negative	0	0

* A positive response was based on a stimulation index above 25.

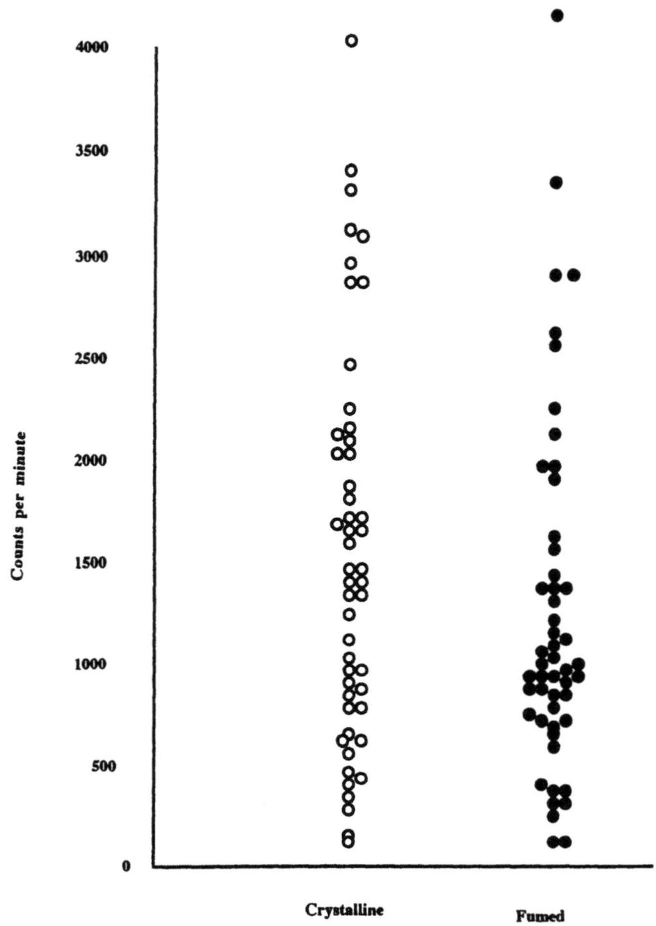

Fig 3. Counts per minute for 50 implant patients stimulated with crystalline and amorphous silica

Table 3. Comparison of stimulation indexes between colloidal silicon dioxide and amorphous silica in ten random normal controls

Amorphous Silica	Colloidal Silicon Dioxide	
	Positive *	Negative
Positive	0	0
Negative	0	10

* A positive response was based on a stimulation index above 25.

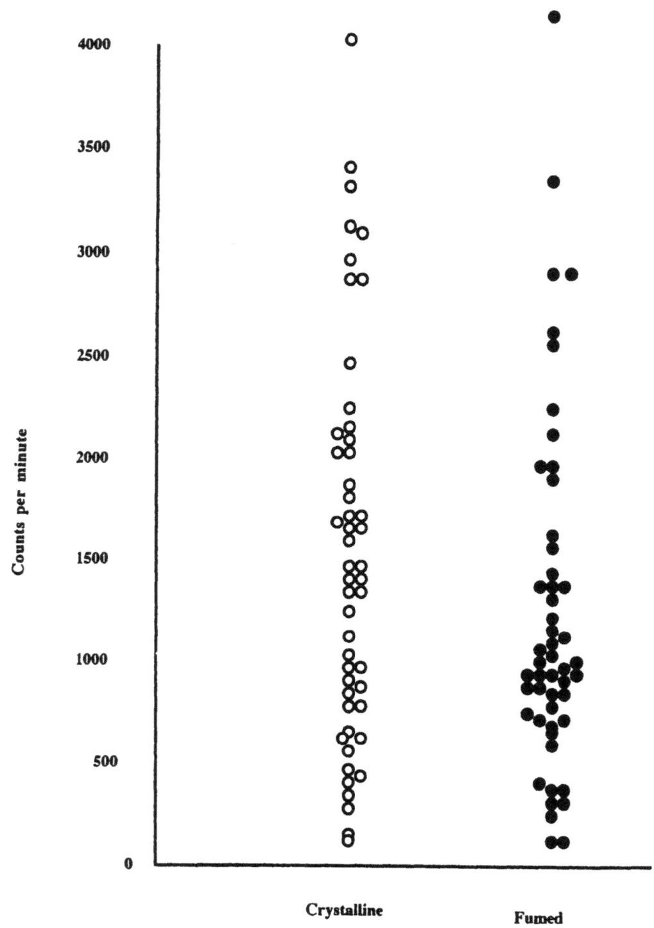

Fig 4. Counts per minute for 51 implant patients stimulated with crystalline and fumed amorphous silica

The cpm of the 51 implant patients' T cells with fumed amorphous silica are shown in Fig. 4. The comparison of SI data with crystalline silica and fumed silica are shown in Table 4. Forty-two patients exceeded the SI of 25 with both forms of silica, whereas, four patients exceeded the SI of 25 with fumed but not crystalline and two patients exceeded the SI of 25 with crystalline but not with the fumed silica. Three patients were below the SI of 25 in both forms of silica. Statistical analysis showed that there was a significant association between the two forms of silica for stimulation, p = 0.01. All ten normal controls tested with crystalline and fumed silica were below the SI of 25 as shown in Table 5.

Table 4. Comparison of stimulation indexes between colloidal silicon dioxide and fumed amorphous silica in 51 random breast implant patients

Fumed Amorphous Silica	Colloidal Silicon Dioxide Positive *	Negative
Positive	42	4
Negative	2	3

* A positive response was based on a stimulation index above 25. Using the Fisher's Exact Test, two-sided p = 0.01, a significant association between the responses.

Table 5. Comparison of stimulation indexes between colloidal silicon dioxide and fumed amorphous silica in ten random normal controls

Fumed Amorphous Silica	Colloidal Silicon Dioxide Positive *	Negative
Positive	0	0
Negative	0	10

* A positive response was based on a stimulation index above 25.

Among the 51 implant patients and the ten normal controls, neither beryllium nor titanium was found to be stimulatory to the lymphocytes (Table 6). There was no significant differences between the controls' and the implant patients' SI for beryllium; however, there was a slight difference with the normal controls being slightly higher than the implant patients when stimulated with titanium, $p = 0.04$. The level of stimulation was very low and these SI are not considered to be significant.

Table 6. Comparison of stimulation indexes between beryllium and titanium for 51 random breast implant patients and ten normal controls

Test Group	Agent Beryllium [a] Mean SI ± SEM	 Titanium [b] Mean SI ± SEM
Normal Controls	1.20 ± 0.13	1.50 ± 0.17
Implant Patients	1 16 ± 0.05	1.18 ± 0.06

[a] No significant differences found, p = 0 7413

[b] Stimulation indexes for normal controls was slightly higher than implant group, p = 0 0417

Discussion

In a retrospective review of 106 patients' records, each patient was reported to have two or more symptoms as described by Bridges et al. [10]. The average number of symptoms was four within a range from two to eight. Among these 106 implant recipients, nearly 93% showed positive T-cell responses which correlates well with findings previously reported [7]. This random selection of implant patients confirms that variations of T-cell response are limited.

The dose response evaluation using a lower concentration of crystalline silica than previously reported [8], had limited effect; however, the specificity would have been lowered to 91.7% rather than the 100% shown in this study at the higher concentration. This means that lower concentrations may affect the outcome even more and levels consistent with those reported previously should be used for future studies.

Antibody to IL2 had little effect on cellular viability but significantly reduced the stimulatory effect of Con A by 98.5% in all patients. The stimulatory effect of crystalline silica also reflected an inhibitory effect by antibody to IL2 by 97-98% even with as little as 2.5 ug/ml of antibody. This clearly shows that T-cells that have memory of silica exposure initiate the proliferative response by production of IL2 which is the classical approach expected by memory cell/lymphocyte recognition. Further studies are planned to evaluate the inhibitory effect at even lower concentrations of antibody. These data also suggest that cytokine blockade may be one consideration in eliminating the immunologic response to silica in these patients.

In the final series of studies, breast implant patients' lymphocytes showed immune reactivity and lymphocyte proliferation to amorphous silica and to fumed silica (Table 2,4). Although some variations occurred, it is clear from these data that antigenic recognition by any of these three forms of silica confirms that the physical variation does not eliminate the antigenic potential. None of the normal controls responded to either amorphous or fumed amorphous silica (Tables 3,5) as described previously with crystalline silica [7]. In addition, specificity of the reaction of silica recognition lymphocytes was confirmed by lack of response to beryllium or titanium (Table 6) and correlates with previous studies [9].

In summary, the reactivity of silicone breast implant recipients was similar to that reported earlier [7,8]. Antibody to IL2 clearly blocked the lymphocyte stimulatory effect and opens the door to understanding the immune response and suggests a potential for blocking such reactions. The form of silica, whether crystalline, amorphous, or fumed amorphous, did not affect the antigenic stimulation of breast implant patients which was not found in normal controls.

References

1. Kossovsky N, Heggers JP, Robson MC (1987) Experimental demonstration of the immunogenicity of silicone-protein complexes. J Biomed Material Res 21:1125-1133
2 Garrido L, Pfleiderer B, Papisov M, Ackerman JL (1993) *In vivo* degradation of silicones. Magn Res Med 29:839-843
3. Pfleiderer B, Ackerman JL, Garrido L (1993) Migration and biodegradation of free silicone from silicone gel-filled implants after long-term implantation. Magn Res Med 30:534-543
4 Krause TJ, Robertson FM, Liesch JB, Wasserman AJ, Greco RS (1990) Differential production of interleukin 1 on the surface of biomaterials. Arch Surg 125:1158-1160
5. Wolfe LE, Lappe M, Peterson RD, Ezrailson EG (1993) Human immune response to polydimethylsiloxane (silicone): screening studies in a breast implant population. FASEB J 7 1265-1268
6 Kossovsky N, Zeidler M, Chun G, Papasian N, Nguyen A, Rajguru S, Stassi J, Gelman A, Spondler E (1993) Surface dependent antigens identified by high binding avidity of serum antibodies in a subpopulation of patients with breast protheses. J Appl Biomaterials 4:281-288
7. Smalley DL, Shanklin DR, Hall MF, Stevens MV, Hannisian A (1995) Immunologic stimulation of T-lymphocytes by silica following use of silicone mammary implants. FASEB J 9.424-427
8. Smalley DL, Shanklin DR, Hall MF, Stevens MV (1995) Detection of lymphocyte stimulation by silicon dioxide Int J Occup Med Toxicol 4:63-69
9. Ojo-Amaize EA, Conte V, Lin HC, Brucker RF, Agopian MS, Peter JB (1994) Silicone-specific blood lymphocyte response in women with silicone breast implants. Clin Diagn Lab Immunol 1:689-695
10 Bridges AJ, Conley C, Wang G, Burns DE (1993) A clinical and immunologic evaluation of women with silicone breast implants and symptoms of rheumatic disease. Ann Intern Med 118:929-936

Immunohistopathology and T Cell Receptor Gene Expression in Capsules Surrounding Silicone Breast Implants

T.P. O'Hanlon, S. Okada[1], L.A. Love[1], G. Dick[2], V.L. Young[3], and F.W. Miller
Molecular Immunology Laboratory, CBER, FDA, Bethesda, MD; [1]Clinical Research and Review Staff, CFSAN, FDA, Washington, DC; [2]Clinical Consultant, Plastic Surgery, NIH, Bethesda, MD; and [3]Division of Plastic Surgery, Washington Univ. Sch. of Medicine, St. Louis, MO

Introduction

Two questions remain central to the silicone debate. The first concerns circumstances under which silicone elicits an immune response, and the second relates to whether silicone-associated immune responses are causally linked with the development of clinical signs and symptoms in certain groups of silicone implant recipients. Several lines of indirect evidence suggest that silicone may act as an immunizing agent. These include a well-characterized foreign body response resulting in the formation of a neo-vascular tissue around implants containing variable numbers and types of inflammatory cells [1], the adjuvant activity of some silicones in animals [2], the detection of elevated levels of silicone-binding immunoglobulins in the sera of some patients [3,4], T cell stimulatory responses induced by some silicones in vitro [5,6], and multiple case reports of autoimmune conditions developing in silicone implant recipients with disease remission following explantation [7].

Silicone implants in the body induce the formation of a complex fibrovascular connective tissue referred to as a capsule. The formation of this periprosthetic neo-tissue is a dynamic process subject to ongoing restructuring. The capsule is an organized, and often multilayered tissue [8,9]. At the implant surface there is usually amorphous proteinaceous material with an adjacent layer of vacuolated, palisading pseudo-synovium containing inflammatory cells. Collagen and fibroblasts form the outermost surface of the capsule.

*Potential conflicts of interest statement: This study was solely supported by FDA internal funds. Drs. O'Hanlon, Okada, Love, and Miller are employees of the FDA; they are not involved in any litigation or profit-making organizations relating to silicone, do not regulate silicone devices, but have been asked to advise FDA advisory committees and personnel on issues relating to breast and other implants. Dr. Dick is a plastic surgeon in solo practice who has implanted and explanted breast implants; he is not involved in any litigation or profit-making organizations relating to silicone. Dr. Young is a plastic surgeon who has implanted and explanted breast implants; he is a consultant to McGhan Medical Corporation and is performing clinical studies of radiolucent breast implants made by Lipomatrix Inc.

These layers, however, differ greatly in thickness and cellular composition from patient to patient for reasons that remain unclear. In an attempt to understand more fully the nature of local immune responses to silicone gel breast implants, we have conducted a preliminary study to develop immunohistochemical and molecular approaches to examine inflammatory cells found in implant capsules.

Immunohistopathology

Sections of capsules obtained during explantation were formalin-fixed and paraffin-embedded for pathologic and immunocytochemical analyses. The fixed tissue sections were evaluated by standard immunocytochemistry using monoclonal antibodies (DAKO Corp.) specific for a variety of immunophenotypic and activation markers (LCA, CD3, CD45RO, OPD4, CD20, CD45R, CD21, VS38c, HAM56, and HLA-DR). Immunohistochemistry was performed by indirect alkaline phosphatase staining using the streptavidin-biotin method according to the manufacturer's instructions (DAKO Corp.).

The cellular phenotypes of the 22 capsules evaluated were heterogeneous, both from capsule to capsule and from different areas within a given capsule. The histopathology ranged from nearly acellular, densely fibrotic, collagenous structures, to areas showing intense inflammation, which were primarily surrounding vacuoles containing a highly refractile, nonpolarizable foreign material consistent with that observed for silicone [10]. The inflammatory infiltrates contained multinucleated giant cells, activated T and B lymphocytes, macrophages, and plasma cells. In some instances, lymphocytes were arranged in follicular patterns with germinal centers. Cellular expression of CD3 (a pan T cell marker), CD45RO (a T cell activation marker), HAM56 (a macrophage-specific marker), and HLA-DR (a marker associated with activated antigen-presenting cells) was most prominent in areas surrounding or adjacent to silicone vacuoles. Some epithelioid cells in the pseudo-synovial layer of the capsules showed strong OPD4 and HLA-DR staining, suggesting activation of cells with phagocytic characteristics. Collectively, the data indicate that the number and type of inflammatory cells vary greatly among different capsules, but when present were usually localized around silicone vacuoles, suggesting an association between silicone release and local immune responses.

Molecular Analyses of T Cell Receptor Gene Expression

Polymerase chain reaction (PCR) technology has provided a rapid and sensitive means of studying T cells infiltrating pathologic tissues [11]. This technology can be used to accurately identify T cell receptor (TCR) genes expressed at sites of disease activity. Studies of TCR gene expression by PCR have proven useful in defining possible pathogenic subsets of T cells within inflammatory lesions [12,13].

The full complement of TCR genes are physically separated into multiple, structurally diverse variable (V), diversity (D), joining (J), and constant (C) gene segments. As T cells mature in the thymus, individual T cells randomly recombine distinct V, D, J, and C gene segments to form functional TCR genes. The mature, cell-surface form of the TCR is encoded by two such independently rearranged TCR genes (designated α and ß). The αß TCR complex recognizes foreign peptide antigens presented in the context of major histocompatibility (MHC) molecules by antigen-presenting cells. The expression of alternative V, D, and J gene segments or families creates among circulating T cells a vast potential for foreign antigen recognition. In many instances, the recognition of structurally similar antigens is mediated by T cells expressing particular TCR gene families [14]. In fact, limited or restricted patterns of TCR gene expression have been described for a variety of human autoimmune diseases [12,13,15,16].

Sections of capsules obtained during explantation were rapidly frozen at -80°C for TCR studies. RNA from frozen capsular tissue (100 mg per capsule) was isolated and cDNA was prepared for PCR assays to determine the pattern of αß T cell receptor V gene expression in each capsule according to established methods [17]. Under the PCR conditions utilized in this study, all the αß TCR V genes surveyed (TCR Vα1-22 and Vß1-24) were consistently detected in control peripheral blood samples (PBL) from a healthy donor (Fig. 1, upper panels). In contrast, the number and identity of TCR Vα and Vß gene families detected in silicone breast implant capsules varied and ranged from the absence of detectable TCR gene expression to the detection of multiple TCR V gene families (Fig. 1, patients 3, 12, and 2 were chosen to illustrate the range and variability of TCR V gene expression in capsules).

Of the 20 frozen capsules analyzed, TCR gene expression was detected in 14 capsules that also showed prominent inflammation in adjacent histological sections. Overall, the number and type of TCR V gene families detected varied from capsule to capsule. Yet, despite this heterogeneity, certain TCR V gene families were frequently detected (TCR Vα 1, 7, 15, 19 and Vβ 5, 6, 7, 12). In some cases, similar patterns of TCR V gene family expression were detected from multiple, physically remote pieces of the same capsule or, as illustrated in Fig. 2, in both the left and right capsules from the same individual. In this example, TCR Vß 5.2, 6, and 7 gene family expression were detected in both the left and right capsule from the same patient. Collectively, the data suggest that at least in certain individuals, antigenic selection may account for observed similarities in TCR V gene expression. We are currently exploring this possibility by direct DNA sequence analysis of the TCR antigen-binding sites associated with these capsule-infiltrating T cells.

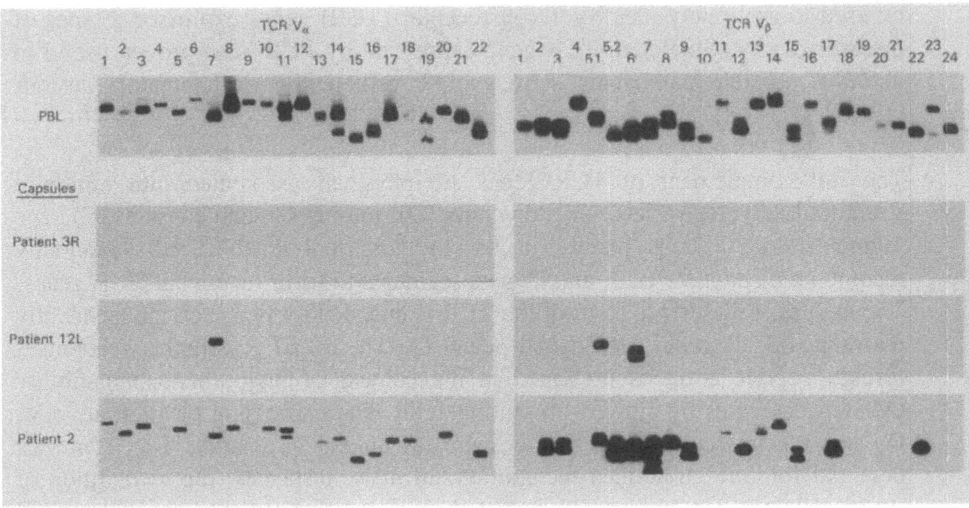

Fig. 1. Representative TCR analyses of silicone breast implant capsules. Shown are results illustrative of the range and variability of TCR V gene expression in capsules from three patients (patients 3, 12, and 2). Analysis of peripheral blood lymphocytes (PBL) from a healthy donor served as a positive control for the detection of all the TCR V gene families surveyed. cDNA samples isolated from capsules and control PBLs were analyzed for the expression of 22 different Vα and 24 different Vß TCR gene families as previously described [17]. The sizes of TCR V gene amplification products detected correspond with that predicted for the respective V gene families. (L, left capsule; R, right capsule)

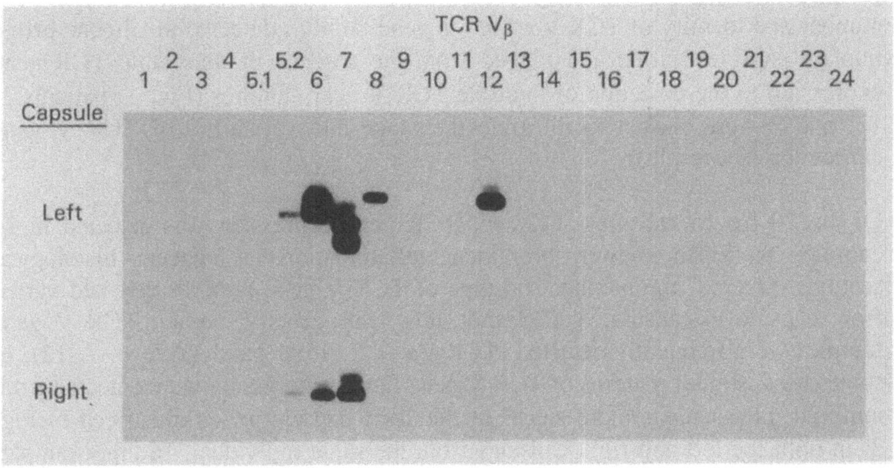

Fig. 2. Representative TCR analyses of silicone breast implant capsules. Shown are results illustrating the similar pattern of TCR Vß genes detected in left and right capsules from the same patient.

Our current study has focused on establishing methodologic approaches for examining the nature and extent of immune responses in silicone breast implant capsules. Preliminary findings indicate that, under certain circumstances, local immune responses induced by silicone involve activation of macrophages, B and T lymphocytes, and perhaps selected TCR utilization. Ongoing and future investigations are directed at correlating these and additional data with the clinical and immunogenetic features of the subjects, the chemical composition of the implants, and other parameters that may influence the character of the body's reactions to silicone. These studies may serve as a first step in understanding the reasons for, and implications of, individual variations in silicone-associated immune responses.

References

1. Kossovsky N, Freiman CJ (1994) Silicone breast implant pathology. Clinical data and immunologic consequences. Arch Pathol Lab Med 118:686-693
2. Naim JO, Lanzafame RJ, van Oss CJ (1993) The adjuvant effect of silicone-gel on antibody formation in rats. Immunol Invest 22:151-161
3. Goldblum RM, Pelley RP, O'Donell AA, Pyron D, Heggers JP (1992) Antibodies to silicone elastomers and reactions to ventriculoperitoneal shunts. Lancet 340:510-513
4. Wolf LE, Lappe M, Peterson RD, Ezrailson EG (1993) Human immune response to polydimethylsiloxane (silicone): screening studies in a breast implant population. FASEB J 7:1265-1268
5. Ojo-Amaize EA, Conte V, Lin H, Brucker RF, Agopian MS, Peter JB (1994) Silicone-specific blood lymphocyte response in women with silicone breast implants. Clin Diag Lab Immunol 1:689-695
6. Smalley DL, Shanklin DR, Hall MF, Stevens MV, Hanissian A (1995) Immunologic stimulation of T lymphocytes by silica after use of silicone mammary implants. FASEB J 9:424-427
7. Houpt KR, Sontheimer RD (1994) Autoimmune connective tissue disease and connective tissue disease-like illnesses after silicone gel augmentation mammoplasty. J Am Acad Dermatol 31:626-642
8. Emery JA, Spanier SS, Kasnic G,Jr., Hardt NS (1994) The synovial structure of breast-implant-associated bursae. Mod Pathol 7:728-733
9. Kasper CS (1994) Histologic features of breast capsules reflect surface configuration and composition of silicone bag implants. Am J Clin Pathol 102:655-659
10. Raso DS, Greene WB, Vesely JJ, Willingham MC (1994) Light microscopy techniques for the demonstration of silicone gel. Arch Pathol Lab Med 118:984-987
11. Panzara MA, Oksenberg JR, Steinman L (1992) The polymerase chain reaction for detection of T-cell antigen receptor expression. Curr Opin Immunol 4:205-210
12. Paliard X, West SG, Lafferty JA, Clements JR, Kappler JW, Marrack P, Kotzin BL (1991) Evidence for the effects of a superantigen in rheumatoid arthritis. Science 253:325-329
13. Oksenberg JR, Panzara MA, Begovich AB, Mitchell D, Erlich HA, Murray RS, Shimonkevitz R, Sherritt M, Rothbard J, Bernard CAA, Steinman L (1993) Selection for T-cell receptor $V\beta$-$D\beta$-$J\beta$ gene rearrangements with specificity for a myelin basic protein peptide in brain lesions of multiple sclerosis. Nature 362:68-70

14. Jorgensen JL, Reay PA, Ehrich EW, Davis MM (1992) Molecular components of T-cell recognition. Ann Rev Immunol 10:835-873
15. Davies TF, Martin A, Concepcion ES, Graves P, Cohen L, Ben-Nun A (1991) Evidence of limited variability of antigen receptors on intrathyroidal T cells in autoimmune thyroid disease. N Engl J Med 325:238-24414
16. O'Hanlon TP, Dalakas MC, Plotz PH, Miller FW (1994) Predominant $\alpha\beta$ T cell receptor variable and joining gene expression by muscle-infiltrating lymphocytes in the idiopathic inflammatory myopathies. J Immunol 152:2569-2576
17. O'Hanlon TP, Dalakas MC, Plotz PH, Miller FW (1994) The $\alpha\beta$ T-cell receptor repertoire in inclusion body myositis: diverse patterns of gene expression by muscle-infiltrating lymphocytes. J Autoimmun 7:321-333

Cellular Reactions to Silicone Implants

Macrophage-Silicone Interactions in Women with Breast Prostheses

N. S. Hardt[1], J. A. Emery[1], G. LaTorre[2], C. Batich[2], and W. E. Winter[1]
[1]Pathology and Laboratory Medicine, University of Florida College of Medicine, [2]Materials Science and Engineering, University of Florida College of Engineering, Gainesville, Florida

Introduction

In order for silicone from breast implants to have an effect on the immune system, it must be demonstrated that cells with the potential for immune system function have access to silicone. It had long been thought that the fibrous capsule surrounding breast prostheses functioned as an effective barrier between the biomaterial and the host. Implants that ruptured were thought to be innocuous to the host as long as the fibrous tissue capsule surrounding the implant was intact. This was termed "contained rupture." Thus, the capsule was thought to prevent the egress of foreign material (Bingham et al. 1988)

However, a puzzling observation was made. In patients with presumably intact capsules and in some cases intact elastomer shells, foreign material with light microscopic characteristics of silicone were found in lymph nodes (Hausner et al., 1978, Tabatowski et al., 1990, Silver et al., 1993). The mechanism by which this transfer of foreign material might occur has undergone recent study.

The Interdisciplinary Research Group on Silicone at the University of Florida, formed in 1991, has made systematic observations on animal models and on human patients undergoing removal of breast prostheses to provide clues to the mechanisms behind such observations. Observations have been recorded from the surface of the elastomer shell, from the cellular constituents of the potential space between the elastomer shell and the implant related capsule (Caffee et al. 1995, in press), from the capsule architecture, and from pericapsular soft tissues (Hardt et al. 1994, Hardt et al. 1995, Emery et al. 1994a, b).

Conflict of Interest Statement:
NH, JE, GL, WW are not involved as plaintiff's or defendant's experts in any implant related litigation. CB has served as an expert witness on behalf of a patient in a case against a manufacturer. None of the authors have a financial interest in a biomaterials company or a laboratory. This research was supported in part by the University of Florida Diagnostic Referral Laboratory and by a grant from the Plastic Surgery Education Foundation.

The observations reported here are limited to those between cellular constituents of the immune system and implant related foreign materials. These observations were made on more than 200 patients undergoing prosthetic explantation with capsulectomy. A few patients with lymphadenopathy requiring biopsy or breast carcinoma requiring axillary lymphadenectomy provided regional lymph nodes for study. The authors make no attempt to link these cellular/foreign material interactions with human disease. However, reasonable hypotheses of a mechanism for such linkage are offered. Establishment of the linkage of immunologic phenomena with disease must be established with detailed mechanistic studies which are beyond the scope of the observations reported here.

Methods

At the time of explantation, the implant capsule was entered using a technique previously described (Caffee et al. 1993). Using a catheter, 10cc of sterile saline was instilled. After gentle agitation, the saline was aspirated and placed in 10cc of modified Eagle's medium. This fluid was spun to prepare cytospins which were stained with Papanicolaou stain (Caffee et al. 1995). These preparations were examined light microscopically, and in selected cases the identity of observed foreign materials was confirmed by applying 4 drops of the aspirate to an infrared crystal for infrared spectroscopy (Hardt et al. 1994).

Fourier transform infrared spectroscopy (FTIR) is an analytical technique which yields information on the molecular level. It allows the identification of unknown compounds since the spectrum obtained is a complex fingerprint that is unique to a specific compound.

Fresh capsular tissue obtained at operation was fixed in 10% buffered formaldehyde and embedded in paraffin. Five micron sections were stained with hematoxylin and eosin or Masson's trichrome stain for light microscopic evaluation. In selected cases the identity of the foreign materials was confirmed using microscopically guided FTIR and or the tissue was fixed in 2.5% glutaraldehyde in 0.1M phosphate buffer (Ph 7.4) for transmission electron microscopy (Emery et al. 1994a).

Results

Intracapsular Space

In all but two cases, washings from the intracapsular space surrounding gel filled implants contained round droplets of refractile foreign material morphologically consistent with silicone. In selected cases, Fourier transform infrared spectroscopy was used to confirm the identity of the foreign material as silicone. The finding of silicone droplets in the washing was corroborated by the finding of silicone in the corresponding capsular tissues. Silicone droplets were observed with gel filled implants, even those with intact elastomer shells at the time of surgery.

Of note, the silicone in the capsular spaces was noted in two forms: intracellular and extracellular. In many cases most silicone droplets were intracellular. The cells containing the silicone were mononuclear macrophage type cells with reduced nuclear cytoplasmic ratios due to the presence of numerous cytoplasmic vacuoles containing droplets of water clear refractile foreign material. In some cases, variable amounts of extracellular silicone were observed. The extracellular silicone droplets were surrounded by amphophilic, amorphous material with the appearance of protein (Fig. 1). In no cases were the extracellular droplets of silicone observed to be "bare" or unaccompanied by the protein.

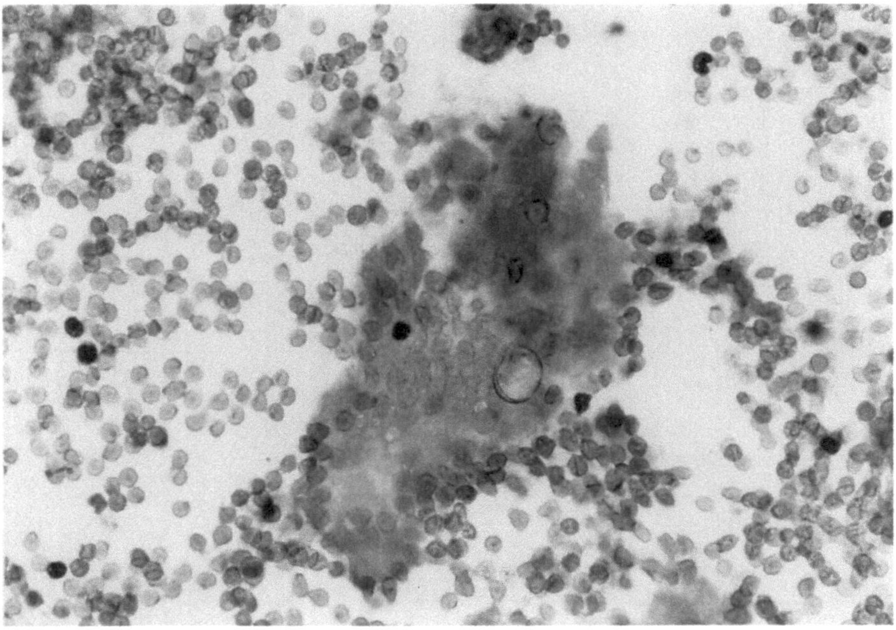

Fig.1 Capsular washing indicating the presence of silicone droplets surrounded by amorphous protein. Most of the cells present in the photomicrograph are red blood cells. A few lymphocytes with scant cytoplasm are present. In the center of the image a large amorphous "cloud" of proteinaceous material surrounds one large and numerous smaller refractile droplets of foreign material resembling silicone. Microscopically directed Fourier transform infrared spectroscopy confirmed that the foreign material seen was silicone. Papanicolaou stain at 400X.

In the patients with no silicone observed in the capsular space or in the implant related capsule (most frequently those with saline filled implants), the cellular constituents of the space were mixed inflammatory cells. Observed were lymphocytes, mononuclear macrophages (without conspicuous vacuoles), and occasional eosinophils and polymorphonuclear leukocytes. Stromal fibroblasts were also observed.

Capsule

The anatomy of the implant related capsule was observed to resemble that of synovial lined joint or bursal spaces. The capsular tissue was predominantly composed of mature collagen with a highly vascularized capillary network. The most superficial layer of cells were vacuolated mononuclear cells resembling those observed free in the capsular space. Often, amorphous proteinaceous material formed the surface of the capsule, and extracellular droplets of refractile foreign material were noted to be embedded there (Fig. 2). In other cases, vacuolated macrophages containing refractile droplets were the most common cell present. Surrounding the vessels of the capillary network were aggregates of mononuclear macrophages containing vacuoles of foreign material.

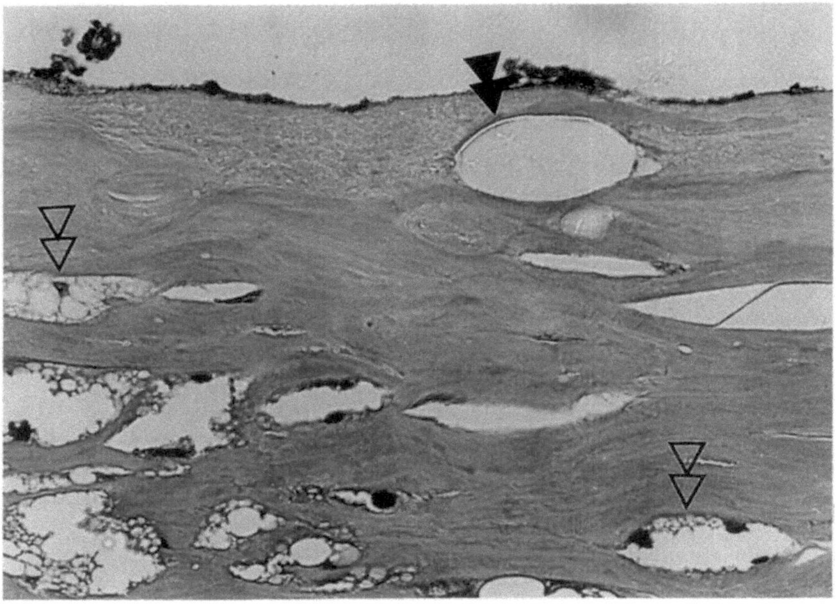

Fig 2 Implant related capsule. The capsule of a patient with silicone surrounded by amorphous protein from the capsular aspirate is shown. The most superficial aspect of the capsule is acellular, with large vacuoles of refractile foreign material surrounded by amorphous protein. This protein is not thought to represent mature collagen, because it is non-refractile and it does not polarize as does mature collagen. The solid arrow indicates the extracellular droplet of refractile foreign material. Most of the foreign material in the photomicrograph is intracellular. Two cells containing multiple vacuoles of refractile foreign material are indicated with hollow arrows. Hematoxylin and eosin at 400X.

In the capsules of textured implants, elastomer shell fragments or polyurethane fragments were incorporated into collagen layers. These shell fragments were usually irregular in shape, and were surrounded by multinucleate histiocytes. Capsules of some gel filled implants had particularly large aggregates of silicone surrounded by multinucleate histiocytes. These were seen deep to the capsule in some patients and were recognized as discrete masses or silicone granulomas. Occasionally lymphoid aggregates were observed just deep to the collagen layers of the capsule, but plasma cells were observed rarely.

Using special stains and transmission electron microscopy, the capsule was remarkable for the absence of a basement membrane or basal lamina. This anatomy allows mononuclear macrophage type cells to freely migrate from the surface to deep soft tissues. This anatomic structure is identical to that of synovium.

Regional Lymph Nodes

In patients with lymph nodes available for review, vacuolated histiocytes were not uncommon. They were usually noted in aggregates, and therefore stood out against a background of lymphocytes (Fig. 3). The histiocyte vacuoles contained refractile droplets of foreign material confirmed to be silicone by FTIR.

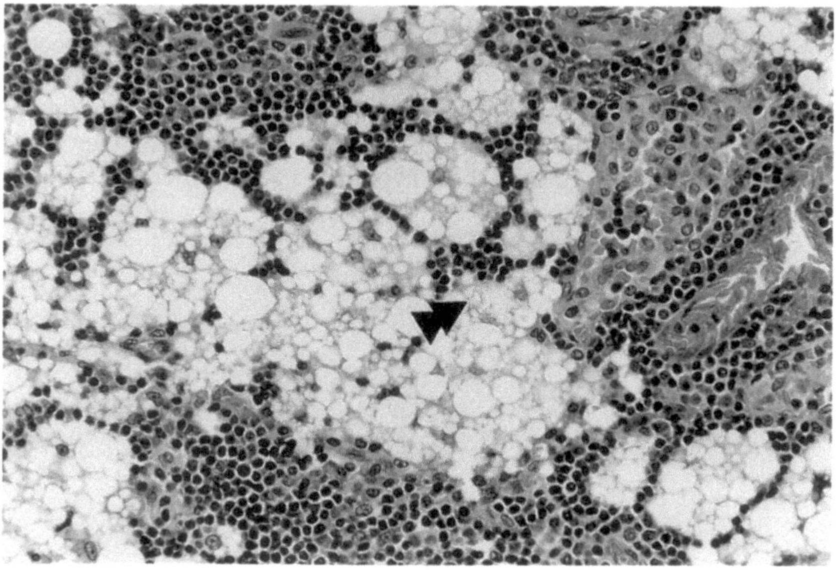

Fig.3 Regional lymph node
A regional lymph node from a patient with a gel filled prosthesis is shown. Large aggregates of foamy macrophages stand out in sharp contrast to the closely packed nuclei of the lymphocytes. The mononuclear macrophages have numerous, variable size round vacuoles expanding the cytoplasm. In some vacuoles remnant refractile foreign material is seen (arrow). This was confirmed to be silicone with FTIR.

Discussion

Breast implant related capsules are far different structurally than other wound healing tissues. They can be regarded as tissue adapted for processing of particulate matter. The specialized surface incorporates foreign materials which also are identified in deeper tissues (Emery et al. 1994b). Due to the absence of a basement membrane, basal lamina, and cell to cell junctions, there is no barrier to the migration of macrophages throughout the tissue. Macrophages move freely to the space surrounding the implant, ingest foreign particulate material, re-enter the tissue moving through capsular layers to subcapsular capillaries and to regional lymph nodes.

The ingestion of silicone by tissue macrophages does not constitute evidence for autoimmune disease related to silicone. For a foreign material such as silicone to stimulate the T-cells of the immune system, an antigen must be involved. It is unlikely that silicone per se is recognized as an antigen by T-cells since it is not composed of peptides or proteins. However, the observation that silicone droplets are surrounded by protein in the capsular space may indicate chemical interaction between silicone and protein. Silicone protein interactions are not unexpected due to the hydrophobicity of the polymer. Hydrophobic surfaces adsorb proteins. Available proteins in the capsular space include constituents of serum and extracellular matrix such as fibrinogen, fibronectin, collagen, immunoglobulin, and albumin.

Silicone protein complexes could have one or more activities with respect to the immune system. They could stimulate cytokine production by macrophages, result in chemical change or denaturation of a self protein or peptide, they could crosslink cell surface adhesion molecules, or they could have superantigen activity. Each of these hypotheses will be addressed (Fig.4).

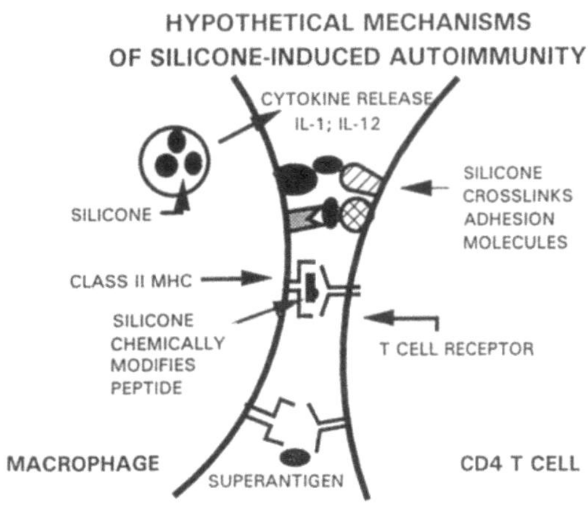

Fig.4 Illustrated hypotheses. Hypothetical interactions between macrophages which have ingested silicone and T-helper cells are illustrated. IL=interleukin, MHC=major histocompatibility complex

For antigens to be recognized by the immune system, they must be perceived by cell-surface receptors. T-cells do not "see" native or soluble antigens. T-cell receptors see antigen-peptide fragments derived through antigen processing and presentation via major histocompatibility complex molecules on macrophages. Complexes between silicone and self proteins could be ingested by tissue macrophages and mononuclear macrophages. Ingested materials come to reside in lysozomes where hydrolysis occurs under the influence of lysosomal enzymes. Small fragments of complexed foreign material and protein might then be available for antigen presentation to the T-cells.

In addition, silicone could stimulate macrophages to release cytokines such as IL-1 or IL-12. These cytokines could enhance an immune response by providing second signals to the T-cell thus preventing anergy to self antigens.

Silicone, known to adsorb proteins, could potentially crosslink adhesion molecules between the surfaces of macrophages and T-cells. This costimulatory signal could commit the T-cell to respond to an otherwise non-immunogenic self-antigen.

A final hypothesis to consider is that silicone or silicone-protein complex could act as a superantigen, crosslinking class II MHC and T-cell receptors. This would trigger recognition of a variety of non-specific antigens that could account for the multisystem ailments of some women with breast implants. Once an anti-self CD4 T-cell is triggered, a Th1 or Th2 response could ensue. Then an autoimmune humoral and/or cell mediated response would be possible.

These hypotheses require investigation which could provide the missing link between histopathologic observations reported here and human disease.

References

Bingham, H.G., Copeland, E.M., Hackett, R. and Caffee, H.H. (1988). Breast cancer in a patient with silicone breast implants after 13 years. Ann Plast Surg 20:236-237.

Caffee HH, Rotatori DS (1993) Intracapsular injection of triamcinolone for prevention of contracture. Plast Reconstr Surg 92:1073-1077

Emery JA, Spanier SS, Kasnic G, Hardt NS (1994a) The synovial structure of breast implant associated bursae. Mod Pathol 7:728-733.

Emery JA, Hardt NS, Caffee H, Spanier SS (1994b) Breast implant capsules share synovial transporting capabilities. Mod Pathol 7:15A.

Hardt NS, Yu LT, LaTorre G, Steinbach B (1994) Fourier transform infrared microscopy used to identify foreign materials related to breast implants. Mod Pathol 7:669-676.

Hardt NS, Yu LT, LaTorre G, Steinbach B (1995) Complications related to retained breast implant capsules. Plast Reconstr Surg 95:364-371

Hausner, R.J., Schoen, F.J., Pierson, K.K. (1978). Foreign body reaction to silicone gel in

axillary lymph nodes after augmentation mammaplasty. Plast Reconstr Surg 62: 381-384.
Silver R.M., Sahn, E.E., Allen J. A., Sahn, S., Greene, W., Maize, J.C., Garen, P.D. (1993). Demonstration of silicon in sites of connective tissue disease in patients with silicone-gel breast implants. Arch Derm 129: 63-68.
Tabatowski K., Elson, C.E., Johnston, W.W. (1990). Silicone lymphadenopathy in a patient with a mammary prosthesis. Acta Cytologica 34:10-14.

Acknowledgements

This work was supported in part by the University of Florida Department of Pathology and Laboratory Medicine Diagnostic Referral Laboratories and by the Plastic Surgery Education Foundation.

Microscopic Techniques and Histologic Findings in Silicone Mammary Implant Capsules and Regional Paranodal Tissues

D. R. Shanklin, M.D., FRSM [1,2] and D.L Smalley, Ph.D. [1]

University of Tennessee, Departments of [1]Pathology and [2]Obstetrics and Gynecology, Memphis, Tennessee 38163

The best known silicone medical devices are mammary implant prostheses. Capsular fibrosis is a common result after use of these devices. An acute inflammatory reaction occurs adjacent to silicone mammary implants shortly after insertion in experimental animals [1-3]. This is expected on the basis of surgical creation of an artificial tissue plane for the prosthesis independent of reaction to silicone by adjacent connective tissues. Vistnes et al. did not quantify the acute reaction after ten days, noting rather that it became minimal by 42 days [3]. The singular difference from a simple surgical plane without foreign material lies in the early formation of a planar capsule, which thickened only slightly with time in the absence of silicone spillage [3]. Vistnes et al. reported thicker capsules both early and late following prosthetic rupture [3]. We have seen few comparable early human tissues but clinical assessments [4-6] have been reported since 1965 [5], shortly after the introduction of silicone devices for human use. Moreover, cAMP as a chemical marker for acute inflammatory reaction has been found in both human and animal material [7]; experimental work has shown comparable cellular responses to intraperitoneal injection of silicones [8].

The 1991 Baltimore Symposium on Silicone in Medical Devices developed consensual frequencies for fully developed capsular fibrosis: 15 per cent with severe, often distorting contracture, 25 per cent with moderate, usually symptomatic, fibrosis, and 40 per cent with palpable induration, or 80 per cent overall [9]. Overt rupture of the devices is common, often after so-called closed capsulotomy [10-13]. Hidden rupture also occurs

Drs Shanklin and Smalley have served as expert witnesses in the past, mainly for claimants and have one active case in mediation. Funding of this and related work has been entirely internal.

[12-15]. Less well appreciated is that silicone gel bleeds from implants [16-19] and that after rupture bulk leakage may migrate to elsewhere in the body [20-23]. This report is to emphasize the microscopic methods which serve to identify and characterize silicone and crystalline silica in tissues post implantation [24,25].

Tissue and Photographic Methods

Tissue samples were received as previously prepared and stained microslides, unstained slides, or paraffin blocks. Sections were stained by hematoxylin and eosin in all instances: in selected cases reticulin stains were performed.

Slides were examined on a Leitz Ortholux microscope which has transmitted, incident, and ultraviolet light capacity. A polarizing filter above the stage operates through a sliding chase; the rotating initial filter is inserted below the condenser when desired. Dark field illumination is achieved by removing the transmission condenser unit and inserting the dark field condenser in its place. These basic attributes are usually found in comparable if more modern instruments.

Color photographic documentation was by the Leitz Orthomat photomicrographic camera integrated with the Ortholux microscope. Representative fields were photographed, usually on Ektachrome EPT 135-36 film (ASA = 160), with a machine setting of ASA 200, the nearest setting available on the timer. This has the effect of reducing exposure time by 20 per cent, which yields a sharper image. The principal alternate film used recently is Ektachrome EPJ 135-36 (ASA = 320; machine setting ASA 400), and infrequently, Kodachrome KPA 135-36, Type A (ASA = 40). Daylight film (Kodak Gold, ASA = 200) works well for screening prints but is less versatile. We found no effective differences in the resulting photographic images; the E-6 process films were chosen mainly because they could be processed locally on a 2-hour schedule. For uniform background color, a Tiffen Protar 82A blue filter (Series # 6) was used in all modalities: transmitted light and polarizing and dark field microscopy. Dark field orientation was confirmed by dropping the special condenser to the lowest position; this removes most of the optical effect, allowing clear field identification and orientation.

Black and white photographic prints were made from the 35 mm color transparencies by a custom photographic laboratory using 70 mm black and white internegatives. Occasionally, direct black and white prints were made using Kodak TMAX film (TMY 135-24, ASA = 400 or TMZ 135-36, ASA = 3200; the latter was possible because the Orthomat unit has a four power adjustment scale even though the nominal highest ASA rating available is 1600).

Identification of Silicone

Foreign material identifiable as silicone is seen in 90 per cent of capsules [26] [Figures 1-4] and in migratory sites [Figures 5-6]. This is mostly silicone gel with occasional fragmented sections of ruptured elastomer shell {Figure 7-8].

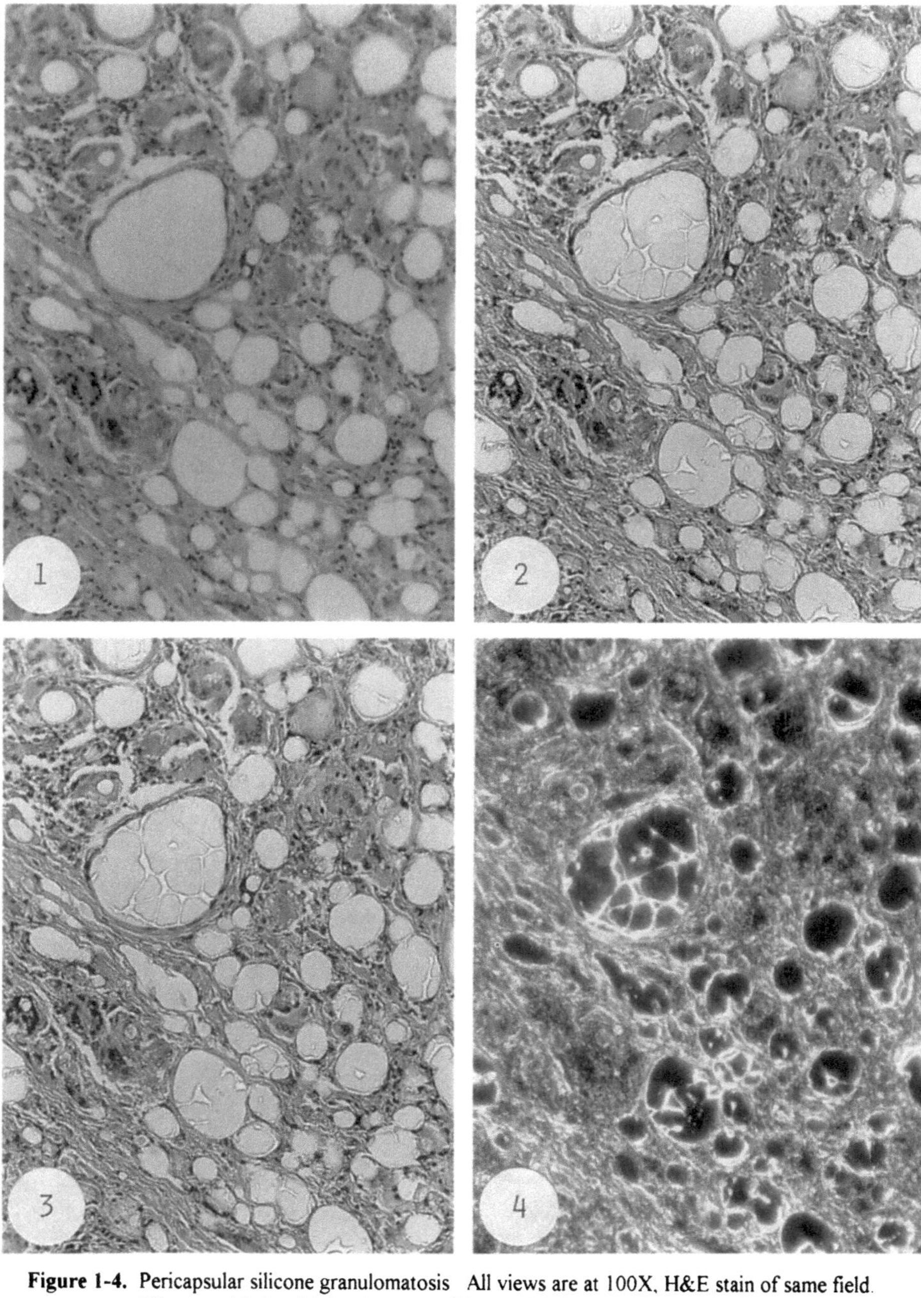

Figure 1-4. Pericapsular silicone granulomatosis All views are at 100X, H&E stain of same field. [1]: normal light with barely perceptible unstained material in largest follicle-like spaces. [2]: substage diaphragm nearly closed. [3]: substage condenser low. [4]: by dark field light. Adjusting either diaphragm or condenser or both adds significant refractility to the silicone; dark field shows bright white silicone gel in the spaces.

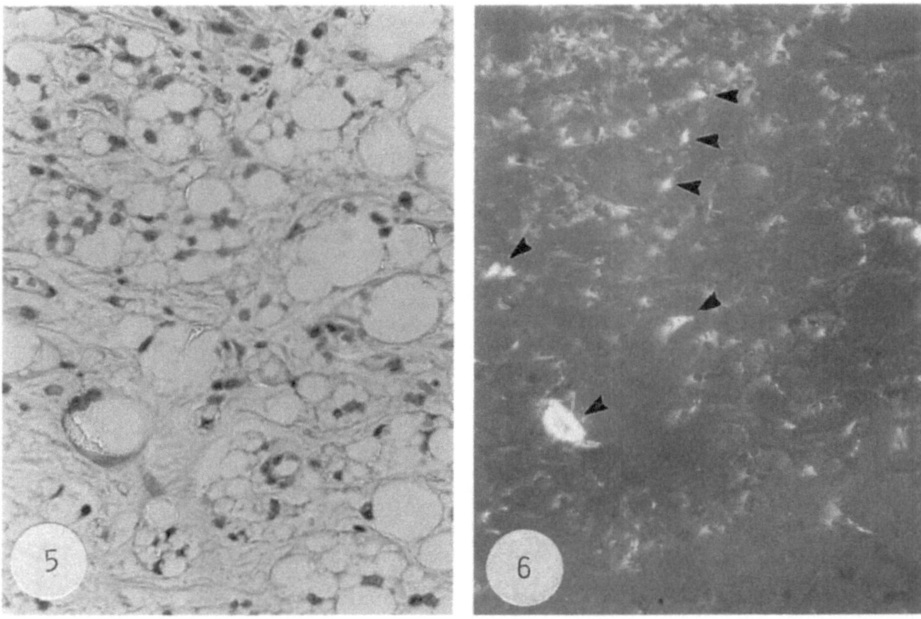

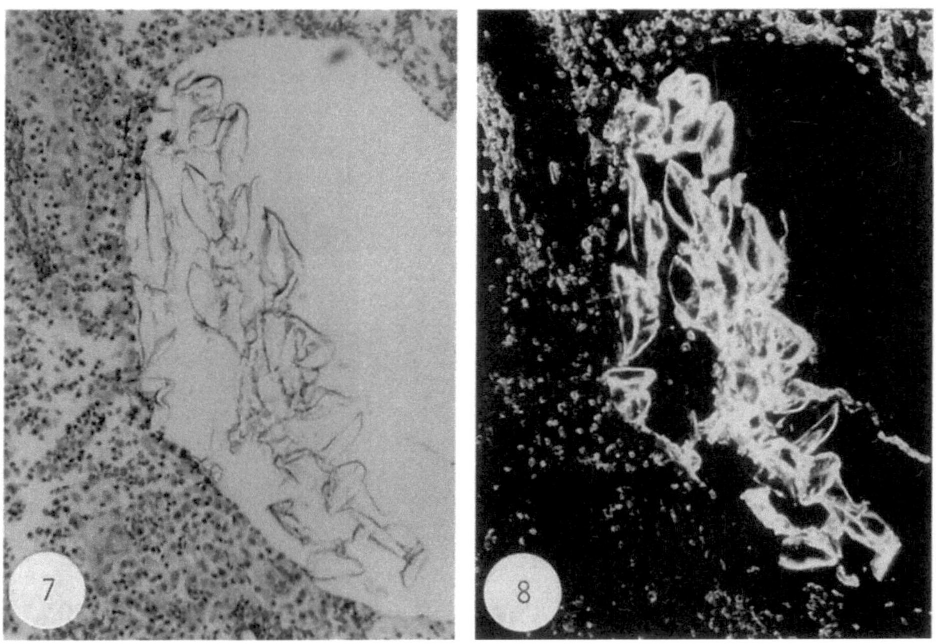

Figures 5-6. Nodular silicone mass in axilla near a lymph node (not shown). Both 200X, H&E stain, same field. [5]: normal light. [6] dark field shows brightened silicone deposits (arrows)

Figures 7-8. Folded, fragmented silicone elastomer shell after rupture trapped in highly cellular inflammatory reaction; both at 100X, H&E stain. [7]: normal light. [8]: dark field light.

Silicone does not stain with either hematoxylin or eosin, a trait shared by many foreign bodies. More importantly, silicone is not dissolved by ordinary tissue fixation or during processing of sections although it may be displaced or fragmented by the microtome. Accordingly, this alien material remains and is readily shown by manipulation of the microscope light source either by lowering the condenser or reducing the aperture of the substage diaphragm or both. These adjustments provide a refractile image with the edges and internal structure often quite dramatically shown. The use of dark field microscopy greatly enhances identification of silicone [27] [Figure 9].

Cellular Findings

Study of more than 350 tissue specimens, total and subtotal capsulectomies, excisions of silicone granulomas, and other biopsies including axillary lymph nodes, indicates a wide range of cellular and tissue reaction, in part dependent on adequacy of tissue samples [26]. Capsular tissue sections contained findings indicative of both local inflammatory and immunological processing. Immune processing is through memory T-lymphocyte cellular responses with a high index of affinity in symptomatic cases [28]. The specific cellular stimulant is silica [28].

The periprosthetic capsule shows thick, hypermature scar (74 per cent of samples), lymphocytic infiltration (90 per cent), focal and florid granulomatosis (63 per cent), and much less often, a few plasmacytes and eosinophils. The quantitative relationships between lymphocytes, granulomas, and silicone in tissue is described in more complete detail elsewhere [26]. Briefly, there is high correlation between lymphocytic response and subsequent granuloma formation [26]. These and other samples showed progressively maturing collagen and some reticulin, lymphocytes, plasmacytes, and macrophages, indicative of an immunopathic process directed back at the capsular tissues themselves. Vistnes et al. described enhancement of elastin in the capsules [3]; we have not examined our material for elastin.

Correlation of Silicone and Cellular Responses

Bulk deposits of silicone, from rupture of mammary prostheses, are strongly correlated with granuloma formation [26]. We found 30 cases with bulk deposits of silicone out of 121 examined for this finding; all had granuloma formation, whereas lesser amounts of silicone were associated with granulomas in 42 out of 79 cases in the same substudy (53.2 per cent) [26]. The bulk deposits are often several millimeters across even after much fragmentation during granuloma formation [Figures 1-4].

Identification of Crystalline Silica

The other principal readily identifiable foreign material in periprosthetic and other tissues in these patients is crystalline silica. An important limitation on optical

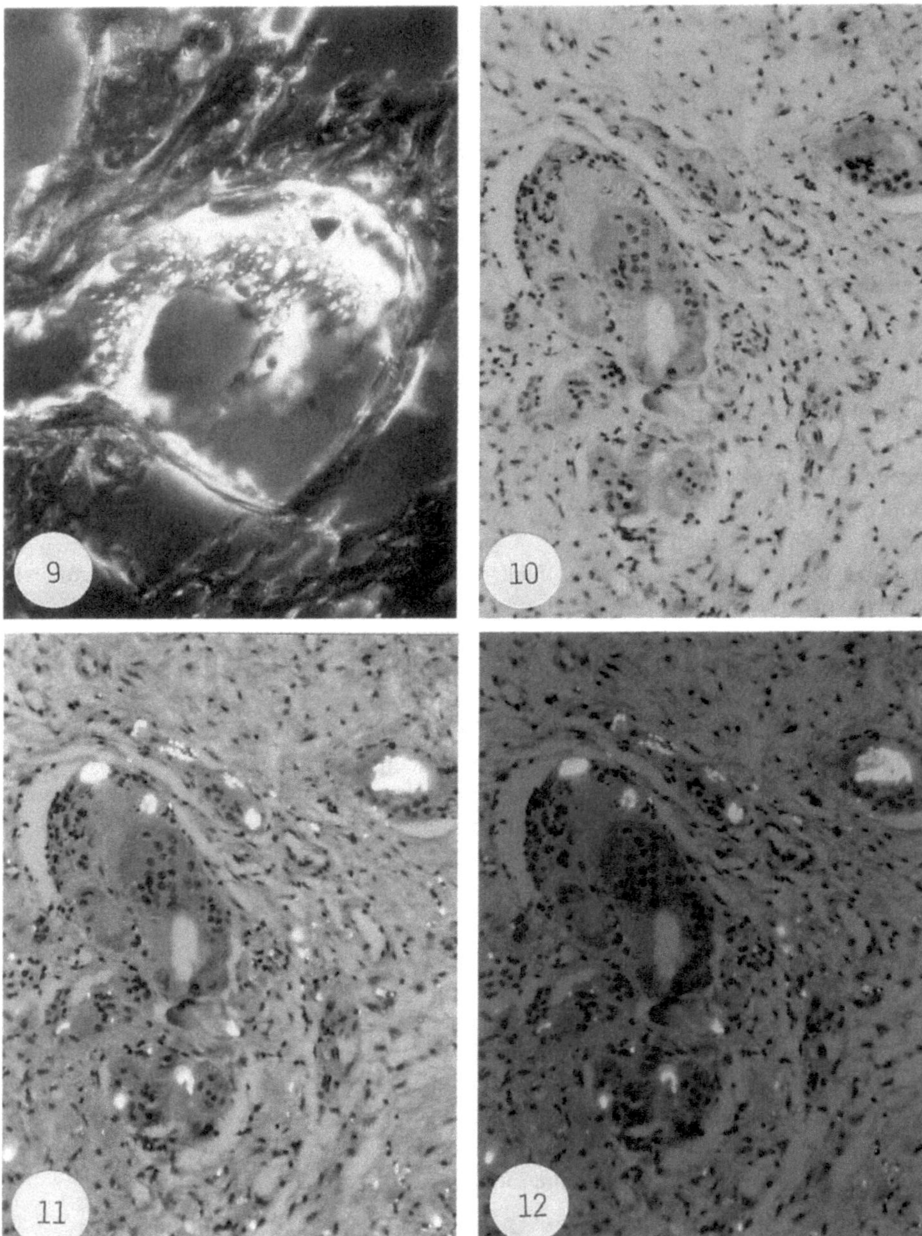

Figure 9. Complex globule of silicone gel, dark field microscopy. 200X H&E. The inner detail of a large globule is well shown. **Figures 10-12.** Polarization of capsular granulomas, same field, 100X, H&E. [10]: normal light. [11]: 45° polarization. [12]: 90° polarization. Full polarization reveals an extensive, complex deposit. Granulomatous silica in periprosthetic capsules is capsular silicosis, diagnostically.

characterization comes from the fact that polarizing microscopy identifies only the crystalline form of silica [29] [Figures 10-12]. Review of two different sets of our material for polarizable crystalloid silica yielded frequencies of 76.2 and 86.7 per cent, rates only slightly lower than those for silicone. Additionally, there is experimental [30], clinicopathologic [31,32], and immunologic evidence [33] that amorphous and fumed amorphous silica are closely if not equally reactive. Presently, the evidence of a pivotal role of silica comes from the demonstration of memory T lymphocytic reactivity [28] which is more sensitive than available means of microscopic identification. What is needed is a method for quantitative estimation of total capsular silica.

Comment

Some 26 per cent of case material has less than thick, hypermature fibrous capsular scar [26]; variations within the samples from individual patients were such that some of the samples in this 26 per cent were there due to the random means by which such materials came to us. Some of the lesser capsules had relatively less cellular reaction but these had rather more mineralization which accounted for 15.7 per of the whole [26]. Accordingly, our samples from mammary capsular region showed the prosthetic:patient interface to consist of cellular fibrous scar, confirming other reports [34-42].

These results are not surprising from a physicochemical perspective [43]; silica does not exist as free molecular silicon dioxide but in tetrahedral matrices of varying density [43]. Amorphous silica is simply a looser matrix of tetrahedra, with a density approximately 83 per cent of α-quartz, the most dense of the polarizable tetrahedral crystalline silicas [43]. Silica, of course, is a noteworthy sclerogen productive of massive fibrotic lesions in the upper lobes in inhalant pulmonary silicosis [44].

References

1. Rees TD, Ballantyne DL, Seidman L, Hawthorne GA (1967) Visceral response to subcutaneous and intraperitoneal injections of silicone in mice Plast Reconstr Surg 39.402-410
2. Rigdon RH, Dricks A (1975) Reaction associated with a silicone rubber gel: an experimental study J Biomed Mater Res 9:645-659
3. Vistnes L, Bentley JW, Fogarty DC (1977) Experimental study of tissue response to ruptured gel-filled mammary prostheses Plast Reconstr Surg 59 31-34
4. Burkhardt BR, Dempsey PD, Schnur PL, Tofield JJ (1986) Capsular contracture: a prospective study of the effects of local antibacterial agents Plast Reconstr Surg 77:919-930
5. Rees TD, Platt JM, Ballantyne DL (1965) An investigation of cutaneous response to dimethylpolysiloxane (silicone liquid) in animals and human--a preliminary report Plast Reconstr Surg 35 131-139
6. Rushton DN, Brindley GS, Polkey CE, Browning GV (1989) Implant infections and antibiotic-impregnated silicone rubber coating J Neurol Neurosurg Psychiat 52 223-229
7. Faga A, Merlino M (1985) cAMP levels in reactive tissues around dimethylpolysiloxane solid implants. Plast Reconstr Surg 76 570-573
8. Champion R, Faulborn J, Bowald S, Erb P (1987) Peritoneal reaction to liquid silicone: an experimental study Graefes Arch Clin Exp Ophthalmol 225:141-145

9. Stratmeyer ME (1991) ed., Silicone in medical devices, HHS Publication FDA 92-4249, Rockville, Maryland, 330 p.
10. de Camara DL, Sheridan JM, Kammer BA (1993) Rupture and aging of silicone gel breast implants. Plast Reconstr Surg 91:828-836
11. Dowden RV (1993) Detection of gel implant rupture: a clinical test. Plast Reconstr Surg 91:548-550
12. Levine RA, Collins TL (1991) Definitive diagnosis of breast implant rupture by ultrasonography. Plast Reconstr Surg 87:1126-1128
13. Rosculet KA, Ikeda DM, Forrest ME, Oneal RM, Rubin JM, Jeffries DO, Helvie MA (1992) Ruptured gel-filled silicone breast implants: sonographic findings in 19 cases. Amer J Roentgenol 159:711-716
14. Brem RF, Tempany CM, Zerhouni EA (1992) MR detection of breast implant rupture. J Comput Assist Tmogr 16:157-159
15. Harris KM, Ganott MA, Shestak KC, Losken HW, Tobon H (1993) Silicone implant rupture: detection with US. Radiology 187:761-768
16. Barker DE, Retsky M, Schulz SL (1981) The new low bleed mammary prosthesis: an experimental study in mice. Aesth Plast Surg 5:85-91
17. Barker DE, Retsky M, Searles SL (1985) New low-bleed implant--silastic II. Aesth Plast Surg 9:39-41
18. Caffee HH (1986) The influence of silicone bleed on capsule contracture. Ann Plast Surg 17:284-287
19. Cohen IK (1984) Leakage of breast prostheses. Arch Surg 119:615 (letter)
20. Bilbey JH, Connell DG (1993) MRI diagnosis of a ruptured breast implant presenting as an infra-clavicular mass. Can Ass Radiol J 44:224-226
21. Leibman AJ, Kossoff MB, Kruse BD (1992) Intraductal extension of silicone from a ruptured breast implant. Plast Reconstr Surg 89:546-547
22. Sanger JR, Kolachalam R, Komorowski RA, Yousif NJ, Maltoub HS (1991) Silicone gel extravasation into the arm: a clinical and experimental correlation of the effect on peripheral nerve, in: Stratmeyer ME, ed. Silicone in medical devices, HHS Publication FDA 92-4249, Rockville, Maryland, pp. 69-76
23. Taupmann RE, Adler S (1993) Silicone pleural effusion due to iatrogenic breast implant rupture. South med J 86:570-571
24. Shanklin DR (1991) Late tissue reactions to silicone and silica: the natural history of silicone-associated diseases with special reference to infections and immunological markers in tissue, in: Stratmeyer ME, ed., Silicone in medical devices, HHS Publication FDA 92-4249, Rockville, Mary-land, pp. 103-125
25. Shanklin DR (1993) Silicone-associated diseases: tissue findings. South Med J 86:S104 (abstract)
26. Shanklin DR, Smalley DL (1995) Quantitative aspects of cellular responses to silicone. Int J Occup Med Toxicol 4:99-111
27. Thomassen RW, Howbert JP, Thompson SW (1960) Transparent colorless emboli associated with dimethylsiloxane as demonstrated by phase microscopy and darkfield illumination. J Histochem Cytochem 8:2-3
28. Smalley DL, Shanklin DR, Hall MF, Stevens MV, Hanissian A (1995) Immunologic stimulation of T lymphocytes by silica after use of silicone mammary implants. FASEB J 9:424-427
29. Goldsmith S, Kopeloff A (1961) Use of polarized-light microscopy as an aid in the diagnosis of silicosis. New Engl J Med 265:233-235
30. Schepers GWH, Durkan TM, Delahant AB, Creedon FT, Redlin AJ (1957) The biological action of Degussa submicron amorphous silica dust (Dow Corning silica). AMA Arch Indus Health 16:125-146
31. Vitums VC, Edwards MJ, Niles NR, Borman JO, Lowry RD (1977) Pulmonary fibrosis from amorphous silica dust, a product of silica vapor. Arch Environ Health 32:62-68
32. Philippou S, Teschler H, Morgenroth K (1992) Lungenfibrose durch Inhalation von amorpher Kieselsaure [Lung fibrosis after inhalation of amorphous silica]. Zentralbl Pathol 138:41-46

33. Shanklin DR, Smalley DL, Hall MF, Stevens MV (1995) T cell-mediated immune response to silica in silicone breast implant patients. Curr Topic Microbiol Immunol
34 Asplund O (1984) Capsular contracture in silicone gel and saline-filled breast implants after reconstruction. Plast Reconstr Surg 73 270-275
35. Brantley SK, Davidson SF, Johnson MB, St. Arnold PB, Das SK (1990) The effects of prior exposure to silicone on capsule formation, histology and pressure. Ann Plast Surg 25:44-47
36. Moufarrege R, Beauregard G, Bosse JP, Papillon J, Perras C (1987) Outcome of mammary capsulotomies. Ann Plast Surg 19:62-64
37. Rudolph R, Abraham J, Vecchione T, Guber S, Woodward M (1978) Myofibroblasts and free silicon around breast implants. Plast Reconstr Surg 62:185-196
38. Thomsen JL, Christensen L, Nielsen M, Brandt B, Breiting VB, Felby S, Nielsen E (1990) Histologic changes and silicone concentrations in human breast tissue surrounding silicone breast prostheses. Plast Reconstr Surg 85:38-41
39 Ravis WD, Balogh K, Abraham JL (1985) Silicone granulomas. report of three cases and review of the literature Human Pathol 16.19-27
40 Troum OM, Mongan ES, Brody GS, Gray JD, Quismorio FP (1987) Immunological function of patients with augmentation mammoplasty (AM). Arthritis Rheum 30:S107 (abstract D96)
41. Wagner H, Beller FK, Pfautsch M (1977) Electron and light microscopy examination of capsules around breast implants. Plast Reconstr Surg 60:49-55
42. Wickham MG, Rudolph R, Abraham J (1978) Silicon identification in prosthesis-associated fibrous capsules Science 199:437-439
43 Bergna HE (1994) Colloid chemistry of silica, an overview, in Bergna HE ed. The colloid chemistry of silica, Amer Chem Soc, Washington DC pp 1-47, especially pp 2-6
44. Ziskind M, Jones RN, Weill H (1976) Silicosis. Amer Rev Res Dis 113.643-665

Autoimmune Antibodies

Antinuclear Antibodies in Apparently Healthy Women with Breast Implants

H. N. Claman, M.D., and A. D. Robertson, Ph.D.
University of Colorado Health Sciences Center, Denver, Colorado USA

There has been much controversy about whether women with breast implants are at increased risk for autoimmune disease, particularly scleroderma [1-7]. Associations between breast implants and autoimmunity have been asserted [8-10] and denied [11-14]. We performed a cross-sectional analysis of two cohorts of women with breast implants who considered themselves healthy together with suitable controls. A serum test for antinuclear antibodies (ANA) was the laboratory marker studied.

Patients and Methods

Women with breast implants were recruited to a special Breast Implant Evaluation Clinic primarily through word of mouth and through the news media. Each woman filled out a detailed questionnaire concerning their implant history and a history of possible illnesses, signs, symptoms and concurrent medications. Each woman had a physical examination by a physician. This report only concerns women with implants who considered themselves healthy; they came to the clinic requesting information about implants. This group is called group 1/0 (meaning the presence of implants = 1 and no symptoms = 0).

Control women were recruited by notices placed in the University Hospital. We requested women without implants who considered themselves healthy. This group is called group 0/0 (meaning no implants = 0 and no symptoms = 0). These women also filled out a questionnaire and had a brief physical examination by a physician.

Two sequential studies were performed and there was no overlap in patients. The results in patients in Study A (the first study) have been published previously [15]. Because the results in these women were unexpected, we decided to repeat the study with new groups of implanted and control women. This is Study B. The full results of Study B are incorporated into a separate paper which is being prepared for publication. Study A and Study B each include additional symptomatic patients, but the purpose here is only to compare the ANA prevalence in two sequential cohorts of apparently healthy women with implants and controls.

Study A had 19 healthy volunteers (=group 0/0) and 38 women with breast implants who felt well (=group 1/0). ANA tests were done at a University-based laboratory. Tests were performed at dilutions of 1:16, 1:64, 1:256, 1:512, etc. A test must have shown staining 1+ at 1:256 to be considered positive in this laboratory. "Trace" readings were ignored.

Study B had 18 healthy volunteers (=group 0/0) and 37 women with breast implants who felt well (=group 1/0). ANA tests were done at a University-affiliated laboratory separate from the laboratory used in Study A. Tests were performed at dilutions of 1:40, 1:80, 1:160, etc. In this laboratory, a test must have shown staining 1+ at a dilution of 1:80 to be considered positive. "Trace" readings were ignored.

In each laboratory, the ANA test was done by indirect immunofluorescence using Hep-2 cells as substrate. In all cases, the laboratory technicians were unaware of the patient's status.

Results (Table 1)

In each study, approximately three-quarters of the women were implanted for cosmetic reasons and the rest had reconstruction. About 90% of the implants were silicone gel or double lumen.

In Study A, women with implants who felt well had an 18% prevalence of a positive ANA test compared to 0% in controls ($p<0.05$). Study B, with different women and a different ANA laboratory, showed that women with implants who felt well had a 35% prevalence of a positive ANA test compared to 6% in controls ($p=0.02$).

As the methods used in the two studies appeared comparable, we combined the results, showing that 27% of 75 apparently healthy women with implants had a positive ANA test compared with 3% in controls ($p=0.002$).

In each study there was no correlation between ANA positivity and patient age, type of implant (saline or silicone gel), or indication for implantation (i.e. cosmesis vs. reconstruction).

Table 1. ANA Tests in Apparently Healthy Women with Implants and in Controls.

Group	Clinical Characteristic	Subjects, Number	Age (yr.) mean ± SD	ANA Positive
		Study A		
0/0	No implants, healthy	19	38.8 ± 8.5	0%
1/0	Implants, healthy	38	45.2 ± 9.0	18%*
		Study B		
0/0	No implants, healthy	18	39.0 ± 7.0	6%
1/0	Implants, healthy	37	45.0 ± 12.0	35%**
		Studies A + B Combined		
0/0	No implants, healthy	37		3%
1/0	Implants, healthy	75		27%***

*p=<0.05 **p=0.02 ***p=0.002

Discussion

Biologic effects of silicone products were discussed at length at the March, 1995, symposium at the National Institutes of Health, and many of these papers are included in this volume. Silicone is doubtless less inert than was believed in the past. How relevant the bioactivity of silicone may be to the question of autoimmune disease is not answered at the moment.

The experimental observations that silicone gel can act as an immunologic adjuvant for antibody production in rats [16] indicates that silicone can stimulate the immune system. In a special strain of mice, silicone gel can induce plasmacytomas [17]. It is not yet clear that these observations are relevant to women with implants of various kinds, although all breast implants have silicone in the capsule if not in the lumen.

Our cross-sectional studies of the prevalence of antinuclear antibodies in women with implants who feel well is one of the very few studies which are not retrospective and which appear to be free of ascertainment bias, as none of the women (controls or implanted subjects) had had a previous ANA and none considered themselves to be ill. Furthermore, the two studies were independent as each concerned different groups of women and the ANA tests were done in different laboratories. Therefore the fact that the findings were similar, namely that implanted women had a significantly higher prevalence of positive ANA tests, lends credence to the concept that this is a meaningful and not a chance result.

The ANA titers were in what might be considered to be moderate or low range for the laboratories concerned; and the ANA patterns were, in general, speckled and not strongly suggestive of any particular autoimmune syndrome.

Lastly, one is faced with the question "What is the biologic significance of a positive ANA test in an apparently healthy woman?" This question is not easy to answer, as ANA tests are not usually run on healthy women. One follow-up study of asymptomatic women with positive ANA tests indicated that in five years following the discovery of antinuclear antibodies, 12% developed signs or symptoms suggestive of autoimmunity [18]. Other data from years ago found that there was a considerable risk of developing SLE or "questionable connective tissue disease" in women (but not men) found to have a chronic biologic false positive (BFP) test for syphilis [19]. As many consider that a BFP test is a serological indication of autoimmunity (but not necessarily of autoimmune disease), a positive ANA in implanted women may possibly be a harbinger of disease itself in the future. In any case, only careful follow-up studies will answer the question, and it is an important question. One hopes that the current climate of medicolegal activity will calm down so that such studies can be done.

Acknowledgments

We wish to thank Drs. Lawrence Ketch, and Richard Hamman, Ms. Susie Stutsman and the staffs of the Adult CRC and UCHSC Breast Center for their assistance, and Ms. Kathryn Utschinski for preparing the manuscript.

Supported in part by NIH AI-34592, NIH RR-00051, and by Dow Corning, Inc.

References

1. Baldwin CM, Kaplan EN (1983) Silicone-induced human adjuvant disease? Ann Plast Surg 10:270-273
2. Sergott TJ, Limoli JP, Baldwin Jr. CM, et al (1986) Human adjuvant disease, possible autoimmune disease after silicone implantation: A review of the literature, case studies, and speculation for the future. Plast Reconstr Surg 78:104-114
3. Endo LP, Edwards NL, Longley S, Corman LC, Panush RS (1987) Silicone and rheumatic diseases. Arthritis Rheum 17:112-118
4. Fock K, Feng P, Tey B (1984) Autoimmune disease developing after augmentation mammoplasty: Report of three cases. J Rheumatol 11:98-100
5. Varga J, Heiman-Patterson TD, Emery DL, Griffin R, Lally EV, Uitto JJ, Jimenez SA (1990) Clinical spectrum of the systemic manifestations of the eosinophilia-myalgia syndrome. Semin Arthritis Rheum 19:313-328
6. Press RI, Peebles CL, Kumagai Y, Ochs RL, Tan EM (1992) Antinuclear autoantibodies in women with silicone breast implants. Lancet 340:1304-1307
7. Bridges AJ, Conley C, Wang G, Burnes DE, Vasey FB (1993) A clinical and immunologic evaluation of women with silicone breast implants and symptoms of rheumatic disease. Ann Int Med 118:929-936
8. Brozena SJ, Fenske NA, Cruse CW, et al (1988) Human adjuvant disease following augmentation mammoplasty. Arch Dermatol 124:1383-1386
9. Gutierrez F, Espinoza LR (1990) Progressive systemic sclerosis complicated by severe hypertension: Reversal after silicone implant removal. Am J Med 89:390-392
10. Kumagai Y, Shiokawa Y, Medsger Jr. TA, Rodnan GP (1984) Clinical spectrum of connective tissue disease after cosmetic surgery: Observation on 18 patients and a review of the Japanese literature. Arthritis Rheum 27:1-12
11. Shons AR, Schubert W (1992) Silicone breast implants and immune disease. Ann Plast Surg 28:491-501
12. Peters W, Keystone E, Snow K, Rubin L, Smith D (1994) Is there a relationship between autoantibodies and silicone-gel implants? Ann Plast Surg 32:1-7
13. Gabriel SE, O'Fallon WM, Kurland LT, Beard CM, Woods JE, Melton III LJ (1994) Risk of connective-tissue diseases and other disorders after breast implantation. N Engl J Med 330:1697-1702
14. Sanchez-Guerrero J, Schur PH, Sergent JS, Liang MH (1994) Silicone breast implants and rheumatic disease: clinical, immunologic, and epidemiologic studies. Arthritis Rheum 37:158-168
15. Claman HN, Robertson AD (1994) Antinuclear antibodies and breast implants. West J Med 160:225-228
16. Naim JO, Lanzafame RJ, van Oss CJ (1993) The adjuvant effect of silicone-gel on antibody formation in rats. Immunological Investigations 22:151-161
17. Potter M, Morrison S, Wiener F, Zhang XK, Miller FW (1994) Induction of plasmacytomas with silicone gel in genetically susceptible strains of mice. J Natl Cancer Inst 86:1058-1065
18. Yadin O, Sarov B, Naggan L, Slor H, Schoenfeld Y (1989) Natural autoantibodies in the serum of healthy women - a five-year follow-up. Clin Exp Immunol 75:402-406
19. Moore JE, Lutz WO (1955) Natural history of systemic lupus erythematosus: an approach to its study through chronic biologic false-positive reactors. J Chron Dis 1:297

Silicone Binding Immunoglobulins in Human Sera

N.R. Rose[1,2‡], M. Landavere[1,2] and R.C. Kuppers[2¶]
Departments of [1]Pathology and of [2]Molecular Microbiology and Immunology, The Johns Hopkins Medical Institutions, Baltimore, Maryland 21205

Abstract

We have evaluated two recently published test procedures for demonstrating antibodies to silicone. Positive control serum samples provided to us by the original authors were positive in our hands, using the methods described. However, serum samples from patients with certain connective tissue diseases but no history of silicone implants were also positive. The question of silicone-specific antibodies remains unresolved.

Introduction

Silicone compounds are widely used to make medical implants and prostheses because they are generally believed to be non-antigenic. Two reports have recently appeared, however, suggesting that antibodies to silicone may appear in individuals who have long-standing silicone implants, including ventricular peritoneal shunts and breast implants [1,2]. The demonstration of antibodies to silicone is complicated by the hydrophobic properties of silicones and the consequent propensity of many serum proteins to adhere non-specifically to silicone surfaces (van Oss; Butler; Kossovsky; in this volume). In order to elucidate the situation, we evaluated two enzyme-linked immunosorbent assays (ELISAs) to demonstrate silicone-specific antibodies described in the recent literature. We tested the sera of women with silicone breast implants who had various symptoms of connective tissue disease (CTD), implanted women with no symptoms, in men and women with CTD symptoms but no implants, and individuals with neither implants nor symptoms.

Materials and Methods

To repeat the method of Wolf *et al.* [1], we obtained coded serum samples, coated ELISA plates, and buffers through the gracious cooperation of Dr. E.G. Ezrailson (Emerald Biomedical Sciences Inc., The Woodlands, TX). The test was carried out exactly following the protocol provided by the company.

The second test procedure was based on that of Goldblum *et al.* [2]. Dr. Goldblum kindly provided three positive serum samples. Initially, the test was carried out exactly as described by these authors, using Silastic tubing. Later, the test was modified as follows. Using an Osborne ¼" punch (Harreson, NJ), silicone disks were cut from sheets of elastomer obtained from Dow Corning (Q7-2383). These disks were then firmly fitted to the bottom of the wells of an Immulon 2 ELISA plate. In repeated tests for leaking, no dye was found seeping between the elastomer and the sides of the wells after 48 hours incubation. The plates were then checked for consistency by measuring absorption in an ELISA plate reader at 450 nm. The mean absorbance was 0.220 ± 0.010 (variation 4.6% or less). The plates were blocked by using 100 µl of 0.05% Tween 20 in phosphate-buffered saline (PBS) for 30 minutes. The blocking solution was removed, the plates were tapped dry, and 100 µl of serum, diluted 1:250 in the blocking buffer, were added to triplicate wells and allowed to incubate for 2 hours. The plates were then washed 5 times with the blocking buffer, using a Skatron automated plate washer adjusted to compensate for the thickness of the elastomer. Goat anti-human IgG (Jackson Immunoresearch Laboratories), 100 µl, diluted 1:10,000, was added to each well for 2 hours. The plates were then washed as before and TMB substrate (KPL), 100 µl added to each well. Plates were read on an ELISA reader at intervals at 6301 nm. Positive and negative control sera were run on each plate. The following formula was used to adjust for plate variations:

$$100/(\text{Positive Control OD}) = X/\text{sample OD}.$$

Serum Samples

Serum samples from women with various symptoms were obtained from Drs. Stanley Klatsky (Johns Hopkins University), Vernon Young (Washington University, St. Louis, MO), and Arch Miller (Tulsa, OK). Serum samples from patients with connective tissue diseases but no history of implantation were obtained from Dr. Grant Anhalt (Johns Hopkins University) and Dr. Gerald Miller (Tulsa, OK). Normal sera were obtained from employees of our own department.

Results

Wolf *et al.* Procedure

Using materials provided to us by Dr. Ezrailson, we first attempted to repeat the results obtained by the Emerald Laboratories [1]. Tested in a blindfolded fashion, we found the absorbencies obtained in our laboratory were well within the accepted allowable limits of error of those obtained at Emerald (**Fig. 1**). These include high, medium and low control samples as well as 9 samples from the Emerald test series.

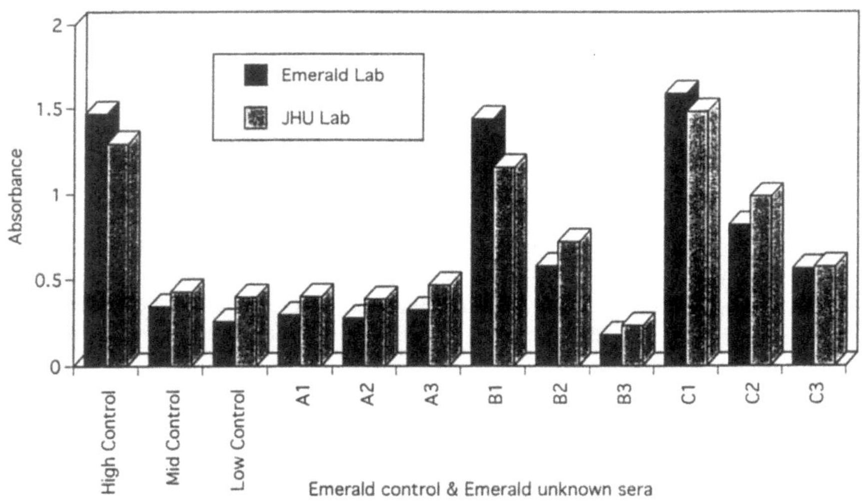

Fig. 1. ELISA method (Wolf *et al.* [1]). Comparison of results obtained by Emerald Laboratories with those obtained in our laboratory at Johns Hopkins University. Plates, reagents and serum samples were provided by Dr. Edward Ezrailson (Emerald Laboratories, Inc.) and tests were carried out in our laboratory in a blinded fashion. Absorbance values obtained by each laboratory are shown.

We next carried out tests using serum samples from individuals with CTD (**Fig. 2**). The high, medium and low control samples obtained from Emerald Laboratories again showed the expected absorbencies as did a sample of normal serum (D.F.) from our own institution. We found that two samples from patients with breast implants who had symptoms of CTD were strongly positive in the assay. Seven samples from patients with scleroderma and five from patients with lupus were tested on the same plates. Many of these serum samples were also strongly positive, giving absorbencies even greater than the high control sample.

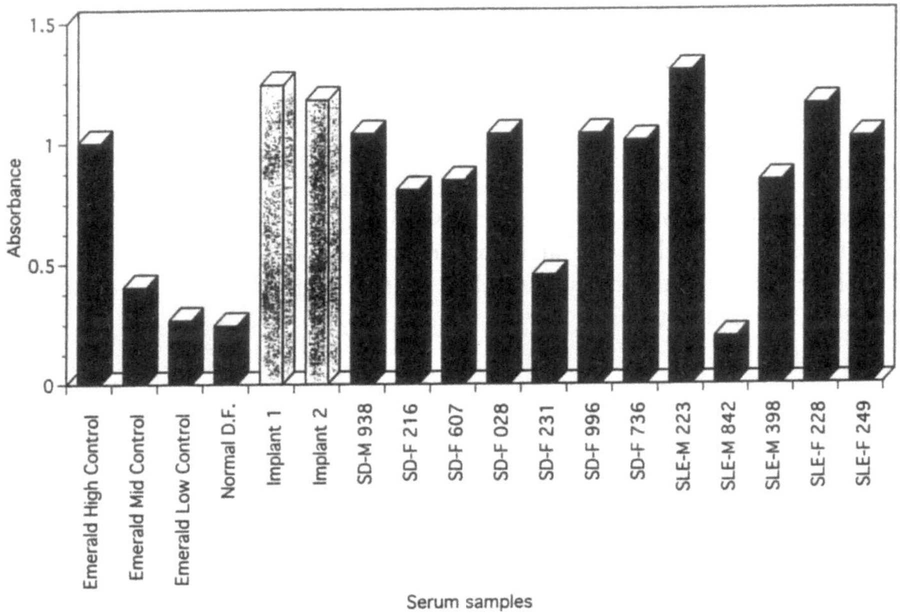

Fig. 2. ELISA method (Wolf *et al.* [1]), using kits provided by Dr. Ezrailson. High, medium and low controls were the same ones shown in Figure 1. Normal serum and two implant sera were taken from our own collection. The remaining sera came from patients diagnosed with CTD: SD = scleroderma; SLE = systemic lupus erythematosus; M = male patient; F = female patient.

Goldblum *et al.* Procedure

ELISAs were next set up to reproduce of the findings of Goldblum *et al.* [2]. In the first study, it was found that absorbencies were unacceptably high, using serum from a normal individual, if no blocking agent was used. We then compared three commonly used blocking agents, bovine serum albumen (BSA) (1%), condensed milk (2%), goat serum (1%) or Tween (0.5%). The best results were obtained using Tween as blocking agent. We, therefore, tested various concentrations of Tween and determined that the optimal concentration was 0.01%. This concentration was used in all washes. We also compared incubation times and found that 2 hours appeared to be optimal.

These investigations were carried out with measured pieces of Silastic tubing as originally described by Goldblum *et al.* However, the use of this material proved to be technically difficult, because the pieces of tubing did not remain in the wells during the washes. We, therefore, developed the method described in Materials and Methods, utilizing disks of silicone elastomer cut to fit tightly in the ELISA wells. In this way, we could carry out the various maneuvers with an automatic plate washer and reader. The results were reproducible with smaller standard deviations than obtained with the pieces of tubing (**Fig. 3**).

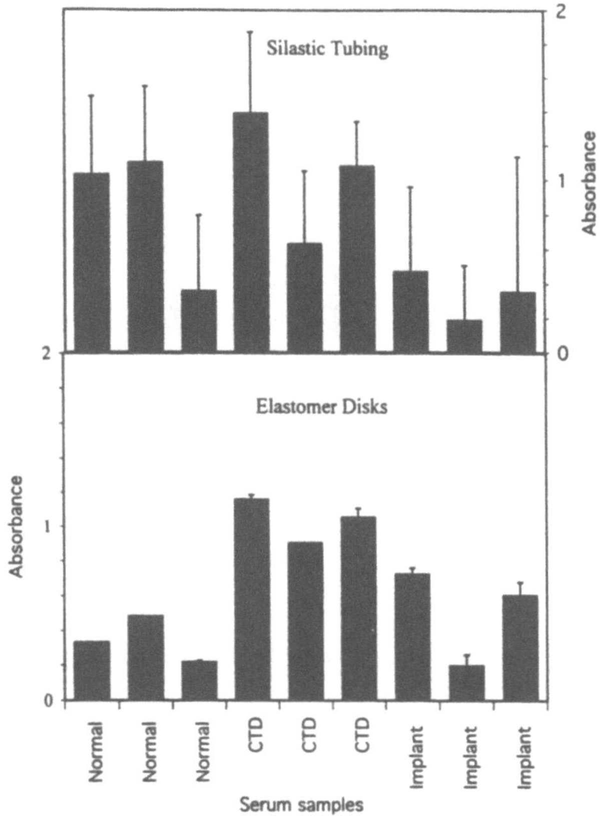

Fig. 3. ELISA method (Goldblum *et al.* [2]). Comparison of silastic tubing and elastomer disks. Methods are described in the text. Bars represent absorbance ± standard deviation.

Three serum samples sent to us by Dr. Goldblum were tested with this modified method (**Fig. 4**). Two samples gave high titers (absorbance >1.0) and one a medium titer (absorbance <1.0 >0.5). To estimate the precision of the method, we tested the same serum samples on three or four different occasions. The results are given in **Fig. 5** and show that the method is acceptably reproducible.

Using this modified method, we examined sera of individuals with and without breast implants and with and without symptoms of connective tissue disease. **Fig. 3** shows the results of one such test. Three normal samples gave low values, whereas two of the three sera from patients with implants were significantly elevated. In this test, all three samples from patients with CTD also showed elevated values.

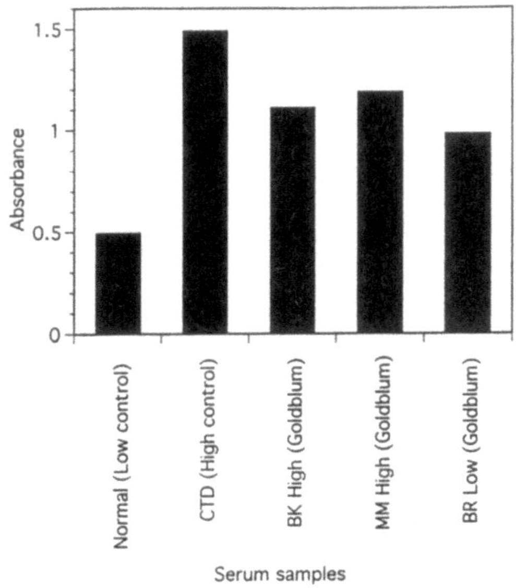

Fig. 4. Modified Goldblum ELISA method. Three standard sera were provided by Dr. Goldblum. CTD = connective tissue disease.

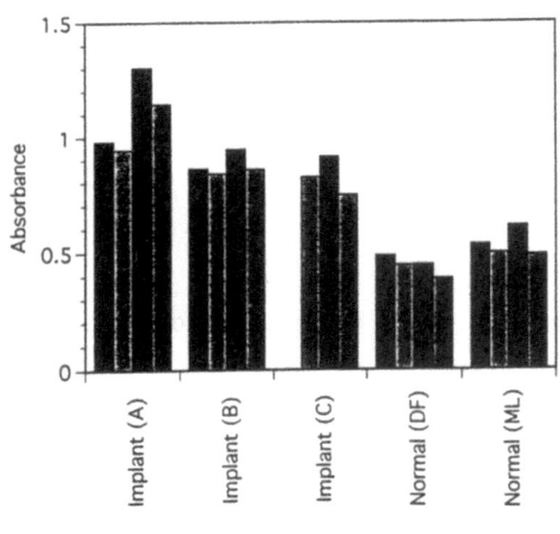

Fig. 5. Modified Goldblum ELISA method. Serum samples from three implant patients and two normal individuals were tested on three or four different occasions.

We then proceeded to compare a large number of serum samples from patients with CTD whom we could confirm had not had silicone implants and from patients with implants with or without symptoms of CTD (**Fig. 6**). Many sera from both populations gave high absorbance values, although the means was significantly higher with the CTD sera. Since a number of other laboratory tests had been carried out on the sera from patients with CTD, we were able to perform correlative studies. A significant correlation (R=0.43) was found between the titer of antinuclear antibody and silicone-binding immunoglobulin. The correlation was highly significant (P=0.006). A significant correlation was also found with the values for anti-SS/A (anti-Ro) of R=0.43, with a probability of P=0.007, but no correlation was obvious with anti-SS/B (anti-La) or anti-DNA.

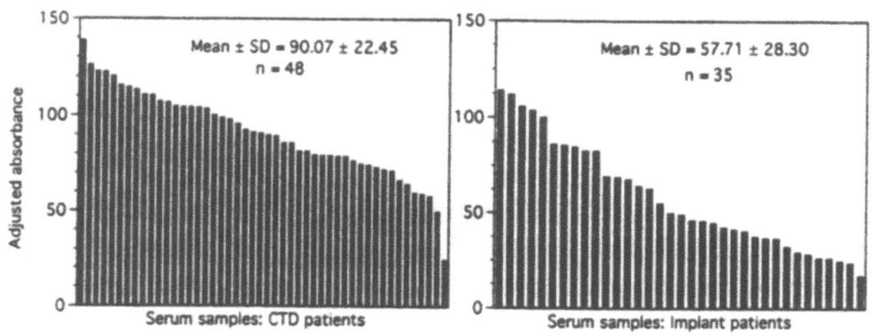

Fig. 6. Modified Goldblum ELISA method. Serum samples tested were from patients with CTD but no history of silicone implants and from implanted patients with or without clinical symptoms.

Finally, we tested the immunoglobulin subclass and found that all three classes of immunoglobulin, IgG, IgA, and IgM, adhered to the silicone elastomer (data not shown).

Discussion

We were able to repeat, in a blinded fashion, the results obtained by Emerald Laboratories with materials and serum samples sent to us by them. We also found, however, that several sera from patients with CTD were positive in the test. A number of explanations are possible. First, the CTD patients may have had silicone implants. This hypothesis is unlikely, especially since some of the highest reactions were found with male subjects. Second, the individuals may have been exposed to silicone in foodstuffs, medications or other sources from the environment. Since silicone is so prevalent, it is difficult to exclude this possibility. Third, the reactions might reflect the elevated immunoglobulin levels found in many patients with CTD. Finally, the reactions might represent the presence of autoantibodies commonly found in many patients with CTD. In order to examine these possibilities, we collected a large number of sera from patients with CTD whose medical records were available and who, under direct questioning, were ensured not to have had silicone implants of any sort. Unfortunately, no further kits were available to us from the manufacturer, so that we have been unable to complete these definitive studies.

Our investigation of the Goldblum procedure also showed that high values are obtained using the serum of patients with CTD, even though there was no history of silicone implant. We arbitrarily divided the values in the two populations (CTD and silicone implant) into those with high values above the median and low values below the median. An analysis of these values shows that high values were present in 60% of CTD patients and 40% of implant patients. The possible explanations for these findings are much the same as those given above.

In view of the fact that these reactions are common among symptomatic women without implants, it seems likely that these tests cannot be used to determine the presence of silicone implants. That there is more binding by the serum of implanted patients may simply represent the elevated immunoglobulin levels in these individuals due to the chronic inflammation induced by the implant.

The ultimate question is whether any of these reactions represent silicone-specific antibody. It is not possible to determine the nature of these silicone-binding immunoglobulins from the information presently available. We must show that the binding is due to the Fab portion of the immunoglobulin molecule and, most important, that it is specific for one of the determinant groups on the silicone elastomer. Both of those experiments have proved to be technically difficult because of the high level of non-specific binding of immunoglobulins by the silicone elastomer.

References

1. Wolf LE, Lappé M, Peterson RD, Ezrailson EG (1993) Human immune response to polydimethylsiloxane (silicone): screening studies in a breast implant population. FASEB J 7:1265-1268
2. Goldblum RM, Pelley RP, O'Donell AA, Pyron D, Heggers JP (1992) Antibodies to silicone elastomers and reactions to ventriculoperitoneal shunts. Lancet 340:510-513

Endnotes

† This study was supported by a grant from the Plastic Surgery Educational Foundation.

‡ Dr. Rose has served as an expert witness for defendants in several legal proceedings involving silicone breast implants.

¶ Present address: SAIC - Life Sciences Operation
5340 Spectrum Drive, Suite N
Frederick, MD 21701

Autoantibodies in Patients with Silicone Implants

A. J. Bridges, J. D. Anderson, D. E. Burns, K. Kemple, J. D. Kaplan, and T. Lorden

Section of Rheumatology, Department of Medicine, University of Wisconsin Hospital and Clinics, William S. Middleton Memorial Veterans Hosptial, Madison, WI 53705

Abstract

We assessed the prevalence of autoantibodies in women with silicone implants and controls. Five hundred consecutive patients with silicone implants, 25 age-matched normal women, 25 women with silicone implants and no rheumatic symptoms, and 100 women with fibromyalgia were tested. Immunofluorescence antinuclear antibodies (ANA) were performed using HEp-2 cells. Subtype autoantibodies were performed by enzyme-linked immunoassay and Western blot. ANA tests were positive in 30% of patients with silicone implants and rheumatic symptoms, 8% of age-matched normal women, 28% of women with silicone implants without clinical symptoms, and 25% of women with fibromyalgia and no silicone implants. The predominant ANA pattern was speckled (55%). ANA subtype testing was positive in 4.8% of patients and none of the controls. We conclude that a larger proportion of women with silicone implants have autoantibodies compared to age-matched asymptomatic women suggesting immune activation in women with silicone implants.

Introduction

Immune disorders are characterized by the development of autoantibodies. Autoantibodies, particularly antinuclear antibodies (ANA), are detected in the majority of patients with connective tissue diseases such as systemic lupus erythematosus (SLE) and scleroderma. Recent reports have described persons with silicone implants who have developed scleroderma and SLE [3,4,6]. Since autoantibodies are suspected to play an important role in the pathogenesis of the connective tissue diseases, the nature of the autoantibodies produced in patients with rheumatic symptoms and silicone implants is important to understand.

Few controlled studies have been reported which have examined this issue. Bridges, et al. evaluated autoantibodies in 156 women with silicone implants and rheumatic symptoms and controls [3]. A greater proportion of patients with silicone implants and rheumatic symptoms had a positive ANA test than women with silicone implants and no symptoms. However, there was no difference in the proportion of patients with a positive ANA when patients with fibromyalgia were compared with the silicone implant group. Patients with silicone implants and connective tissue disease had a positive ANA test in 45% of cases.

Claman, et al. studied 131 patients with silicone implants and controls [4]. Patients with silicone implants, with or without symptoms, had a higher prevalence of autoantibodies than controls without implants. Peters, et al. studied 200 patients with breast implants and found a prevalance of autoantibodies of 26.5% which did not significantly differ from controls [6].

In attempt to better understand autoantibody production in women with silicone implants, we performed autoantibody testing in a large series of patients with silicone implants and controls.

Materials and Methods

Subjects: Consecutive patients (n=500) with silicone implants referred to three rheumatologists and one pulmonologist for evaluation of rheumatic and pulmonary symptoms were entered into the study. Age-matched control subjects included normal women (n=25), women with silicone implants without clinical symptoms (n=25), and women with fibromyalgia (diagnosis based on American College of Rheumatology criteria) who did not have silicone implants (n=100) [10].

Immunologic studies: ANA testing was performed using HEp-2 cells as tissue substrate (Sanofi Diagnostics Pasteur Inc., Chaska, MN). Serum ANA titers greater than or equal to 1:80 were considered positive. Testing for antibodies to double stranded DNA (ds-DNA) was performed by indirect immunofluorescent technique using Crithidia luciliae as substrate (Sanofi Diagnostics Pasteur Inc., Chaska, MN). Titers of anti-ds-DNA antibody greater than 1:10 were considered positive. Testing for antibodies to Sm, ribonucleoprotein (RNP), SSA/Ro, SSB/La, Scl-70, and Jo-1 antigens were performed by enzyme-linked immunoassay (Sanofi Diagnostics Pasteur Inc., Chaska, MN). The presence of autoantibodies to cellular antigens was further assessed by Western blot using MOLT-4 cells as substrate [2]. Human sera were used at a dilution of 1:100. Each experiment included standard sera that detected Sm, U1RNP, Scl-70, centromere, PM-Scl, Jo-1, SSA/Ro and SSB/La polypeptides.

Statistics: Kruskal-Wallis and Chi-square tests were used to examine the data for statistically significant differences between groups.

Results

Patient and control subjects:
Patients (n=500) with silicone implants ranged in age from 22-72 years, with a mean of 44 years. The mean age of the controls was 45 years. Thirty percent of the patients with silicone implants and symptoms of rheumatic disease had a positive ANA test greater than or equal to 1:80. Negative immunofluorescence was found in 62.5% of patients and immunofluorescence at a serum dilution of 1:40 was found in 7.5% of patients. The ANA titers are shown in Table 1.

Table 1

Antinuclear Antibodies in Women with Silicone Implants

	ANA TITERS				
	≥1:80	1:160	1:320	1:640	≥1:1280
Normal controls n=25	2(8)	1(4)	0	0	0
Assymptomatic women with silicone implants n=25	7(28)	2(8)	2(8)	1(4)	0
Women with fibromyalgia without implants n=100	25(25)	5(5)	4(4)	3(3)	2(2)
Symptomatic women with silicone implants n=500	150(30)	60(12)	15(3)	15(3)	35(7)

(%)

Antinuclear antibodies were found in 8% of age-matched normal women (n=25), 28% of women with silicone implants without clinical symptoms (n=25), and 25% of women with fibromyalgia and no silicone implants (n=100) (Table 1). Patients with silicone implants were more likely to have a positive ANA than normal controls without implants ($p<.05$). The proportion of patients with silicone implants and a positive ANA did not differ from the proportion of fibromyalgia patients with a positive ANA (30% vs 25%, $p>.05$). Patients with fibromyalgia without silicone implants were more commonly ANA positive than normal controls (25% vs 8%, $p<.05$).

The ANA patterns of women with silicone implants and ANA titers greater than 1:40 were: 55% speckled, 34% homogeneous, 10% nucleolar and 1% cytoplasmic. In contrast, the controls were 42% speckled and 58% homogeneous. A speckled or nucleolar pattern was found more frequently in patients with silicone implants but this did not reach statistical significance ($p>.05$).

Subtype autoantibody testing was positive in 4.8% of patients with silicone implants and rheumatic symptoms. Nineteen patients (3.8%) were positive for anti-SSA/Ro antibodies. Nine of the patients who were positive for anti-SSA/Ro antibodies also had anti-SSB/La antibodies, one had anti-Jo-1 antibodies and one had anti-Scl-70 antibodies. Five patients had anti-RNP antibodies and one patient had anti-Sm antibodies. One of these patients also had anti-double stranded DNA antibodies. None of the controls (asymptomatic without silicone implants, asymptomatic with silicone implants, or fibromyalgia without silicone implants) showed positive results for subtype autoantibody testing.

Discussion

The goal of this study was to assess the proportion of women with silicone implants who have autoantibodies. The findings suggest that women with silicone implants are more likely to have a positive ANA test than normal controls. In addition, it does not appear to matter whether the patients were symptomatic or not since 28% of the women with silicone implants and no rheumatic symptoms had a positive ANA test.

These findings are consistent with previous investigations regarding autoantibodies in women with silicone implants [3,4]. Bridges, et al. and Claman, et al. have published controlled studies of autoantibodies in women with silicone implants. Their results suggested that autoantibodies are found in women with silicone implants in 20-35% of cases with a higher prevalence of autoantibodies in patients with implants than controls. Peters, et al. found autoantibodies in 26.5% of patients with silicone implants; however, this proportion did not significantly differ from controls [6].

The meaning of a positive ANA test in the women with silicone implants is unclear. Patients with well-defined connective tissue diseases such as SLE and scleroderma are invariably ANA positive [7]. The relatively small proportion of silicone implant patients who are positive by ANA testing (30%) suggests that these patients do not have the serologic pattern seen in classic connective tissue diseases. It is possible that the autoantibody reactivity detected by the immunofluorescence test in patients with silicone breast implants is from polyclonal immunoglobulin activation or an adjuvant effect associated with silicone implants.

Approximately 25% of patients with fibromyalgia in this study were found to be ANA positive. This is consistent with findings of other reports which described a positive ANA test in a small proportion of patients with fibromyalgia [1,5,10]. The results of this study also showed that the proportion of patients with fibromyalgia and a positive ANA test was significantly higher than the proportion of normal controls with a positive ANA test. This finding is curious because fibromyalgia is considered to be a noninflammatory disorder which should be ANA negative. An abnormality of the hypothalamic-pituitary-adrenal axis in fibromyalgia may lead to low level immune activation and autoantibody formation in fibromyalgia [11]. Thyroid disorders of an autoimmune basis may also lead to a positive ANA test in fibromyalgia [1].

Patients with classic SLE often have autoantibodies directed to a few distinct intracellular proteins, specifically the ribonuclear proteins: Sm, RNP, SSA/Ro and SSB/La [8]. Autoantibodies to these proteins were found in a small proportion of patients with silicone implants in this study. Most of these patients were found to have SLE or Sjogren's syndrome after full rheumatologic evaluation (data not shown). This supports the specificity of these tests for connective tissue diseases.

In summary, a larger proportion of women with silicone implants have autoantibodies when compared with age-matched normal women suggesting immune activation in women with silicone implants. A 25% prevalence of a positive ANA test in patients with fibromyalgia without silicone implants suggests that further study of the immune system in this group of patients is warranted.

References

1. Bridges A (1993) Fibromyalgia antinuclear antibodies and clinical features of connective tissue disease. Clin Exp Rheumatol 11:696-697.
2. Bridges A, Anderson J, Wang G, Johnson J, Sharp G (1995) Comparison of hemagglutination, immunodiffusion and immunoblotting methods for detecting autoantibodies to small nuclear ribonucleoproteins (Sm and RNP). Lab Med 26:150-156.
3. Bridges AJ, Conley C Wang G, Burns D, Vasey F (1993) A clinical and immunologic evaluation of women with silicone breast implants and symptoms of rheumatic disease. Ann Intern Med 118:929-936.
4. Claman HN, Robertson AD (1994) Antinuclear antibodies and breast implants. West J Med 160:225-228.
5. Dinerman H, Goldenberg DL, Felson DT (1986) A prospective evaluation of 118 patients with fibromyalgia syndrome: Prevalence of Raynaud's phenomenon, sicca symptoms, ANA, Low complement, and Ig deposition at the dermal-epidermal junction. J Rheumatol 13:368-373.
6. Peters W, Keystone E, Snow K, Rubin L, Smith D (1994) Is there a relationship between autoantibodies and silicone-gel implants? Ann Plast Surg 32:1-7.
7. Press RI, Peebles CL, Kumagai Y, Ochs RL, Tan EM (1992) Antinuclear autoantibodies in women with silicone breast implants. Lancet 340:1304-1307.
8. Tan EM. (1989) Antinuclear antibodies: diagnostic markers for autoimmune diseases and probes for cell biology. Adv Immunol 44:93-151.
9. Sternberg EM (1993) Hypoimmune fatigue syndrome response? J Rheumatol 20:418-421.
10. Wolfe F, Smythe HA, Yunus MB, et al (1990) The American College Of

Rheumatology 1990 criteria for the classification of fibromyalgia. Arthritis Rheum 33:160-172.

11. Yunus MB, Hussey FX, Aldag JC (1993) Antinuclear antibodies and connective tissue disease features in fibromyalgia syndrome: a controlled study. J Rheumatol 20:1557-1560.

Conflict of Interest Statement: The authors of this study have served as consultants on the issue of silicone and immune dysfunction. Dr. Bridges is a co-investigator on a study funded in part by the Plastic Surgery Education Foundation.

Clinical and Laboratory Features of Patients with Scleroderma and Silicone Implants

T. Field, MD PhD and A. J. Bridges, MD

Section of Rheumatology, Department of Medicine, University of Wisconsin Hospital, Madison, WI 53792

Abstract

We reviewed the available clinical and laboratory data from 56 patients with scleroderma and silicone implants from the English medical literature and 19 cases which have not been previously reported. The average age of onset of scleroderma was 43.6 $\pm$ 10 years (range 20-73). Patients had silicone implants for an average of 9 $\pm$ 4 years prior to the development of scleroderma (range 1-32). Most patients had limited scleroderma (41%). Twenty three percent had intermediate scleroderma and 36% had diffuse scleroderma. Clinical findings included: Raynaud's phenomenon in 77%, esophageal dysfunction in 53%, and pulmonary involvement in 47%. Cardiac and renal involvement were uncommon. Antinuclear antibodies by immunofluorescence were found in 83 percent of patients. The immunofluorescence pattern was speckled in 53%, centromere in 31% and nucleolar in 9%. Other antibodies (Scl-70, RNP, SSA/Ro, PM-Scl) were found in only a small proportion of patients. A clinical, serologic and immunogenetic comparison of patients with silicone implants and scleroderma and patients with idiopathic scleroderma is needed to better understand the pathogenesis of this disorder.

Introduction

A major concern of patients with silicone breast implants is the possible association of silicone exposure with connective tissue disease. At the present time there are no epidemiologic data which establish a direct link between silicone and rheumatic disease. However, scleroderma appears to be overrepresented among the published reports of patients with silicone breast implants and rheumatic disease [3,23].

There are data to suggest that the derivatives of elemental silicon, silica and silicone, can "trigger" the immune system and cause fibrotic and connective tissue diseases, specifically scleroderma [10,21]. Indeed, chronic exposure to silica dust in miners is associated with a 25-110 fold increase in the development of scleroderma [10]. In attempt to better understand the clinical features of patients with silicone implants and scleroderma, we reviewed the literature and an additional 19 cases that have not been previously reported.

Materials and Methods

Diagnostic criteria: The diagnosis of scleroderma was made if the patient met criteria for progressive systemic sclerosis according to American College of Rheumatology criteria or CREST (calcinosis, Raynaud's phenomenon, esophageal dysmotility, sclerodactyly and telangiectasia) syndrome [17]. Skin sclerosis was subdivided into diffuse, intermediate or limited cutaneous involvement according to Barnett [2]. Patients were considered to have CREST syndrome when two clinical manifestations were present along with anti-centromere antibodies or three clinical manifestations [18].

Patients: Records of patients with silicone implants and scleroderma which had not been previously reported were solicited from physicians and attorneys for review. Records of 50 patients were sent to the authors for review. Fifteen patients met criteria for scleroderma or CREST as defined above. Four additional patients were evaluated by the author for a total of 19 new cases of scleroderma.

Literature review: A comprehensive list of publications was obtained from medline searches and a manual review of the manuscripts and abstracts written in English was performed. In addition, all abstracts presented at the American College of Rheumatology meetings were reviewed. Clinical data was available on 56 scleroderma patients with silicone implants and unavailable on 25 scleroderma patients with silicone implants.

Results

New Cases of Scleroderma and Silicone Implants

Table 1 shows the clinical features of the 19 unreported patients with scleroderma and silicone implants. Eighteen patients had silicone gel breast implants and one patient had silicone injections into the leg. Thirteen patients underwent augmentation, four patients had mastectomy for fibrocystic breast disease, and one patient had reconstruction for breast cancer. The average age at implantation/injection was 36 ± 8 years and the average post-surgery time until the diagnosis of scleroderma was 12 ± 6 years.

Table 1 Clinical Features of Patients with Scleroderma and Silicone Implants

CLINICAL FEATURES

Pt	Age at Implant	Age at Dx	Skin	Rayn	Pulm	Cardiac	GI	Calcinosis	Autoantibodies
1	35	46	D	+	-	+	-		1:1280 Sp
2	47	48	D	+	ILD	+	+	+	1:640 H
3	31	41	I	+	ILD	-	+	+	1:1280 Sp, Scl-70
4	28	34	L	+	-	-	-	-	1:80 Sp
5	31	43	I	+	↓DLCO	+	+	-	1:320 nuc
6	39	59	L	-	-	-	+	-	1:80 Sp
7	28	35	L	+	↓DLCO	-	-	-	1:1280 cent
8	23	33	L	+	-	-	-	-	1:160 Sp
9	42	49	L	+	-	-	+	-	1:2560 cent
10	45	53	L	+	↓DLCO	-	+	+	1:160 cent
11	28	34	I	+	-	-	+	+	1:640 cent
12	42	55	L	+	-	-	+	-	1:1280 cent, RNP
13	32	51	L	+	-	-	+	-	1:1280 cent
14	31	33	L	+	-	-	-	-	1:1280 cent
15	41	48	L	+	-	-	-	-	1:1280 cent
16	40	50	L	+	-	-	-	-	1:640 nuc Scl-70
17	33	53	L	+	ILD	-	+	-	Negative
18	29	61	D	+	ILD	-	+	-	1:40 Sp
19	27	39	I	+	-	-	-	-	1:320 Sp

Pt = patients
Dx = diagnosis
Rayn = Raynaud's phenomenon
I = Intermediate
Pulm = pulmonary involvement
ILD = interstitial lung disease
DLCO = diffusing capacity
L = Limited Skin Involvment
GI = esophageal involvement
H = homogeneous
Sp = speckled
nuc = nucleolar
cent = centromere
D = diffuse

Most patients had limited skin involvement (63%) (Table 1). Raynaud's phenomenon was common (95%). Esophageal dysmotility defined by abnormal barium swallow or motility study was found in 58%. Pulmonary dysfunction was found in 37% characterized by interstitial lung disease (4 patients) and diminished diffusion capacity (3 patients). Pericardial effusion was seen in 3 patients. No patient had renal dysfunction.

Anti-centromere antibodies were found in 8 patients (Table 1). Anti-Scl-70 antibodies were found in 2 patients. On patient had a negative antinuclear antibody (ANA) test and one patient had a low titer result (1:40). Seven patients had moderately high ANA titers of speckled pattern.

All patients have been explanted. Two patients died; one from scleroderma cardiac disease and one from pulmonary infection. One third of the patients improved post-explantation.

Review of the Literature: Scleroderma and Silicone Implants

Table 2 combines the information reported on 56 cases from the literature and the additional 19 patients presented above [1,3,4,5,6,7,9,13,16,19,20,23,24,27]. The average age of onset of scleroderma was 43.6 ± 10 years with a range of 20-73 years. The average length of time post-implantation to the development of scleroderma was 9 ± 4 years with a range of 1-21 years.

Table 2 Clinical Features of 75 Patients with Scleroderma and Silicone Implants

Age at implantation: 43.6 ± 10 years (range 20-73 years)	
Interval to diagnosis: 9 ± 4 years (range 1-21 years)	
Skin involvement	
Diffuse	27(36%)
Intermediate	17(23%)
Limited	31(41%)
Raynaud's phenomenon	58(77%)
Esophageal dysfunction	40(53%)
Pulmonary dysfunction	35(47%)
Decreased DLCO	19(25%)
Interstitial lung disease	11(15%)
Both	5 (7%)
Cardiac involvement	3 (4%)
Calcinosis	3 (4%)
Renal dysfunction	1 (1%)
Antinuclear antibodies	62(83%)
Speckled	40(53%)
Centromere	23(31%)
Nucleolar	7(9%)
Scl-70	7(9%)
RNP	3 (4%)
SSA/Ro	1 (1%)
PM-Scl	1 (1%)

Skin examination showed diffuse scleroderma in 27 (36%), intermediate scleroderma in 17 (23%), and limited scleroderma in 31 (41%). Raynaud's phenomenon was found in 77% and esophageal dysfunction defined by abnormal barium swallow or motility study in 53%. Pulmonary dysfunction was found in 47%, with diminished DLCO as the most common abnormality. Calcinosis, renal and cardiac involvement were uncommon.

Antinuclear antibodies were found in 83% of patients. A speckled pattern was most common (53%). Anti-centromere antibodies were found in 31%. A nucleolar pattern on ANA testing was found in 9%. Anti-Scl-70 antibodies were found in 7 patients and anti-RNP antibodies were found in 3 patients.

Discussion

In 1979, the first report of connective tissue disease associated with cosmetic surgery was published in the English literature [12]. Investigators from Japan described four patients with scleroderma. Since that time numerous investigators have described patients with silicone implants who have developed scleroderma [1,3,4,5,6,7,9,13,16,19,20,23,24,27]. This manuscript is a review of the literature and presentation of the clinical findings of 19 additional patients with scleroderma and silicone implants.

Patients with silicone implants and scleroderma appear to have some atypical clinical and serologic features which differ from idiopathic scleroderma abstracted from the medical literature. Idiopathic scleroderma is accompanied by Raynaud's phenomenon in greater than 95 percent of patients [14,25] whereas only 77 percent of patients with scleroderma and silicone implants had Raynaud's phenomenon. Eighty-three percent of patients with scleroderma and silicone implants had a positive ANA test while most studies report that nearly 100 percent of patients with scleroderma have a positive ANA test [8,26]. There were 44 patients with diffuse or intermediate cutaneous scleroderma and silicone implants and only 7 had anti-Scl-70 antibodies. Antibodies to Scl-70 are found in 30 percent to 100 percent of patients with diffuse and intermediate cutaneous scleroderma [8,14,18]. Anti-centromere antibodies predominated in the patients with scleroderma and silicone implants reported in this study. Thus, certain clinical and serologic features of patients with scleroderma and silicone implants appear to differ from patients with idiopathic scleroderma.

In series of patients with silicone implants which have been examined for connective tissue disorders, the proportion of patients with scleroderma appeared to be over-represented [3,23]. This is an important finding. Since the Food and Drug Administration (FDA) hearings, significant media attention has been given to the silicone implant dilemma. Thousands of women have presented to rheumatologists for evaluation of diverse rheumatic signs and symptoms. Yet, the proportion of patients with scleroderma has remained larger than the proportion with rheumatoid arthritis [3,23,24]. Since rheumatoid arthritis is approximately 500 times more common than scleroderma in the population at large, the overrepresentation of scleroderma and under-representation of rheumatoid arthritis in series of patients with silicone implants is an important finding.

Preliminary reports of an epidemiologic study of the prevalence of silicone implants among patients with scleroderma, however, do not support an association [11,29]. Investigators at 3 referral centers reviewed 141 cases of scleroderma with disease onset prior to 1990 to determine the number of patients who had silicone implants placed prior to the onset of scleroderma. The mean disease duration in the scleroderma group was 9 years. One patient with scleroderma had silicone implants placed prior to disease onset (0.7%).

Unfortunately, the study design did not account for the latency time between implantation and the development of scleroderma. The study did not take into account that the average length of time to the development of scleroderma after reconstructive surgery with silicone implants is approximately 9 years [3,23,24]. Since the group of patients with scleroderma evaluated by the investigators had their disease approximately 9 years before the date of the study, and taking into account an average of 9 years from implantation to development of scleroderma, the study design should have compared the incidence of implantation in the scleroderma group with the incidence of implantation in the general population prior to 1972-4. The number of implants placed prior to 1972-4 is much smaller that the estimate of silicone implants in the general population used by the investigators (0.65-2%). These design problems greatly limit the ability of the study to answer questions about the relationship between scleroderma and silicone implants.

Recently, Levine and Ilowite described 6 breast-fed children of mothers with silicone implants with esophageal dysmotility similar to that seen in patients with scleroderma [15]. Although there was significant referral and selection bias in the sample tested, the manometric findings were distinctly unusual for children. No skin manifestations of scleroderma were described suggesting the patients had isolated gastrointestinal dysfunction. Isolated organ system findings, typically called "scleroderma-sine scleroderma" may be incomplete expressions of a fibrosing-illness [22]. These findings and the strong relationship between silica exposure and scleroderma give further support to the importance of defining the relationship between scleroderma and silicone implants.

In summary, the number of cases of scleroderma in patients with silicone implants continues to rise. The years of delay between implantation and disease (latency) make investigation of this issue difficult. Any epidemiologic study will need to consider disease latency. It will also be important to compare the clinical, serologic and immunogenetic features of patients with scleroderma with and without implants.

Conflict of Interest Statement: The authors of this study have served as consultants on the issue of silicone and immune dysfunction. Dr. Bridges is a co-investigator on a study funded in part by the Plastic Surgery Education Foundation.

References

1. Appleton BE, Lee P (1993) The Development of systemic sclerosis (scleroderma) following augmentation mamoplasty. J Rheumatol 20:1052-1054
2. Barnett AJ, Miller MH, Littlejohn GO (1988) A survival study of patients with scleroderma diagnosed over 30 years (1953-1983): The value of a simple cutaneous classification in the early stages of the disease. J Rheumatol 15:276-283
3. Bridges AJ, Conley C, Wang G, Burns DE, Vasey FB (1993) A clinical and immunologic evaluation of women with silicone breast implants and symptoms of rheumatic disease. Ann Intern Med 118:929-36
4. Brozena SJ, Fenske NA, Cruse CW, Espinoza CG, Vasey FB, Germain BF, Espinoza LR (1988) Human adjuvant disease following augmentation mammoplasty. Arch Dermatol 124:1383-6
5. Claman HN, Robertson AD (1994) Antinuclear antibodies and breast implants. West J Med 160:225-228
6. Cuellar MF, Scopelitis E, Citera G, Gutierrez M Silveira LH, Espinoza LR (1993) A prospective clinical evaluation of 300 women with silicone breast implants (SBI). Arthritis Rheum 36:C192
7. Englert HJ, Howe GB, Penny R, Brooks P (1994) Scleroderma and Silicone Breast Implants. Brit J Rheum 33:397-399
8. Giordano M, Valentini G, Migliaresi S (1986) Different antibody patterns and different prognoses in patients with scleroderma with various extent of skin sclerosis. J Rheumatol 13:911-916
9. Gutierrez FJ, Espinoza LR (1990) Progressive systemic sclerosis complicated by severe hypertension: reversal after silicone implant removal. Am J Med 89:390-2
10. Haustein UF, Ziegler V (1985) Environmentally induced systemic sclerosis-like disorders. Int J Dermatol 24:147-51
11. Hochberg MC, White B, Steen V, Medsger TA, Weisman M, Wigley FM (1993) The association fo augmentation mammoplasty with systemic sclerosis: preliminary results from a case-control study. Arthritis Rheum 36:196
12. Kumagai Y, Abe C, Shiokawa Y (1979) Scleroderma after cosmetic surgery. Arthritis Rheum 22:532-7
13. Lee SS, Liln HY, Wang SR, Tsai Cy, Liu HN (1994) Scleroderma after silicone augmentation. Mammoplasty: Report of a case. J Formos Med Assoc 93:66-70.
14. LeRoy EC, Black C, Fleischmajer R (1988) Scleroderma (Systemic Sclerosis): Classification, Subsets and Pathogenesis. J Rheumatol 15:202-205
15. Levine JJ, Iiowite T (1994) Sclerodermalike esophageal disease in children breast-fed by mothers with silicone breast implants. JAMA 271:213-216
16. Marik PE, Kark AL, Zambakides A (1990) Scleroderma after silicone augmentation mammoplasty. A report of 2 cases. S Afr Med J 1990; 77:212-213.
17. Masi AT, Rodnan GP, Medsger TA, Altman RD Jr, D'angelo WA, Fries JF (1980) Preliminary criteria for the classification of systemic sclerosis (scleroderma). Arthritis Rheum 23:581-590
18. Masi AT (1988) Classification of systemic sclerosis (Scleroderma): Relationship of cutaneous subgroups in early disease to outcome and serologic reactivity. J Rheum 15:6:8894-898.
19. Osborn TG, Lawrence JM, Madson KL, Ghosh S, Moore TL (1992) Silicone gel breast implants: Spectrum of rheumatologic complaints. Arthritis Rheum 35:S162
20. Press RI, Peebles CL, Kumagai Y, Ochs RL, Tan EM (1992) Antinuclear autoantibodies in women with silicone breast implants. Lancet 340:1304-1307
21. Reiser KM, Last JA (1979) Silicosis and fibrogenesis: fact and artifact. Toxicology 13:51-72
22. Rodnan GP, Fennell RH Jr (1962) Progressive systemic sclerosis sine scleroderma. JAMA 180:665-670

23. Spiera H (1988) Scleroderma after silicone augmentation mammoplasty. JAMA 260:236-8
24. Speira H, Kerr LD (1993) Scleroderma following silicone implantation: A cumulative experience of 11 cases. J Rheumatol 20:958-961
25. Steen VD, Powell DL, Medsger TA (1988) Clinical Correlations and Prognosis Based on Serum Autoantibodies in Patients with Systemic Sclerosis. Arthritis Rheum 31:196-203
26. Tan EM, Rodnan GP, Garcia I (1980) Diversity of antinuclear antibodies in progressive systemic sclerosis. Arthritis Rheum 23:617-624
27. Varga J, Schumacher HR, Jimenez SA (1989) Systemic sclerosis after augmentation mammoplasty with silicone implants. Ann Intern Med 111:377-83
28. Vasey FB, Havice D, Bocanegra T (1992) Clinical manifestations of fifty consecutive women with silicone breast implants and connective tissue disease. Arthritis Rheum 35:S212
29. Wigley FM, Miller R, Hochberg MC, Steen V (1992) Augmentation mammoplasty in patients with systemic sclerosis: data from the Baltimore scleroderma research center and Pittsburgh scleroderma data bank. Arthritis Rheum 35:S46

Re-Evaluation of Autoantibodies and Clinical Overview of Silicone-Related Disorders

E.M. Tan[1], R.L. Ochs[1], Y. Kumagai[2], M.L. Cuellar[3] and L.R. Espinoza[3]
[1]Autoimmune Disease Center, The Scripps Research Institute, La Jolla, CA., [2]Imaichi Hospital, Tokyo, Japan and [3]Section of Rheumatology, LSU School of Medicine, New Orleans, LA.
Supported in part by NIH grants AI34594 and DK49413. This is publication No. 9344-MEM from The Scripps Research Institute

Introduction

In a recent study to characterize antinuclear autoantibodies (ANAs) in women with silicone breast implants [1], it was reported that in 11 patients who had symptoms and signs that met criteria for defined autoimmune diseases such as scleroderma and systemic lupus erythematosus, all had the presence of ANAs which on further characterization could be shown to be antigen-antibody systems characteristic of idiopathic autoimmune diseases. Silicone breast implant patients who had the diagnosis of scleroderma had antibodies such as anti-Scl-70 (DNA topoisomerase I), anti-RNA polymerase I and anti-centromere protein antigens CENP-A and B. These antigen-antibody systems had been shown previously to be present in patients with the spontaneous form of scleroderma or with the CREST (calcinosis, Raynaud's phenomenon, esophageal dysmotility, sclerodactyly, telangiectasia) subset of scleroderma. Silicone breast implant patients who had the diagnosis of systemic lupus erythematosus or mixed connective tissue disease also had characteristic antigen-antibody systems present in the spontaneous forms of these diseases, including antibodies to double-stranded DNA, Sm antigen and small nuclear ribonucleoprotein (snRNP) antigens. These findings showed that both clinically as well as in immune response parameters, patients with silicone breast implants who had diagnoses such as scleroderma and lupus could not be regarded as unique compared to those with the spontaneous form of these diseases.

EMT, RLO, and MLC have no conflicts of interest. LRE has participated as an expert witness on behalf of plaintiffs in silicone breast implant litigation cases.

An important publication in this field was a study reported by Kumagai *et al.* in 1984 [2]. Heretofore, there had been isolated reports of individual or limited numbers of cases with silicone-related disorders. This publication was more comprehensive, describing clinical and serological findings in 18 patients studied at the Division of Rheumatology, Juntendo University Hospital in Tokyo from 1970 to 1981. These 18 patients were classified into two major groups, group 1 with defined connective tissue diseases and group 2 with symptoms, signs and laboratory abnormalities related to one or another connective tissue disease, but with insufficient criteria for definitive diagnoses. In group 1, there were 11 patients, five of whom had the diagnosis of scleroderma, one with the diagnosis of localized morphea, two with the diagnosis of mixed connective tissue disease and three with the diagnosis of rheumatoid arthritis. Of interest with reference to the findings reported in 1992 [1], the Japanese studies showed that antinuclear antibodies were present in only three of the 11 patients, two of whom had mixed connective tissue disease and one had rheumatoid arthritis. These results would tend to suggest that in contrast to the naturally-occurring systemic autoimmune disorders, patients with silicone breast implants were lacking in the immune responses present in the idiopathic form of these diseases.

Of the eleven patients in group 1 of the Japanese study [2], ten of the eleven original sera were available for re-evaluation. Only three of the seven patients in group 2 who had undefined connective tissue diseases were available for further study. In addition, some sera were available from silicone breast implant patients in Japan who had been studied at other medical centers. All these sera were re-evaluted with current techniques for determining antinuclear antibodies and their immunological specificities. These studies included ANA determination on tissue culture cell substrates by immunofluorescence microscopy and defining specificities of antibodies by Western blotting.

It is well recognized that silicone-related disorders are manifested as a wide variety of clinical symptoms [3-5]. Only a small number of patients can be defined as typical connective tissue disorders such as scleroderma, lupus, Sjogren's syndrome, mixed connective tissue disease or rheumatoid arthritis. On the other hand, the majority of patients have symptoms which do not meet established criteria for these diseases. In this report, we describe findings in a large number of patients with silicone breast implants who fall into categories which appear to belong to diseases such as fibromyalgia and chronic fatigue syndrome.

MATERIALS AND METHODS

Detection and Determination of ANA Specifities

Indirect immunofluorescence was done on commercially prepared HEp-2 cell slides (Bion, Park Ridge, Ill) as described [1]. Briefly, all sera were assayed at a starting dilution of 1/40 and when positive, they were further studied at serial doubling dilutions. Antibody specificities were determined by a combination of immunodiffusion and Western blots. In immunodiffusion, standard sera containing precipitating antibodies (anti-Sm, anti-nRNP, anti-Scl-70 and anti-SS-A/Ro, SS-B/La) were used as positive reference antibodies. For Western blotting, MOLT-4 whole cell extracts were used as the antigen and human sera were used at a dilution of 1/100. In every experiment, standard sera containing antibodies that blotted Sm antigens, nRNP antigens, Scl-70 (DNA topoisomerase I), CENP-A and B, and SS-A/Ro, SS-B/La were run simultaneously.

Patients and Diagnostic Criteria

Patients in the second part of this report were referrals to the LSU Medical Center Rheumatology Clinic and all had a complete history and physical examination. Diagnosis of the different connective tissue diseases was based on the following criteria: 1982 Revised Criteria of the American College of Rheumatology (ACR) for the Classification of Systemic Lupus Erythematosus [6]; the 1980 criteria of the ACR for scleroderma [7]; the 1990 ACR criteria for fibromyalgia [8]; the 1987 revised criteria for the diagnosis of rheumatoid arthritis [9]; the criteria for chronic fatigue syndrome [10].

Results

The re-evaluation of autoantibodies in the sera of Japanese patients with silicone breast implants is presented in Tables 1 and 2. Table 1 shows the data from patients personally evaluated by Kumagai et al. at Juntendo University [2]. In group 1, sera from ten of the eleven original patients were available for the current studies. The table shows that all of these patients had injections of silicone or paraffin directly into the breasts. Column 3 of Table 1 shows the diagnoses given to these patients. They include mixed connective tissue disease, rheumatoid arthritis, diffuse scleroderma and limited scleroderma. In group 2, with undefined autoimmune disorders, patients had the diagnosis of human adjuvant disease. Column 4 shows the original ANA determinations on these patients and it is seen that three patients out of the ten with defined autoimmune disorders had positive antinuclear antibodies whereas all the others, including those with undefined autoimmune disorders in group 2, were negative for ANAs. In the original study, the ANA determination used rat liver sections as the substrate in indirect immunofluorescence. Currently, tissue culture cells (particularly the HEp-2 cell line) are being used as the standard substrate for ANA determinations in immunofluorescence microscopy. With this technique nine of the ten patients with defined autoimmune disorders were positive for antinuclear antibodies with the exception of patient 9, with rheumatoid arthritis, who was negative. In addition, one patient (#13) of the three with undefined autoimmune disorders had antinuclear antibodies. The next column shows that the majority of the antinuclear antibodies could be defined in terms of immunological specificities. Of particular interest were the findings that patients with the diagnosis of scleroderma had antibodies such as anti-Scl-70 and anti-centromere proteins CENP-A and -B, features which are characteristic of the antibody specificities in the spontaneous forms of scleroderma. Patients who carried the diagnosis of systemic lupus erythematosus or mixed connective tissue disease had antibodies to Sm, double-stranded DNA and to nuclear RNP, respectively, features which are characteristic of the antibodies seen in spontaneous SLE and MCTD. It is also of interest that the patient with undefined autoimmune disorder who carried the diagnosis of human adjuvant disease (patient #13) had antibodies which were identified as anti-Sm, anti-nuclear RNP and anti-double-stranded DNA, immune response specificities which would be consistent with the diagnosis of SLE.

TABLE 1. Breast Augmentation Patients: Kumagai Series

Patient	Implant Type	Diagnosis	Original ANA Titer	Recheck ANA Titer	ANA ID or WB kDa
Defined Autoimmune Disorders GROUP 1					
1	SIL IN	MCTD	1:640	1:320	Sm, nRNP
2	PAR IN	MCTD/SS/ PBC	1:320	1:160	nRNP, SS-A, Mitocho
3	SIL IN	RA/HT	1:40	1:80	Sm, nRNP, SS-A
4	PAR IN	d-Scl	neg (-)	1:80	46,90
5	PAR IN	l-Scl	-	1:80	Scl-70, 85
6	PAR IN	l-Scl/SLE	-	1:160	Sm, nRNP, ds DNA
7	PAR IN	l-Scl/HT	-	1:320	CENP-A/B, 76
8	PAR IN	l-Scl-M	-	1:320	CENP-A/B
9	SIL IN	RA	-	-	-
10	SIL IN	RA	-	1:160	-
Undefined Autoimmune Disorders GROUP 2					
11	SIL IN	HAD	-	-	-
12	SIL IN	HAD	-	-	-
13	?	HAD	-	1:160	Sm, nRNP, ds DNA

Abbreviations: HAD=human adjuvant disease, HT=Hashimoto's thyroiditis, IN-injection, M=morphea, PAR-paraffin, PBC=primary biliary cirrhosis, Sil=silicone, SS=Sjogren's syndrome

Representative Western blots, which were used to identify the specificities of these antinuclear antibodies, are shown in Figure 1. Lanes 1 and 2 show the absence of any reaction of two normal sera against the MOLT-4 cell extracts used as the antigen preparation. Lane 3 is a reference serum for anti-Scl-70 and the arrowheads show the 100 kDa DNA topoisomerase I antigen and the 70 kDa degradation product, Scl-70. Lane 4 is the serum from patient #5 of Table 1, showing identical reactivity as the reference serum. Lane 5 is a reference serum with the arrowheads showing antibody reacting with CENP-A (19 kDa) and CENP-B (80 kDa). Lanes 6 and 7 are sera from patients 7 and 8, respectively, in Table 1 showing identical reactivities with CENP A and CENP-B compared to the reference sera. Lane 10 is a reference serum with the arrowheads showing reactivities with the 70 kDa antigen of U1 nuclear RNP and the B/B' antigens of Sm (28/29 kDa). Lanes 8 and 9 of this figure are from patients 6 and

3, respectively. Patient #6 carried the diagnosis of limited scleroderma/SLE, whereas patient #3 carried the diagnosis of rheumatoid arthritis/Hashimoto's thyroiditis. In addition to antibodies which blotted antigens consistent with lupus (B/B' Sm) and 70 kDa nuclear RNP, there were other reactivities present in these two sera. Some of these might have been against the SS-A/Ro antigen. Lane 11 is a reference serum for antibodies to the SS-A/Ro and SS-B/La antigens denoted by arrowheads. It can be seen that patients 6 and 3 also showed antibodies to these antigens.

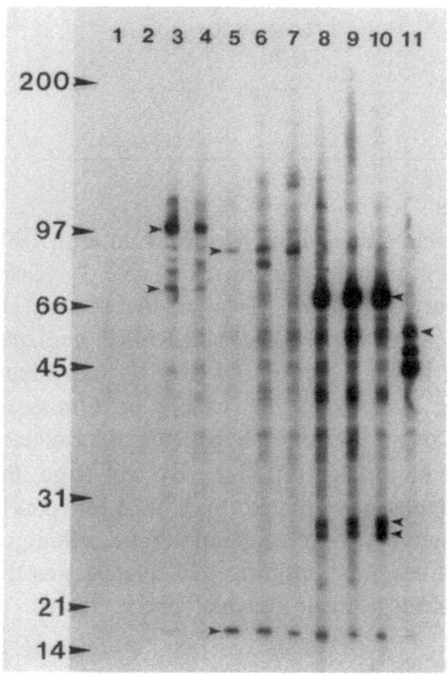

Fig. 1. Western blot analysis. MOLT-4 (a T lymphocyte cell line) whole cell extracts were used as antigens in SDS-PAGE gel electrophoresis and Western blot studies with the following sera: Lanes 1 and 2, normal human sera. Lane 3 reference anti-Scl-70 serum reacting with the 100 kDa DNA topoisomerase I antigen and the 70 kDa Scl-70 antigen (arrowheads). Lane 5 is reference serum reacting with CENP-A (19 kDa) and CENP-B (80 kDa), both marked by arrowheads. Lane 10 depicts reference serum reacting with 70 kDa U1 RNP (arrowhead) antigen and the 28/29 kDa B/B' antigen. Lane 11 is reference serum reactive with 60 kDa SS-A/Ro and 48 kDa SS-B/La (arrowheads). The other lanes are patients in Table 1, lane 4 is patient #5, lanes 6 and 7 are patients #7 and #8 and lanes 8 and 9 are patients #6 and #3, respectively.

The results of the studies depicted in Table 1 show that with improved techniques for the detection of antinuclear antibodies and for characterization of the immunological specificities, silicone-related disorders in the Japanese patients reported in 1984 who were classified as having defined autoimmune disorders also had immune responses which were similar to those seen in the spontaneous forms of these diseases.

Table 2 depicts the data on ten other patients with silicone-related disorders who were from clinical centers other than Juntendo University and had been reported previously by other investigators. In three group 1 patients who had the diagnosis of MCTD and SLE, patients 1 and 2 had antinuclear antibodies whose specificities fit the clinical diagnosis. In addition, in a group of patients with undefined autoimmune disorders, there were several patients whose antibody specificities are those which are encountered in certain spontaneous autoimmune disorders.

TABLE 2. Breast Augmentation Patients: Other Japanese Patients

Patient	Implant Type	Diagnosis	Original ANA Titer	Recheck ANA Titer	ANA ID or WB kDa
Defined Autoimmue Disorders GROUP 1					
1	SIL IN	MCTD	neg (-)	1:320	nRNP, SS-A, 31,44,52
2	SIL IN	SLE	-	1:320	nRNP, SS-A 52,60,66
3	?	SLE	-	-	-
Undefined Autoimmune Disorders GROUP 2					
4	PAR IN	HAD	-	-	-
5	PAR IN	HAD	-	1:80	Sl/Ki 33,70
6	?	HAD	-	1:160	SS-A 49,70
7	SIL IN	HAD	-	1:80	33,70
8	?	HAD	-	1:160	SS-A 46,70,80
9	?	HAD	-	-	-
10	PAR IN	HAD	-	-	-

Clinical Findings in LSU Cohort of Patients

Three hundred patients with breast implants seen at LSU Medical Center in 1991 were analyzed and clinical parameters of these patients presented in Table 3. There were a total of 300 patients and all except two were women. Two hundred seventy six patients had silicone gel implants and the remaining 24 had saline-filled implants. Augmentation mammoplasty was the reason for implants in 209 (69.6%) individuals and reconstructive mammoplasty following mastectomy for cancer or fibrocystic disease in 91 (30.4%). It can be seen from Table 3 that all these patients had evidence of encapsulation (75.6%) or implant rupture or leakage (26.3%). By and large, the overwhelming majority of women with implants exhibited ill-defined or poorly characterized rheumatic complaints with the majority complaining of fatigue, arthralgia, myalgia and skin rash. Only 2% of patients had frank arthritis. Of interest was the observation that approximately 24% of the patients had hair loss or alopecia.

TABLE 3. Clinical Parameters in Silicone Breast Implants

Manifestation	N=300
Age (years)	44.4 (25-69)
Fatigue	68%
Arthritis	2%
Raynaud's	4.3%
Sicca symptoms	12.6%
Hair loss/alopecia	24.1%
Augmentation mammoplasty	69.6%
Reconstructive mammoplasty	30.4%
Implant to symptoms (years)	6.8 (0.5-19)
Evidence of encapsulation	75.6%
Implant rupture or leakage	26.3%

Defined connective tissue disorders such as scleroderma, SLE or rheumatoid arthritis were diagnosed in 13.2% of the patients. Two hundred and fifty of the 300 patients (83.3%) had clinical manifestations suggestive of some connective tissue disorder. In these 250 patients, fatigue was the predominant complaint in 170 (68%). When these 170 patients with fatigue were further analyzed, 46/170 (27%) fulfilled the criteria for chronic fatigue syndrome [10] and 79/170 (43.4%) fulfilled criteria for fibromyalgia [8].

Discussion

An unusual opportunity was available in this study, in which sera from a cohort of Japanese patients with silicone-related disorders reported in 1984 was re-evaluated for antinuclear antibodies. With an immunofluorescence technique using tissue culture cells (HEp-2) as substrate, which is the standard substrate currently used for such analysis, it was found that those patients who were diagnosed in 1984 as having defined autoimmune diseases such as scleroderma, lupus and mixed connective tissue disease did indeed have high titers of antinuclear antibodies and the specificities of the ANAs were in agreement with ANA specificities found in the respective diseases of idiopathic etiology. Therefore, results of the present study confirmed the studies reported in 1992 [1] that the autoimmune responses of silicone-related disorders fulfilling criteria for defined autoimmune diseases were similar to those of idiopathic etiology. These findings raise the following questions. When patients with silicone-related disorders develop the clinical manifestations of scleroderma, lupus and other autoimmune disorders, is this causally related to the silicone implants or could these patients have spontaneously developed such autoimmune disorders? Many investigators have attempted to answer these questions, but because the development of defined autoimmune disorders are rare events, epidemiological studies have not been definitive because of the lack of biostatistically significant numbers of patients studied [3-5]. One feature, however, appears to suggest a cause and effect relationship with silicone implants and this is the repeated observation of a predominance of scleroderma over other more prevalent autoimmune disorders such as systemic lupus erythematosus, Sjogren's syndrome and rheumatoid arthritis [1,2].

In a larger study of a cohort of 300 patients (this paper), it was observed that undefined connective tissue disorders was by far the more common clinical picture and further analysis showed that a high percentage of these patients fulfilled diagnostic criteria for fibromyalgia [8] and chronic fatigue syndrome [10].

References

1. Press RI, Peebles CL, Kumagai Y, Ochs RL, Tan EM (1992) Antinuclear autoantibodies in women with silicone breast implants. Lancet 340:1304-1307

2. Kumagai Y, Shiokawa Y, Medsger TA Jr, Rodnan GP (1984) Clinical spectrum of connective tissue disease after cosmetic surgery. Arthritis Rheum 27:1-12
3. Bridges AJ, Conley C, Wang G, Burns DE, Vasey FB (1993) A clinical and immunologic evaluation of women with silicone breast implants and symptoms of rheumatic disease. Ann Intern Med 118:929-936
4. Spiera RF, Gibofsky A, Spiera H (1994) Silicone gel filled breast implants and connective tissue disease: an overview. J Rheumatol 21:239-245
5. Sanchez-Guerrero J, Schur PH, Sergent JS, Liang MH (1994) Silicone breast implants and rheumatic disease. Clinical, immunologic, and epidemiologic studies. Arthritis Rheum 37:158-168
6. Tan EM, Cohen AS, Fries JF, et al (1982) The 1982 revised criteria for classification of systemic lupus erythematosus. Arthritis Rheum 25:1271-1277
7. Subcommittee for scleroderma criteria of the American Rheumatism Association (1980) Diagnostic and therapeutic criteria committee: preliminary criteria for the classification of systemic sclerosis (scleroderma). Arthritis Rheum 23:581-590
8. Wolfe F, Smythe HA, Yunus MB, et al (1990) The American College of Rheumatology 1990 criteria for the classification of fibromyalgia. Arthritis Rheum 33:160-172
9. Arnett FC, Edworthy S, Block DA (1987) The 1987 revised ARA criteria for rheumatoid arthritis. Arthritis Rheum 30:S17
10. Schluederberg A, Straus SE, Peterson P, Blumenthal S, Komaroff AL, Spring SB, Landay A, Buchwald D (1992) Chronic fatigue syndrome research. Definition and medical outcome assessment. Ann Intern Med 117:325-331

Development of Scleroderma-like Syndrome in Tsk/+ Mice Is Not Enhanced by Silicone Administration

C. Frondoza,[1] L. Jones,[1] N.R. Rose,[1¶] A. Hatakeyama,[2] R. Phelps,[2] and C. Bona[2¶]

Johns Hopkins Depts. of Orthopaedic Surgery, of Molecular Microbiology and Immunology, and of Pathology, [2]Mt. Sinai School of Medicine Dept. of Microbiology and Immunology

Abstract

The possible role of silicone in the pathogenesis of a scleroderma-like syndrome is still unresolved. It has been proposed that silicone escaping from breast implants potentiates the progression of the disease. To clarify whether silicone enhances development of fibrotic skin lesions and autoantibodies, we tested its effect on tight skin (TSK/+) mice. TSK/+ mice spontaneously develop skin fibrosis and characteristic autoantibodies which resemble human scleroderma. The results of the present study indicate that silicone administration does not enhance development of skin fibrosis nor synthesis of autoantibodies to RNA polymerase and topoisomerase in TSK/+ mice.

Introduction

An association has been proposed between the development of connective tissue disorders and exposure to silicone in breast implant patients [1-2]. One of these connective tissue disorders is a scleroderma-like syndrome [3-8]. Scleroderma is a fibrotic disease which displays two distinct pathological features: (a) fibrotic cutaneous lesions and (b) production of characteristic autoantibodies [3-18].

Studies on breast implant cases demonstrated lesions characterized by fibrosis and cellular infiltrates consisting of macrophages and fibroblasts [1-8]. There was also marked proliferation of endothelial cells. Small arteries were

There was also marked proliferation of endothelial cells. Small arteries were observed to undergo myxomatous degeneration. Internal organs were seen to be infiltrated with mononuclear cells with marked vasculitis.

The scleroderma-like syndrome noted in silicone breast implant cases has been associated with autoimmune responses. Hypergammaglobulinemia (IgG) and elevated antibody titers of rheumatoid factor, nuclear antibodies, and antibodies to low molecular weight RNA and RNA polymerase protein (RNAP) complex were detected [12]. Antibodies against fibrillarin [13], topoisomerase I (SCL-70 [14], and centromere antigens, interstitial (type I) and basement membrane (type IV) collagen were also reported [15-18]. Many of these cases with circulating antibodies had activated lymphocytes [18-19].

The question of whether silicone also enhances the development of a scleroderma-like syndrome has not yet been experimentally tested. To help clarify the role of silicone in the pathogenesis of a scleroderma-like syndrome, we have utilized the TSK/+ mouse model. TSK/+ mice have been shown to develop lesions consisting of dermal fibrosis and autoantibodies to topoisomerase and RNA polymerase [20-24]. TSK/+ mice as an experimental model also has the advantage in that normal littermates are available for use as controls. In the same litter, the TSK/- mice differ genotypically only by the TSK mutation and do not develop cutaneous hyperplasia. The disease developed by TSK/+ mice is related to a single gene defect and is not associated with other alterations of immune system [20-21].

The aim of the present study was to determine whether silicone potentiates the development of fibrosis and production of characteristic autoantibodies in TSK/+ mice. By defining the effect of silicone on the onset and severity of the cutaneous hyperplasia and synthesis of autoantibodies, the role of silicone in the development of a scleroderma-like disease in recipients of silicone breast implants may be better defined.

Materials and methods

Four groups of one month old (20-25 g, n=6) TSK+ and five of their normal pa/pa littermates were injected subcutaneously (sc) with 0.1 ml of: (1) low molecular weight polydimethylsiloxane (Dow Corning 360 Medical fluid, 1000 centistoke viscosity, LMW-PDMS), (2) high molecular weight (Dow Corning Q7-2159A gel, HMW-PDMS), (3) incomplete Freunds adjuvant (IFA) or (4) Hanks' balanced salt solution (HBSS) in the dorsal neck area and ventrally in the upper chest region. These regions have been noted to display skin lesions in TSK mice [20]. Prior to injection, mice were bled from their retroorbital plexus. Sera were obtained for determination of antibody against RNA polymerase, topoisomerase and bovine serum albumin using radioimmunoassay [25-26]. Samples of skin, kidney and liver were fixed, paraffin embedded and analyzed by light microscopy.

Data were analyzed with computational assistance from CLINFO, sponsored by National Institutes of Health grant RR00035. The experimental results were analyzed using one-way analysis of variance. Neuman-Keuls multiple group comparisons were made and statistical significance was accepted at the $P < 0.05$ level.

Results

Histological analyses

Phenotypically normal TSK/- pa/pa littermates (20/20) showed no evidence of hyperplasia nor significant pathological changes after injection with HBSS, LMW-PDMS or HMW-PDMS. Lipid vacuoles of varying sizes were observed beneath the panniculus carnosus which were surrounded by histiocytic infiltrate. TSK/+ mice (24/24) developed cutaneous hyperplasia one month after injection of HBSS, LMW-PDMS, HMW-PDMS or IFA. TSK/+ mice injected with HBSS demonstrated slight thickening of the dermis and increased cellularity. The hyperplastic connective tissue beneath the panniculus carnosus formed a hypercellular band above the adipose tissue. Skin samples from TSK/+ mice that received LMW-PDMS showed macrophages containing lipid-like vacuolated materials. Large lipid vacuoles were evident throughout the deeper dermis. TSK/+ mice which received HMW-PDMS showed similar thickening of the dermis and the peri-panniculus carnosus connective tissue. There were no significant differences in the histologic characteristics of the silicone injected TSK/+ mice compared to those that received HBSS or IFA.

Kidney, spleen, or liver samples taken from TSK/+ or TSK/- mice injected with HBSS, IFA or silicone (LMW-PDMS, HMW-PDMS) did not show pathological changes.

Circulating antibodies

TSK/+ mice demonstrated circulating antibodies to BSA and autoantigens associated with the scleroderma-like syndrome (RNAP and toposimerase I). Baseline circulating antibody levels against all three tested antigens in TSK/+ mice were significantly higher ($P<0.01$) than those of their TSK/- littermates. To determine whether silicone administration modulates circulating antibody levels, pre- and post- injection antibody activities were determined as described in Methods. The levels of antibody to BSA were not significantly different to the levels prior to injection with HBSS, silicone or IFA (Fig. 1). The antibody levels to autoantigens RNAP (Figure 2) and topoisomerase I (Figure 3) were also not significantly different to the antibody levels prior to or after injection of contol saline IFA or silicone.

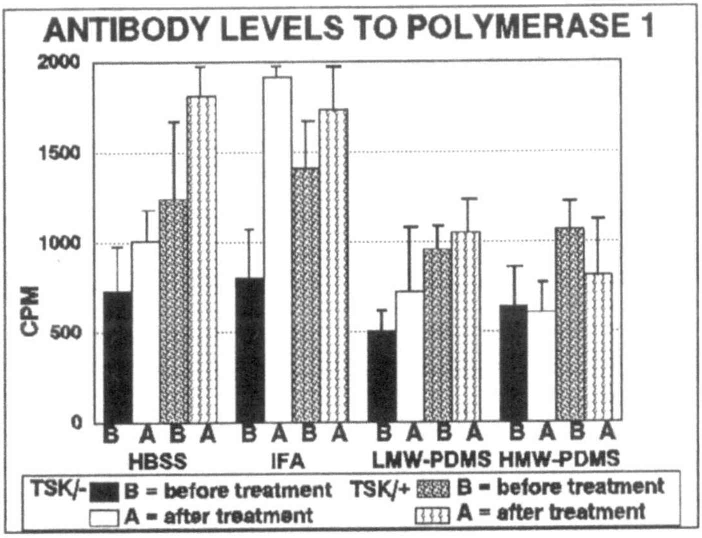

Fig. 1. Antibody levels to BSA in TSK/-pa/pa and TSK/+ mice. Each bar represents the average antibody levels from five pa/pa mice and six TSK/+ mice $\pm$ SD one month after HBSS, LMWPDMS, HMWPDMS or IFA administration.

Discussion

Earlier studies have indicated that silicone induces a fibrotic and granulomatous response in the tissue surrounding silicone implants [1-8]. However, it remains unclear as to whether silicone potentiates the progression of the fibrotic sequence to a scleroderma-like syndrome. In the present study, we demonstrate for the first time that silicone did not potentiate the development of a scleroderma-like syndrome in TSK/+ mice. Exposure to silicone did not exacerbate skin hyperplasia nor did it enhance the production of autoantibodies to RNAP and topoisomerase.

The failure of silicone gel and oil to influence the extent of skin fibrosis in TSK/+ mice may be due to their lack of effect on the distribution of cellular infiltrates. Previous investigation documented the role of macrophages and fibroblasts in the development of fibrosis [27-33]. The failure of silicone gel and oil to influence the extent of skin fibrosis in TSK/+ mice may be accounted for by their lack of effect on the distribution of macrophages. Tissue macrophages play a role in the development of fibrotic syndrome by producing cytokines which regulate fibroblast proliferation and collagen synthesis [27-33]. Fibroblasts

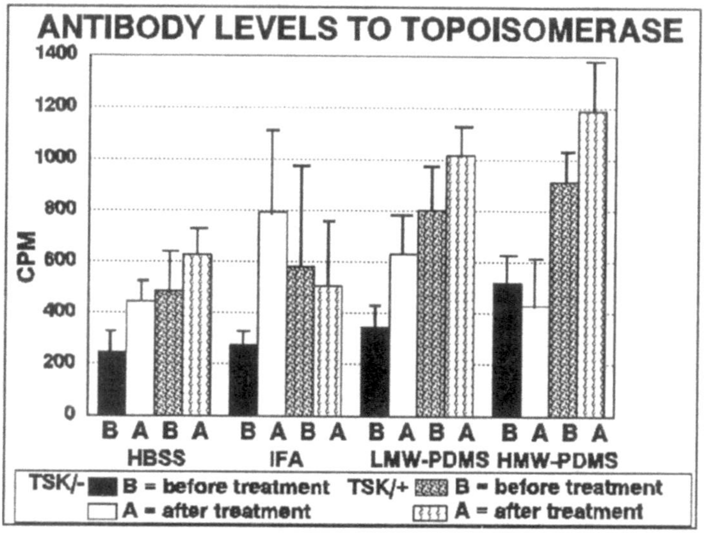

Fig. 2. Antibody levels to RNAP in TSK/-pa/pa and TSK/+ mice. Each bar represents the average antibody levels from five pa/pa mice and six TSK/+ mice ± SD one month after HBSS, LMWPDMS, HMWPDMS or IFA administration.

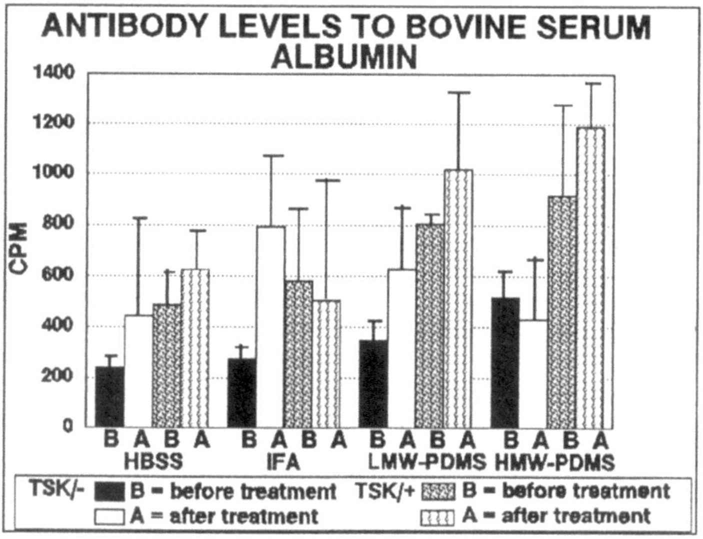

Fig. 3. Antibody levels to topoisomerase in TSK/-pa/pa and TSK/+ mice. Each bar represents the average antibody levels from five pa/pa mice and six TSK/+ mice ± SD one month after HBSS, LMWPDMS, HMWPDMS or IFA administration.

produce skin connective tissue composed of collagen type I and the minorcollagen type III. Changes in the amounts, as well as the type, of collagen being made would result in a change in connective tissue matrix. It is possible that dermal fibroblasts in TSK/+ mice may not be responsive to silicone and are therefore not capable of proliferating or producing the fibrotic collagenous tissue.

Since silicone did not induce increased levels of circulating antibodies it may not be involved in the development of the scleroderma-like syndrome. A distinctive feature of the scleroderma-like syndrome is hypergammaglobulinemia and production of autoantibodies. Studies showed that fifty percent of scleroderma patients exhibited elevated IgG. Others had elevated titers of rheumatoid factors (25-33% of cases) and antinuclear antibodies against self antigens (40% of cases) [9-26]. The antibodies detected were directed against low molecular weight RNA and RNA polymerase I protein complex [10]. Circulating antibodies were also observed against fibrillarin, a 34kd protein of the U3-RNP particles [12]. Others had high titers of autoantibodies against SCL70 (topoisomerase I) while anti-centromere antibodies are regularly found in patients with CREST syndrome [13-14]. Antibodies to interstitial (type I) and basement membrane (type IV) collagen were also identified [16-17].

Based on our observation that silicone did not potentiate development of skin fibrosis and production of autoantibodies in mice, it appears unlikely that silicone is a major predisposing factor in the evolution of the scleroderma-like disease.

References

1. Seleznick MJ, Martinez-Osuna P, Espinoza LR, Vasey FB (1991) Is silicone associated with connective tissue disease? J Florida Med Assoc 78: 85-87
2. Spiera RF, Gibofsky A, Spiera H (1994) Silicone Gel Filled Breast Implants and Connective Tissue Disease: An Overview. Rheumatology 21: 239-245
3. Marik PE, Kark AL, Zambakides A (1990) Scleroderma after silicone augmentation mammoplasty. SAM J 77: 212-213
4. Sahn EE, Garen PD, Silver RM, Maize JC (1990) Scleroderma following augmentation mammoplasty. Arch Dermatol 126: 1198-120257.
5. Varga J, Jimenez SA (1990) Augmentation mammoplasty and scleroderma: Is there an association? Arch Dermatol 126: 1220-1222
6. Englert HJ, Howe GB, Penny R, Brooks P (1994) Scleroderma and Silicone Breast Implants. Br J Rheumatol 33: 397-399
7. Sergott TJ, Limoli JP, Baldwin Jr. CM, Laum DR (1986) Human adjuvant disease, possible autoimmune disease after silicone implantation: A review of the literature, case studies, and speculation for the future. Plast Reconstr Surg 78: 104-114
8. Spiera H (1988) Scleroderma after silicone augmentation mammoplasty. JAMA. 260: 236-238
9. Morse JJ, Spiera H (1992) Autoimmune diseases, immunoglobulin isotypes and lymphocyte subsets in 30 females with breast augmentation mammoplasty. Arthritis Rheum 35: S65
10. Silvira LH, Sandifer M, Cuellar ML, Osuna PM, Scopelitis B, Espinoza LR (1992) Serum antinuclear antibodies in women with silicone breast implants. Arthritis Rheum 35: S66

11. Chen Z-Y, Silver RM, Ainsworth SK, Dobson RL, Maricq TR (1984) Association between fluorescent antinuclear antibodies, capillary patterns and clinical features in scleroderma spectrum disorders. Am J Med 77:812-822

12. Stetler DA, Rose KM, Wenger ME, Berline CM, Jacob S (1982) Antibodies to distinct polypeptides of RNA polymerase I in sera from patients with rheumatic autoimmune disease. Proc Natl Acad Sci (USA) 79: 6499-7503

13. Okano X, Steen VD, Medsger TA (1992) Autoantibody to K3 nucleolar ribonucleoprotein (fibrillarin) in patients with systemic sclerosis. Arthritis Rheum 35: 95-100

14. Shero JH, Bordwell B, Rothfield NI, Earnshaw WC (1986) High titers of autoantibodies to topoisomerase I (ScL-70) in sera from scleroderma patients. Science 231: 737-740

15. Tuffanelli DL, McKeon F, Leinsmith DAM, Burnham TK, Kirschner M (1983) Anticentromere and anticentriole antibodies in the scleroderma spectrum. Arch. Dermatol 119: 560-566

16. Mackel AM, Delustro F, Harper FE, Leroy RC (1982) Antibodies to collagen in scleroderma. Arthritis Rheum 25: 522-531

17. Peltoen J, Kahari L, Uilto J, Jimenez SA (1990) Increased expression of type VI collagen genes in systemic sclerosis. Arthritis Rheum 33: 1829-1835

18. Broughton A, Thrasher JD (1993) Autoantibodies associated with silicone breast implants Clin Chem 39: 1139

19. Claman HN, Robertson AD (1994) Antinuclear antibodies and breast implants. West J Med 160: 225-228

20. Green MC, Sweet HO, Bunker LE (1976) Tight-Skin, a New Mutation of the Mouse Causing Excessive Growth of Connective Tissue and Skeleton. Am J Pathol 82: 493-511

21. Jimenez SA, Millan A, Bashey RI (1984) Scleroderma-like alterations in Collagen Metabolism occurring in the TSK (Tight Skin) mouse. Arthritis Rheum 27: 180-185

22. Bocchieri MH, Heuriksen PD, Kasturi KN, Muryoi T, Bona CA, Jimenez SA (1991) Evidence for autoimmunity in tight skin (TSK/+) mouse model progressive systemic sclerosis. Arthritis Rheum 34: 599-605.

23. Muryoi T, Kasturi KN, Kafina MJ, Cram DS, Harrison LC, Sasaki T, Bona CA (1992) Antitopoisomerase I monoclonal autoantibodies from scleroderma patients and tight skin mouse interact with similar epitopes. J Exp Med 175: 1103-1109

24. Bocchieri MH, Christner PJ, Henriksen PD, Jimenez SA (1993) Immunological Characterization of (Tight Skin/NZB)F1 Hybrid Mice with Connective Tissue and Autoimmune Features Resembling Human Systemic Sclerosis. J Autoimmunity 6: 337-351

25. Shibata S, Muryoi T, Saitoh Y, Brumeanu TD, Bona CA, Kasturi KN (1993) Immunochemical and Molecular Characterization of Anti-RNA Polymerase I Autoantibodies Produced by Tight Skin Mouse. J Clin Invest 92: 984-99229.

26. Phelps RG, Daian C, Shibata S, Fleischmajer R, Bona CA (1993) Induction of Skin Fibrosis and Autoantibodies by Infusion of Immunocompetent Cells from Tight Skin Mice into C57BL/6 Pa/Pa Mice. J Autoimmunity 6: 701-718

27. Brantley SK, Davidson SF, St. Arnold PS, Johnson MB, Talbot PJ, Grogan JB, Cuchens MA, Hsu HS, Das SK (1990) Assessment of lymphocyte response to silicone. Plast Reconstr Surg 86: 1131-1137

28. White Needleman B, Wigley TM, Stair RW (1992) Interleukin-1,interleukin-2, interleukin-4, interleukin-6, tumor necrosis factor alpha and interferon gamma levels in sera from patients with scleroderma. Arthritis Rheum 35: 67-92

29. Das SK, Johnson M, Ellsaesser C, Brantley SK, Johnson SG (1992) Macrophage interleukin-1 response to injected silicone in a rat model. Ann Plast Surg 28: 535-537

30. Kovacs, EJ (1991) Fibrogenic Cytokines: The role of Immune Mediators in the Development of Scar Tissue. Immunol Today 12: 17-23

31. Kahari VM, Heino J, Vuorio E (1987) Interleukin-1 increases collagen production and messenger RNA levels in cultured skin fibroblasts. Biochim Biophys Acta 929: 142-147

32. Varga J, Rosenbloom J, Jimenez SA (1987) Transforming growth factor ß (TGFB) causes a persistent increase in steady-state amounts of type I and type III collagen and fibronectin mRNAs in normal human dermal fibroblasts. Biochem J 247: 597-604

33. Loppnow H, Flad HD, Durrbaum I, Musehold J, Fetting R, Ulmer AJ, Herzbeck H, Brandt E (1989) Detection of interleukin-1 with human dermal fibroblasts. Immunobiol 179: 283-291

¶Dr. Rose has served as expert witness on behalf of defendants in several legal proceedings involving silicone breast implants. He has also served as consultant for Mentor Corporation, a manufacturer of breast implants.

Comparative Epitope Mapping of Antibodies to Collagen in Women with Silicone Breast Implants, Systemic Lupus Erythematosus and Rheumatoid Arthritis

M.J. Rowley[1], A.D. Cook[1], I.R. Mackay[1], S.S. Teuber[2,3], and M.E. Gershwin[2*].
[1]Centre for Molecular Biology and Medicine, Monash University, Clayton, Victoria, Australia.
[2]Department of Internal Medicine, Division of Rheumatology, Allergy and Clinical Immunology, University of California at Davis, School of Medicine, Davis, California, USA.
[3]Department of Veterans Affairs Northern California System of Clinics, Pleasant Hill, California, USA.

Abstract

Previous work has shown that women with silicone gel breast implants have an increased frequency of autoantibodies to collagen types I and II. 70 women without a specific autoimmune disease, using criteria of the American College of Rheumatology, but who had silicone breast implants were studied for the presence of serum antibodies to native and denatured human types I and II collagen by ELISA. 82 women with systemic lupus erythematosus (SLE), 94 women with rheumatoid arthritis (RA), and 133 healthy controls were also studied. There was a high frequency of autoantibodies to collagen in each of the groups when compared to the healthy controls. The specificities of these antibodies were found to differ markedly when examined by immunoblotting using peptides derived by cyanogen bromide digestion of the collagens. Sera from women with silicone implants reacted with multiple peptides of type I collagen in an individual-specific manner, but sera from women with SLE or RA reacted weakly with a restricted range of peptides. Against type II collagen, sera from women with RA reacted strongly with multiple peptides, while sera from women with silicone implants or SLE reacted only weakly or not at all. The patterns of reactivity against collagens by sera from women with silicone implants suggest that silicone can act as an adjuvant to enhance the immunogenicity of type I collagen.

Introduction

Exposure to silicone used in breast augmentation has been clinically linked to both local granulomatous reactions and systemic autoimmune disease [1-6], though the latter is controversial. Women who seek medical advice for rheumatic disease symptoms after breast implants may already be in a prodromal phase of an autoimmune disease unrelated to their implant. We entertain the possibility

*M.E. Gershwin has served as an expert witness for plaintiff's attorneys in breast implant litigation. This presentation is based on work published in the Journal of Autoimmunity 1994;8:777-787.

that silicone is capable of actually initiating an autoimmune process, either by a local adjuvant effect [7], or by causing denaturation of host molecules with ensuing enhancement of their immunogenicity [8,9]. If autoimmunity were to result from exposure to silicone, then the connective tissues most closely associated with the implant should be involved, and particularly collagens since these are the most abundant and form the major structural components of the extracellular matrix. Collagens are immunogenic in animals, and antibodies to various collagens are present in human serum in several diseases, particularly those of autoimmune origin [10-15]. In our experience [15], the most frequent reactivities to collagen are seen in SLE in which type I collagen is the main reactant and RA in which type II collagen is the main reactant.

In a previous study on 46 consecutive self-referred patients with silicone breast implants, antibodies to native and/or denatured type I or type II human collagen were detected in 16 women (35%) [16]. Accordingly, we developed the present study [17] to ascertain the relative frequencies of autoantibodies to collagen in women with breast implants versus patients with SLE or RA, and whether the epitope specificity of such antibodies differed from that present in the spontaneously ocurring autoimmune diseases. A differing epitope specificity of the antibodies would indicate that autoantibodies associated with silicone breast implants could be dissociated from prodromal or actual expressions of SLE or RA.

Methods

Patients. Antibodies to collagen were examined in women who presented to the University of California, Davis with concerns about their implants. Patients were excluded from the study if they carried an established diagnosis of a known autoimmune disease, particularly SLE, RA or scleroderma using criteria of the American College of Rheumatology, and also patients who had previously undergone injection of bovine collagen or had their implants removed. The 70 women in the study ranged in age from 26 to 66 years, mean 45.1 years, and the mean duration of the silicone gel breast implants ranged from 2 to 28 years, mean 13.3 years. Five women had dual lumen implants exclusively, the rest had single lumen gel-filled implants either currently or in the past. Only 5 (7.1%) of the 70 subjects felt entirely well. The other 65 reported symptoms that included fatigue, myalgias, and arthralgias. Six (8.6%) had Raynaud's phenomenon, but this preceded implantation in only one patient. The reasons for prosthesis implantation were after subcutaneous mastectomy for fibrocystic disease (5 cases), after prophylactic mastectomy (2 cases), after mastectomy for breast cancer (2 cases), and for cosmetic augmentation (61 cases). Forty-nine (70%) of 70 women had a history of moderate to severe capsular contracture. Twenty-six (37.1%) of 70 women had experienced one or more ruptured implants. Thirty (42.9%) women had undergone more than one augmentation because of either contracture or rupture. These 70 women accounted for the use of more than 200 individual breast implants.

The controls for this study included 43 generally healthy Californian women (2 of whom had osteoarthritis) of the same age distribution and from the same geographic area as the women with breast implants and 90 Australian blood donors of either sex.

Rheumatoid factor and antinuclear antibody. Rheumatoid factor (RF) was measured by nephelometry. A level of ≥ 60 IU was scored as a positive test. Antinuclear antibody (ANA) was titrated by immunofluorescence on HEp2 cells using a polyvalent antiserum reactive against IgG heavy and light chains (Immuno Concepts, Sacramento, California, USA). A titer of ≥ 1:80 was scored as a positive test.

Preparation of Collagens and Cyanogen Bromide (CB) Peptides. Human type I collagen was obtained commercially (Sigma, St. Louis, MO, USA), dissolved in 0.5M acetic acid, and reprecipitated with 5% NaCl before use. Bovine type I collagen and human type II collagen were prepared as described [13]. Cyanogen bromide digestion by the method of Scott and Veis [18] was accomplished using 3 mg of purified collagen dissolved in 1 ml of 70% (v/v) formic acid which contained 50 mg of cyanogen bromide. Since collagen peptides do not run according to their molecular weight in SDS-PAGE, peptides of type I collagen were identified by comparison with published densitometric scans of type I CB peptides [18] and with human type I CB peptide standards (a gift of Dr. J. Bateman, Department of Paediatrics, Royal Children's Hospital, Parkville, Victoria, Australia). N-terminal sequencing of selected polypeptides confirmed identification. The bands sequenced were identified as CB7, CB8 and CB6 from $\alpha 1(I)$. Peptides of type II collagen were identified by comparison with human type II CB peptide standards and published type II CB peptides maps [19,20].

Antibody Detection by ELISA. Antibodies to each collagen type were measured by ELISA as described [16,17]. To allow for non-specific binding of immunoglobulins to the plates, the optical density obtained in the absence of collagen was subtracted from that obtained in wells coated with collagen. Results were expressed in terms of the number of standard deviations above the mean of the 10 blood donors tested in the same assay. A serum was considered to contain an elevated level of antibodies to collagen if the value was greater than the mean plus 3 standard deviations of the healthy controls.

Immunoblotting of CB Peptides. Antibodies to CB peptides of collagen were detected by immunoblotting [15]. Human type II collagen was used as the standard antigen, but to conserve human type I collagen, bovine type I collagen was used after it was clearly determined that sera that contained antibodies to type I collagen reacted similarly with human and bovine collagen. Sera were diluted 1:400 and incubated approximately 16 hr. at 4°C with the strips. Bound antibodies were detected using enhanced chemiluminescence (Amersham Inc., USA), according to the manufacturer's instructions. Positive control sera were obtained from a patient with silicone implants, with a known reactivity with each of the peptides of type I collagen, and from a patient with RA with a known reactivity with each of the major peptides of type II collagen.

Statistical Analysis. Statistical comparisons employed Chi square analysis in 2x2 contingency tables. One way ANOVA was used for comparison of continuous variable patient characteristics. Results were considered significant if $P \leq 0.05$.

Results

Antibodies to rheumatoid factor and nuclear antigens. For the patients with RA, RF was measured in 82 and 56 (68%) were positive at the time of the test; only 5 of the 82 patients had been consistently seronegative over previous testing. ANA was measured in 84 patients with RA and 27 (32%) were positive. For the 82 patients with SLE, ANA titer was > 1:80 at the time of testing in 58 (71%). The SLE sera were not tested for RF. Of the women with silicone breast implants, none had a positive RF and 19 (27%) had a positive ANA (Table 1).

Table 1. Frequencies of antibodies to native and denatured type I and II collagens measured by ELISA and positive ANA or RF assays in women with silicone breast implants, in women with SLE, RA and in healthy controls.

Group	No.	TYPE I COLLAGEN Antibody to:			TYPE II COLLAGEN Antibody to:			ANA ≥1:80	RF
		Native	Denat.	Either	Native	Denat.	Either		
Silicone (SI)	70	10 (14%)[1]	16 (23%)	18 (26%)	6 (9%)[2]	13 (19%)	16 (23%)	19 (27%)	0
SLE	82	18 (22%)	NA[3]	NA	6 (7%)	NA	NA	58 (71%)	NA
RA	94	5 (5%)	18 (19%)	22 (23%)	22 (23%)	17 (18%)	34 (36%)	27 (32%)	56 (68%)
Controls:									
Donors	90	1 (1%)	2 (2%)	3 (3%)	2 (2%)	4 (4%)	4 (4%)	NA	NA
Women	43	0	1 (2%)	1 (2%)	0	0	0	NA	NA

[1]Frequency of antibodies to native type I collagen (Chi squares). SI vs. RA: $P \leq 0.049$; SI vs. SLE: N.S.; RA vs.SLE: $P \leq 0.0011$

[2]Frequency of antibodies to native type II collagen (Chi squares). SI vs. RA: $P \leq 0.0125$; SI vs. SLE: N.S.; RA vs. SLE: $P \leq 0.0044$

[3]NA - not available. Antibodies to denatured collagen in the SLE sera were not measured, as these sera were known to have been repeatedly frozen and thawed, a procedure that can lead to an apparent increase in the levels of antibodies to denatured collagen [21].

Antibodies to collagen. The frequencies of antibodies to native or denatured type I and type II collagen were significantly elevated in women with implants, women with SLE and women with RA when compared to both populations of healthy controls. Specifically, antibodies to native and/or denatured collagen were present in 29 (41%) of the 70 women with breast implants (Chi squares, $P < 0.0001$), and 23 (28%) of 82 women with SLE (among whom only antibodies to native collagen were compared, Chi squares, $P < 0.0001$) and 45 (48%) of the 94 women with RA (Chi squares, $P < 0.0001$) compared to only 8 (6%) of the 133 healthy controls. Of women with silicone implants, those with antibodies to collagen did not differ significantly from women without such antibodies with respect to age, years with implants, history of capsular contracture, rupture, incidence of positive ANA, number of implant surgeries or total IgG value [17].

Although the overall frequencies of antibodies to collagen were elevated in each of the study groups, the relative frequencies of antibodies to native type I and type II collagens differed (Table 1). Thus, antibodies to native type I collagen were significantly more frequent in women with breast implants (14%) and with SLE (22%), than in those with RA (5%) (Chi squares, $P < 0.05$ and $P < 0.001$), whereas antibodies to native type II collagen were significantly more frequent in RA (23%), than in the other two groups, 9% and 7% (Chi squares, $P < 0.01$ and $P < 0.005$).

Patterns of Reactivity to CB Peptides. There was good correlation between reactivity by ELISA and reactivity by immunoblotting on CB peptides of type I or type II collagen; 52 of 58 sera (89.7%) that reacted with native or denatured type I collagen by ELISA reacted with one or more CB peptides of type I collagen, and 37 of 56 sera (66.1%) that reacted with native or denatured type II collagen by ELISA reacted with one or more CB peptides of type II collagen.

Most sera from each study group that contained antibodies to type I collagen by ELISA reacted with several polypeptides by immunoblotting, but there were patterns of reactivity specific for each group (Table 2). Sera from the patients with breast implants showed variable individual-specific patterns of reactivity with multiple peptides, not all of which could be identified (Figure 1). On the other hand, 39 of 40 (98%) sera from women with SLE or RA showed a similar pattern and intensity of reaction with several bands that were taken to represent reactivity with CB8 from $\alpha 1$ (I) (Table 2), and one was non-reactive. CB8 itself was identified from N-terminal sequencing, and the higher molecular weight bands were taken to represent known products of incomplete cleavage of CB5-CB8 [18]. This reactivity with CB8 was infrequent in sera from women with breast implants, being observed in only 3 of 18 (17%).

The frequencies of reactivity with other type I CB peptides in the three study groups are shown in Table 2. For the women with breast implants that had antibodies to type I collagen by ELISA, 5 sera (28%) were unreactive by immunoblotting. Nine of the remaining 13 sera reacted with CB6 from $\alpha 1$ (I), and 5 also reacted strongly with a low molecular weight component, possibly CB2-4 and CB4-5. Sera from patients with SLE and RA reacted weakly with all peptides other than CB8, but 6 of 18 sera from patients with SLE reacted with CB3 from $\alpha 1$(I), and 5 sera from patients with SLE, and 4 from patients with RA reacted with the low molecular weight component.

Table 2. The frequencies of reactivity against type I cyanogen bromide peptides by Western blotting in women with a positive ELISA to type I collagen.

Group	No.	Cyanogen bromide peptides α2(I): CB4 (%)	α1(I): CB7 (%)	CB8 (%)	CB6 (%)	CB3 (%)	CB2-4/4-5 (%)	Unreactive (%)
Silicone	18	11	17	17	50	17	28	28
SLE	18	6	6	94	11	33	28	6
RA	22	5	0	100	23	0	18	0

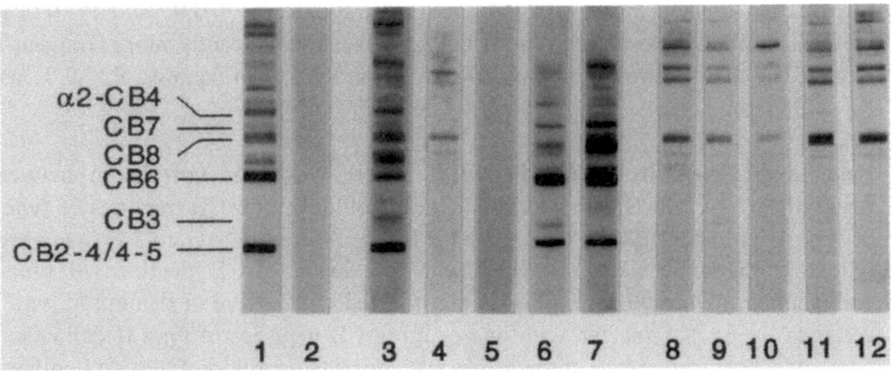

Fig. 1. Western blot profile of type I collagen ELISA positive sera against CB peptides of type I collagen. Lane 1: positive control serum (silicone implant patient). Lane 2: normal serum. Lanes 3-7: silicone implant patient sera. Lanes 8, 9: SLE patient sera. Lanes 10-12: RA patient sera.

Sera from women with breast implants were rarely reactive by immunoblotting to type II collagen; only 6 of the 16 sera (37.5%) that reacted by ELISA were reactive by immunoblotting, 5 with CB10.5 and 2 with CB11. All 6 (100%) ELISA-reactive sera from women with SLE, and 25 of 34 (74%) ELISA-reactive sera from women with RA were reactive by immunoblotting (Table 3). Most unreactive sera contained antibodies to denatured collagen only. Sera from patients with RA showed strong, individual-specific patterns of reactivity with multiple peptides, whereas reactivity with sera from women with breast implants, or SLE was generally weaker (Figure 2). However, there were no significant differences between groups in the peptides recognized. The overall combined frequencies for the three groups were 64% (36 sera) reactive to CB10.5, 27% (15 sera) for CB11, 9% (5 sera) for CB8 and 5% (3 sera) for the low molecular weight peptides CB9, 7 and CB12 (Table 3).

Table 3. The frequencies of reactivity against cyanogen bromide peptides by Western blotting in women with a positive ELISA to type II collagen.

Group	No.	Cyanogen bromide fragment: CB10,5 (%)	CB11 (%)	CB8 (%)	CB9,7/12 (%)	Unreactive (%)
Silicone	16	31	13	0	0	63
SLE	6	100	50	33	0	0
RA	34	74	29	9	9	26

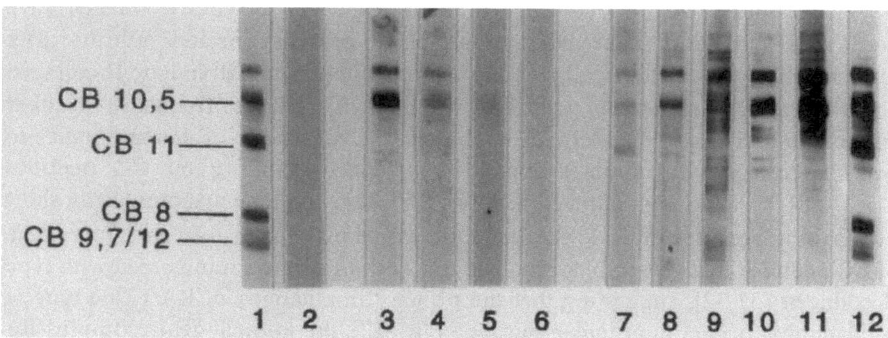

Fig. 2. Western blot profile of type II collagen ELISA positive sera against CB peptides of type II collagen. Lane 1: positive control serum (RA). Lane 2: normal serum. Lanes 3-6: silicone implant patient sera. Lanes 7, 8: SLE patient sera. Lanes 9-12: RA patient sera.

Discussion

Collagens are a family of extracellular matrix molecules with each having a characteristic molecular structure of three polypeptides (α-chains) with long regions of triple helix in which the structure is strictly dependent on glycine at every third position. Of those used in this study, type I collagen occurs throughout the body, and is a major component of the fibrous tissue in the peri-implant milieu of the breast, whereas type II occurs predominantly in hyaline cartilage. Of the women with silicone breast implants, 18 (26%) had autoantibodies to native or denatured type I collagen by ELISA and 16 (23%) to type II collagen. The pattern of reactivity by Western blotting in these women suggested that type I collagen was the primary immunogen, in that the most frequent reactant was type I collagen and sera gave strong individual-specific patterns of reactivity with a range of CB peptides. Antibodies to type II collagen occurred less frequently, and most sera either did not react at all by immunoblotting or reacted weakly and only with CB10.5. The pattern of reactivity to collagens type I and II and the frequency of RF and ANA differed strikingly from those ascertained for women with RA or SLE.

ELISA or solid phase radioimmunoprecipitation assays have been used to survey the frequency of antibodies to different collagens, including type I, in various diseases [10,12-14,22,23]. However, there are hitherto no reports on the epitope-specificity of the antibodies nor the capacity for cross-reactivity among different collagen types. In one study of epitope-specificity of antibodies to type I collagen in patients who developed a reaction after receiving injections with bovine type I and III collagens for cosmetic purposes [24], there were positive reactions to intradermal testing in 1% before treatment and 2% thereafter; among those who did react serum antibodies to bovine collagen were demonstrable to various CB peptides throughout the molecule, most frequently to α1-CB6, and the pattern of reactivity to CB peptides of bovine collagen was very similar to that observed in the present study using human type I collagen. However, there was no cross-reactivity between bovine and human collagens [24].

In contrast to type I collagen, immune responses to type II collagen have been well studied in man and animals since animals develop arthritis after immunization with type II collagen [25], and antibodies to native type II collagen occur in 10-20% of patients with RA [10-12,22,26], and less frequently in other autoimmune diseases [11,14,15,23]. The epitope specificity of autoantibodies to type II collagen has been examined by Western blotting on CB peptides [15,27,28], by ELISA on purified peptides [29], or by epitope mapping using short overlapping peptides [30]. In RA there are varied patterns of reactivity to a range of CB peptides, with resemblance to patterns seen in animals immunized with type II collagen [31,32], suggesting that the primary immunogen in RA is the type II collagen that occurs in articular cartilage. In SLE, the immunogenic stimulus for antibodies to collagen is quite uncertain; the fact that antibodies are demonstrable to the pericellular collagens type IV and V [14] and the collagen-like region of C1q [33], particularly in association with vasculitis or renal disease, suggests that one of these antigens may constitute the primary immunogen in SLE.

The similar specificity of antibodies to human collagen in women with breast implants and antibodies occurring after injections with bovine collagen, make it seem likely that the stimulus for the anticollagen response is immunization to collagen in the breast tissue itself, consequent to local inflammation involving collagen deposition and adjuvant effects of the implant materials [7,34-36].

The clear differences in epitope reactivity of antibodies to type I and type II collagen in women with implants and those with either RA or SLE, together with the differing frequencies of RF and ANA in the three groups makes it unlikely that symptomatic women with breast implants are in a prodromal phase of either of these autoimmune diseases, and moreover, the few retrospective epidemiological studies published to date have not shown any increase in prevalence of "classical" autoimmune diseases in women with breast implants [37, 38]. In fact, silicone breast implants are more associated with various non-specific symptoms and an increased frequency of antinuclear autoantibody reactivities without recognized disease specificity [6,39,40], in line with our present findings that antibodies to collagen in women with breast implants have an epitope specificity different from that of the antibodies to collagen demonstrable in some cases of RA or SLE. We therefore conclude that antibodies to collagen in women with breast implants are a manifestation of adjuvant effects of silicone on the immune response to local peri-implant autoantigens.

REFERENCES

1. Mikuz G, Hoinkes G, Propst A, Wilflingseder P (1984) Tissue reactions with silicone rubber implants (morphological, microchemical, and clinical investigations in humans and laboratory animals). In: Macromolecular Biomaterials. G.M. Hartings and P. Ducheyne, Eds. CRC Press, Inc. Boca Raton, Florida 239-249
2. Travis WD, Balogh K, Abraham JL (1985) Silicone granulomas: report of three cases and a review of the literature. Human Pathol 16:19
3. Van Nunen SA, Gatenby PA, Basten A (1992) Post-mammoplasty connective tissue disease. Arthritis Rheum 25:694-697
4. Spiera H, Dubin Kerr L (1992) Scleroderma following silicone implantation: a cumulative experience of 11 cases. J Rheumatol 20:958-961
5. Bridges AJ, Conley C, Wang G, Burns E, Vasey FB (1993) A clinical and immunologic evaluation of women with silicone breast implants and symptoms of rheumatic disease. Ann Intern Med 118:929-936
6. Press RI, Peebles CL, Kumagai Y, Ochs RL, Tan EM (1992) Antinuclear autoantibodies in women with silicone breast implants. Lancet 340:1304-1307
7. Naim JO, Lanzafame RJ (1993) The adjuvant effect of silicone gel on antibody formation in rats. Immunol Invest 22:151-161
8 Seleznick MJ, Martinez-Osuna P, Espinoza LR, Vasey FB (1991) Is silicone associated with connective tissue disease? J Florida MA 78:85-87
9. Kossovsky N, Zeidler M, Chum G, Papasian N, Nguyen A, Rajguru A, Stassi J, Gelman A, Sponsier E (1993) Surface dependent antigens identified by high binding avidity of serum antibodies in a subpopulation of patients with breast prostheses. J Applied Biomaterials 4:281-288
10. Stuart JM, Huffstutter EH, Townes AS, Kang AH (1993) Incidence and specificity of antibodies of types I, II, III, IV, and V collagen in rheumatoid arthritis and other rheumatic diseases as measured by 125I-radioimmunoassay. Arthritis Rheum 26:832-840
11. Choi EKK, Gatenby PA, McGill NW, Bateman JF, ColeWG, York JR (1988) Autoantibodies to type II collagen: occurrence in rheumatoid arthritis, other arthritides, autoimmune connective tissue diseases, and chronic inflammatory syndromes. Ann Rheum Dis 47:313-319
12. Charriere G, Hartmann DJ, Vignon E, Ronziere MC, Herbage D, Ville G (1988) Antibodies to types I, II, IX and XI collagen in the serum of patients with rheumatic diseases. Arthritis Rheum 31:325
13. Rowley MJ, Gershwin ME, Mackay IR (1988) Collagen antibodies in juvenile arthritis and adult rheumatoid arthritis: differences in levels and type-specificity. J Rheumatol 15:289-293
14. Moreland LW, Gay RE, Gay S (1991) Collagen autoantibodies in patients with vasculitis and systemic lupus erythematosus. Clin Immunol Immunopathol 60:412-418
15. Rowley MJ, Mackay IR, Brand CA, Batemen JF, Chan D (1992) Epitope specificity of antibodies to type II collagen in rheumatoid arthritis and systemic lupus erythematosus. Rheumatol Int 12:65-68
16. Teuber SS, Rowley MJ, Yoshida SH, Ansari AA, Gershwin ME (1993) Anti-collagen autoantibodies are found in women with silicone breast implants. J Autoimmunity 6:367
17. Rowley MJ, Cook AD, Teuber SS, Gershwin ME (1994) Antibodies to collagen: comparative epitope mapping in women with silicone breast implants, systemic lupus erythematosus and rheumatoid arthritis. J Autoimmunity 7:775-789
18. Scott PG, Veis A (1976) The cyanogen bromide peptides of bovine soluble and insoluble collagens. Connect Tissue Res 4:107
19. Bornstein P, Sage H (1980) Structurally distinct collagen types. Ann Rev Biochem 49:957
20. Miller EJ, Rhodes RK (1982) Preparation and characterization of the different types of collagen. Methods Enzymol 82:51-59

21. Woodruff T, Cook A, Rowley M, Mackay I (1994) Antibodies to type II collagen in human serum: storage effects and role of IgM anti-idiotype inregulation. J Rheumatol. 21:197
22. Clague RB, Shaw MJ, Holt PJL (1980) Incidence of serum antibodies to native type I and type II collagens of patients with inflammatory arthritis. Ann Rheum Dis 39:201-206
23. Gioud M, Meghlaoui A, Costa O, Monier JC (1982) Antibodies to native type I and type II collagens detected by an enzyme linked immunosorbent assay (ELISA) in rheumatoid arthritis and systemic lupus erythematosus. Collagen Rela. Res 2:557-561
24. Ellingsworth LR, DeLustro F, Brennan JE, Sawamura S, McPherson J (1986) The human immune response to reconstituted bovine collagen. J Immunol 136:877-882
25. Trentham DE, Townes AS, Kang AH (1977) Autoimmunity to type II collagen: an experimental model of arthritis. J Exp Med 146:857-869
26. Rowley M, Tait B, Mackay IR, Cunningham T, Phillips B (1986) Collagen antibodies in rheumatoid arthritis. Significance of antibodies to denatured collagen and their association with HLA-DR4. Arthritis Rheum 29:174
27. Buckee C, Morgan K, Ayad S, Collins I, Clague RB, Holt PJL (1990) Diversity of antibodies to type II collagen in patients with rheumatoid arthritis: detection by binding to α-chains and to cyanogen bromide peptides. Br J Rheumatol 29:254-258
28. Cook AD, Rowley MJ, Stockman A, Muirden KD, Mackay IR (1994) Specificity of antibodies to type II collagen in early rheumatoid arthritis. J Rheumatol (In Press)
29. Terato K, Shimozuru Y, Katayama K, Takemitsu Y, Yamshita I, Mitayatsu M, Fujii K, Sagara M, Kobayashi S, Goto M, Nishioka K, Miyasaka N, Nagai Y (1990) Specificity of antibodies to type II collagen in rheumatoid arthritis. Arthritis Rheum 33:1493-1500
30. Worthington J, Turner S, Brass A, Morgan K (1993). Epitopes on the CB-11 peptide of type II collagen recognized by antibodies from patients with rheumatoid arthritis. Br J Rheumatol 32:658-662
31. Terato K, Arai H, Shimozuru Y, Fukada T, Tanaka H, Watanabe H, Nagai Y, Fijimoto K, Okubo F,. Cho F, Hongjo S, Cremer MA (1989) Sex-linked differences in susceptibility of cynomolgus monkeys to type II collagen-induced arthritis. Arthritis Rheum 32:748-754
32. Cremer MA, Terato K, Watson EC, Griffiths MM, Townes AS, Kang AH (1992) Collagen-induced arthritis in rats. J Immunol 149:1045-1053
33. Wener MH, Uwatoko S, Mannik M (1989) Antibodies to the collagen-like of C1q in sera of patients with autoimmune rheumatic diseases. Arthritis Rheum 32:544-551
34. Arkles B, Redinger P (1983) Silicones in biomedical applications. In: Biocompatible Polymers, Metals, and Composities. Szycher M, Ed. Technomic Publishing, Lancaster, PA, USA 749-768
35. Picha GJ, Goldstein JA (1991) Analysis of the soft-tissue response to components used in the manufacture of breast implants: Rat animal model. Plast Reconstr Surg 87:490-500
36. Mancino D, Bevilacqua, N (1977) Adjuvant effect of amorphous silica on the immune response to various antigens in guinea pigs. Int Arch Allergy Appl Immunol 53:97-103
37. Weisman MH, Vecchione TF, Albert D, Moore LT, Mueller MR (1988) Connective-tissue disease following breast augmentation: a preliminary test of the human adjuvant disease hypothesis. Plast Reconstr Surg 82:626-630
38. Gabriel SE, Melton JE, Woods JE, O'Fallon WM, Kurland LT (1993) Silicone-containing breast implants and connective tissue diseases: a population-based retrospective cohort study. Arthritis Rheum 36:S70
39. Tenenbaum SA, Silveira LH, Martinez-Osuna P, Cuellar ML, Garry RF, Espinoza LR (1992) Identification of a novel autoantigen recognized in silicone-associated connective tissue disease. Arthritis Rheum. 35:S73
40. Bridges AJ, Lorden T (1993) Sicca syndrome in women with silicone implants: absence of serum autoantibodies. Arthritis Rheum 36:S70

The Prevalence of Autoantibodies in Symptomatic and Asymptomatic Patients with Breast Implants and Patients with Fibromyalgia

S. Silverman[1,2,3], O. Gluck[4], D. Silver[2,3], J. Tesser[4], D.Wallace[2,3], K. Neumann, A. Metzger[2,3,5], and R. Morris[5].

[1]West Los Angeles VA, [2]UCLA School of Medicine, [3]Cedars Sinai Medical Center, Los Angeles, CA, [4]The Arizona Rheumatology Center, Ltd. Phoenix, AZ and [5]Rheumatology Diagnostic Laboratories, Inc., Los Angeles, CA.

Correspondence: Please address all reprint requests to Dr Silverman at the Rheumatology Division, W11J, DVA WLA, 11301 Wilshire Blvd., Los Angeles, CA 90073.

Conflicts of interest: Two of the authors (SS and DS) have been asked to serve as expert witnesses for plaintiff attorneys. One of the authors has been asked to serve as expert witness for defense attorneys (SS). The patients studied in this manuscript were both self referred and referred by attorneys.

Introduction

Patients with silicone breast implants have been reported to have a variety of autoantibodies including antinuclear antibodies[1], abnormal western blots[2,3], antibodies to silicone surface associated antigens[4] and anticollagen antibodies[5]. Reports of the prevalence of antinuclear antibodies have ranged from 20% to as high as 58%[6,7,8,9]. We hypothesized that this wide range may be due to practice site and geographic differences or small sample size and we will therefore report data on over 3000 symptomatic women. Recently Bridges reported a high prevalence of antinuclear antibodies in patients with fibromyalgia using a Hep2 technique[10]. We hypothesized the increased prevalence of antinuclear antibodies in symptomatic women with breast implants could not be explained by an increased prevalence of fibromyalgia. Clinicians have found a high prevalence of sicca symptoms in patients with silicone breast implants[9]. We hypothesized that these sicca symptoms would not be associated with classic autoantibodies of antiRo and antiLa.

Objectives

The objectives of our study were to:

1. Extend prior observations to a large group of symptomatic women.
2. Study the prevalence of antinuclear antibodies of symptomatic women with breast implants in different practice sites and geographic sites.
3. Study the prevalence of other autoantibodies (specifically anti-Ro, anti-La, as well as anti thyroid microsomal, rheumatoid factor, anti DNA) and complement levels (C3, C4).
4. Compare the prevalence of antinuclear antibodies in symptomatic women with breast implants to asymptomatic women with breast implants, and healthy controls.
5. Compare the prevalence of antinuclear antibodies in symptomatic women with breast implants to symptomatic women with an atypical rheumatic disease, fibromyalgia.
6. Identify if the prevalence of autoantibodies in symptomatic women with breast implants could be explained by an increased prevalence of fibromyalgia in the cohort.

Methods

ANA was performed using a Hep2 immunofluorescence assay. Anti-DNA antibodies were performed using a radioimmunoassay using the Farr assay. Anti-centromere antibodies were detected using an immunofluorescence technique. Anti-thyroid microsomal antibodies were detected using an ELISA immunoassay. C3 and C4 components of complement and rheumatoid factor were detected using nephelometry. Anticardiolipin antibodies and antibodies to SS-A (Anti-Ro) and SS-B (Anti-La) were detected using an ELISA immunoassay.

Sicca symptoms were asked by interview using the European criteria[11]. Schirmer's test was considered positive if there was less than 8mm tear secretion in either eye at 5 minutes.

The presence of fibromyalgia was assessed by the ACR operational criteria for fibromyalgia (1990)[12].

Patient populations

We studied the incidence of antinuclear antibodies (ANA) in 3184 consecutive symptomatic patients with breast implants(SXBI); 984 from 4 university affiliated rheumatology practices in Los Angeles and 2200 from one rheumatology group practice in Phoenix and compared them to 40 age matched controls, 37 asymptomatic women with breast implants and 100 consecutive patients who met ACR criteria for fibromyalgia but who did not have silicone exposure from one Los Angeles site and 100 from the Phoenix site for a total of 200 patients. The symptomatic women with breast implants were all seen during the period 1993-1994. The asymptomatic women were women who were seen during 1994 by the Phoenix group practice as women who were "concerned" but who had no symptoms or signs suggestive of a silicone related disorder as judged by a rheumatologist.

Incidence of Positive ANA in the five practices

The overall prevalence in all five sites of positive ANA at 1:40 was 59.6% and 35.2 % at 1:80. The prevalence of positive ANA(>1:80) varied at the five different sites from a low of 31.7 % to a high of 59.4 % and is shown below in Table 1.

Table 1. Prevalence of positive ANA in symptomatic women with breast implants in five practice sites.

	N	%≥1:40	%≥1:80	>1:160
LA Wallace (LAW)	128	87.5	59.4	39.1
LA Metzger (LAM)	39	56.4	43.5	25.2
LA Neumann (LAN)	187	48.1	33.2	18.7
LA Silverman/Silver(LAS)	630	60.4	41.1	25.1
Phoenix	2200	57.0	31.7	13.7
Overall	3184	59.6	35.2	17.6

Prevalence of Positive ANA in the the three control groups

The incidence of positive ANA >1:80 was similar in both the fibromyalgia population (28%) and the symptomatic women with breast implants (35%) as shown in Table 2. Both groups had increased incidence compared to the healthy controls (5%) and the asymptomatic women with breast implants (3%). However, the mean ANA titer was higher in the symptomatic women with breast implants (mean titer of 255) versus the breast implant patients with FM (mean titer of 114).

Table 2. Prevalence of Positive ANA in the control groups

		Percent ANA Positive	
	n	>1:80	>1:160
Healthy Controls	40	5%	0
Fibromyalgia Controls	200	28%	12.8%
Asymptomatic Women with Breast Implants	37	3%	0
Symptomatic Women with Breast Implants	3184	35%	17.6%

The ANA patterns were similar in both the symptomatic patients with breast implants (SXBI) and in the patients with fibromyalgia (FM). Speckled : 52% SXBI, 54% FM; Homogeneous: 38.3% SXBI and 43% FM. However, the SXBI patients had increased incidence of atypical patterns such as nucleolar (8.2%), atypical speckled(0.8%), spindle (0.8%) and centromere patterns(0.8%) as compared to the FM patients nucleolar (2 %), atypical speckled and spindle (0%) and centromere (0.8%).

Prevalence of other autoantibodies in the symptomatic women

Despite a high incidence of sicca symptoms (60%) and a high incidence of positive Schirmers tests (40%) in the Los Angeles subset there was a low incidence of anti- Ro and anti-La antibodies (0.4%) in the SXBI patients overall.

Anticardiolipin antibodies were studied in 392 symptomatic women with silicone breast implants and positive antinuclear antibodies at one of the Los Angeles site and were IgG (6.4%) or IgM (5.6%) and rarely IgA (1.5%). The anticardiolipin antibodies were IgG and IgM (1.0%), IgG and IgA (0.3%) and IgM and IgA (0.3%). There was low incidence of rheumatoid factor in SXBI patients (3.7%). SXBI patients with positive ANA had a low incidence of anti-DNA (0.6%), a low incidence of anti-Sm (0.2%) and anti-RNp (0.6%). They often had low C3 (20.4%) and low C4 (10.5%). Anticentromere antibodies were present in 4.6%. The increased prevalence of autoantibodies in symptomatic women could not be explained by thyroid disease. Only 11.7% of our patients had elevated antithyroid microsomal antibodies.

Prevalence of fibromyalgia

The prevalence of fibromyalgia in patients with silicone breast implants was assessed using the ACR criteria in 2 of the Los Angeles sites (LAS and LAW) and the Phoenix site and was found to range from 11% to 25%.

Discussion

In summary, although both the symptomatic women with silicone breast implants and the women with fibromyalgia, an atypical rheumatic disease, showed an increased prevalence of antinuclear antibodies as compared to healthy controls , there is both an increased mean antibody titer and an increased frequency of atypical patterns in the symptomatic women with silicone breast implants. Furthermore, an increased prevalence of fibromyalgia on the symptomatic women cannot explain the increased antinuclear antibodies prevalence as less than 25% of the patients met ACR criteria for fibromyalgia. Other classical connective tissue diseases such as RA (<1%) and SLE (1%) were rare. Our study confirms variability in prevalence of antinuclear antibodies at different practices and geographic sites.

Our study showed that the prevalence of antinuclear antibodies was increased in symptomatic women versus asymptomatic women and healthy controls and differs from other studies reported which show no difference between asymptomatic and symptomatic women. Our asymptomatic women were "concerned" women who had no symptoms or signs as judged by a rheumatologist as opposed to the "healthy" women of Claman[1] who were not examined by a rheumatologist.

The high prevalence of sicca symptoms despite a low incidence of Sjogrens autoantibodies suggests a a non-immunologic mechanism for their sicca symptoms.

References

1. Claman H., Robertson AD (1994) Antinuclear antibodies and breast implants. Western J Med 1994; 160:225-8
2. Ress RI, Peebles CL, Kumagai Y, Ochs RL, Tan EM (1992). Antinuclear antibodies in women with silicone breast implants. Lancet 340(8831):1304-7
3. Bridges AJ (1994) Autoantibodies in patients with silicone implants. Sem Arth Rheum 24(1) (Suppl);54-60
4. Bridges AJ, Conley C, Wang G, Burns DE, Vasey FB (1993). A clinical and immunological evaluation of women with silicone breast implants and symptoms of rheumatic disease. Annals of Int Med 118(12):929-936

5. Kossovsky N, Zeidler M, Chun G, Papasian N, Nguyen A, Rajguru S, Stassi J, Gelman and Sponsler E. (1993) Surface dependent antigens identified by high binding avidity of serum antibodies in a subpopulation of patients with breast prostheses. J Appl Biomaterials 4: 281-288
6. Teuber SS, Rowley MJ, Yoshida SH, Ansari AA and Gershwin ME.(1993) Anticollagen autoantibodies are found in women with silicone breast implants. J Autoimmunity 6(3); 367- 77
7. Solomon G (1993) A clinical and laboratory profile of symptomatic women with silicone breast implants. Sem Arth Rheum 24 (1 Suppl 1) 29-37
8. Borenstein D (1994) Siliconosis: A spectrum of illness. Sem Arth Rheum 24 (1 Suppl 1) 1-7
9. Cuellar ML, Stein Jr TW, Espinoza LR, Tan EM, Ochs RL. Prevalence of antinuclear antibodies in women with silicone breast implants (SBI): clinical associations. Arth Rheum37: (Suppl) S207, abs 663
10. Freundlich B, Altman C, Sandorfi N, Greenberg M, and Tomaszewski J. A profile of symptomatic women with silicone breast implants: A Sjogrens like syndrome. Sem Arth Rheum 24 (1 Suppl 1) 44-53
11. Bridges AJ. (1993) Fibromyalgia, antinuclear antibodies and clinical features of connective tissue disease. Clin Exp Rheum 11: 696-697
12. Vitali C, Bombardieri S, Moutsopoulos HM, Balestrieri G, Bencievelli W, Bernstein RM. Bjerrum KB, Braga S, et al.(1993) Preliminary criteria for the classification of Sjogren's syndrome. Results of a prospective concerted action supported by the European community. Arth Rheum 36(3): 340-7
13. Wolfe F, Smythe HA, Yunus MB, Bennett RM, Bombardier C, Goldenberg DL, Tugwell P, Campbell SM, Abeles M, Clark P et al.(1990) The American College of Rheumatology 1990 criteria for the classification; of fibromyalgia. Report of the Multicenter Criteria Committee. Arth Rheum 33(2):160-172

Monocyte/Macrophage Infiltrates in the Salivary Glands of Women with Silicone Breast Implants

B. Freundlich[1,2], N. Sandorfi[1], C. Altman[3], and J.Tomaszewski[2]
[1]The Graduate Hospital, Philadelphia, PA [2]University of Pennsylvania, Philadelphia, PA, [3]The Pennsylvania Institute, Philadelphia, PA

The use of silicone breast implants for cosmetic purposes has been prohibited by the Food and Drug Administration since April, 1992. Reports from the Japanese in the 1970's and 80's suggested that silicone exposure could lead to both classic and non-classic connective tissue disease (Kumagai et al.1979, 1984). Questions about the safety of these devices has led tens of thousands of women to seek medical attention. We began to see these women in early 1992 before the ban was imposed.

From the first 24 women that were seen at the University of Pennsylvania it was noted that a prominent and recurrent complaint was mucosal dryness. The sensation of dry sandy eyes and dry mouth along with other connective tissue like symptoms such as polyarthralgias, Raynaud's phenomenon and alopecia was reminiscent of Sjogrens Syndrome. Five patients with symptoms suggestive of Sjogrens Syndrome underwent minor salivary gland biopsies to assess whether the typical histologic changes of Sjogrens could be identified.

These studies demonstrated the presence of inflammatory infiltrates in thesalivary glands (Freundlich 1994). Four of these patients had clusters of mononuclear cells in the interstium compatible with a histologic diagnosis of Sjogrens according to Chisholm and Mason (1968). The most prevalent cell in these infiltrates upon immunohistologic phenotyping was the CD68 positive monocyte/macrophage. These cells could occasionally be seen invading the ductal epithelium of the salivary glands. This phenotype was different from that which is characteristically found in patients with Sjogrens Syndrome. In those patients the CD4 lymphocyte helper cell is the predominant infiltrating cell. There also appeared to be an increase in HLA-DR staining cells in both the infiltrates and in the epithelium of the women with implants. This is a non-specific finding that can be seen in both Sjogrens and chronically inflamed tissue (Lindhal 1985, Moutsopoulous 1986).

To further expand upon these initial observations we studied salivary glands from age and sex matched healthy control volunteers. Frozen sections from labial salivary glands were phenotyped with immunoperoxidase biotintylated monoclonal antibodies (Hsu 1981). Positive labeled cells were counted and expressed per mm^2. The results are partially presented in Table 1 (full manuscript in preparation). Controls and patients had similar small numbers of CD3 and CD19 (Abs from Becton Dickinson:Mountainview,

---

* Potential conflict of interest disclosure: One of us (BF) has received funds for oral presentations to plainftiff andf defense attorneys and written letters for patients with impalnts for the global settlement.

Cal) positive cells, however, CD68 and HLA-DR (Abs from Dako Corp:Carpinteria, Cal.) stained cells were significantly increased among the patients .

Table 1. Cell infiltrate phenotype of labial salivary glands (per mm^2) in women with silicone breast implants compared with healthy controls

Antibody Specificity:	CD3	CD19	CD68	HLA DR
Patients				
1	483	11	1338	2111
2	641	41	2059	3608
3	15	45	2116	3701
4	89	7	914	3499
5	53	69	3432	2860
mean	256	35	1972*	3155*
Controls				
1	252	20	338	259
2	71	5	437	139
3	97	16	235	112
4	7	37	239	160
mean	107	16	312	168

*significant p<.05 (T test)

An example of a salivary gland mononuclear cell infiltrate from a patient can be seen in Figure 1. Specimens from a patient and a healthy control tested with a monoclonal antibody to HLA-DR can be seen in Figure 2 and 3. The darker outlined cells have reacted to the immunoperoxidase labelled antibody.

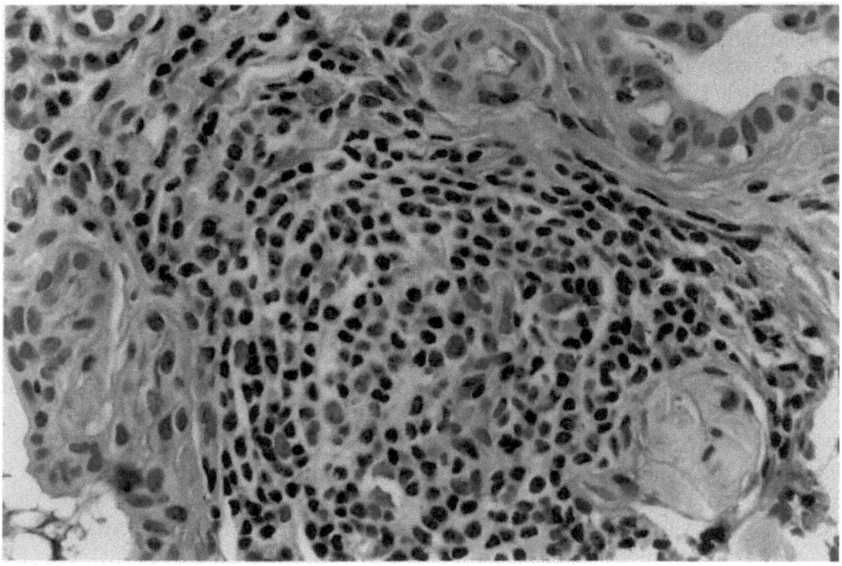

Figure 1. An H&E stained minor salivary gland from an implant patient with dense interstitial infiltratge and active destruction (Mag X 50)

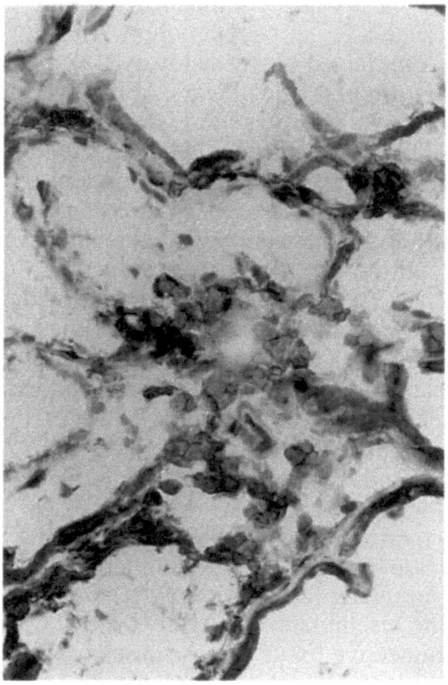

Figure 2. Minor salivary gland stained with Ab to HLA-DR from an implant patient. Darkened cells have bound Ab (Mag X 100)

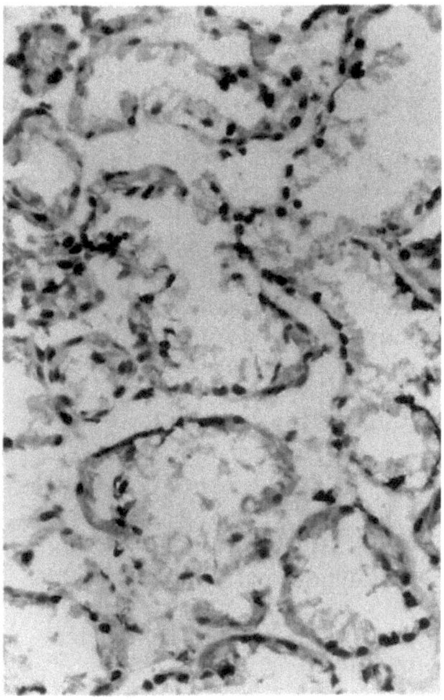

Figure 3. The same as Fig. 2 with a specimen from a healthy control (Mag X 50)

The initial clinical impression that mucosal dryness was a prominent feature in women with silicone breast implants was borne out with a larger patient cohort. In the first 220 patients examined by one of us (BF) 55% complained of dry sandy eyes, almost all of whom used eye drops on a regular basis in the form of artificial tears. Fifty seven percent of patients complained of a dry mouth. A positive Schirmer's test (<5 mm) for eye dryness was found in 28% of patients. Enlarged parotid glands could be palpated in only 1 case while cervical adenopathy was noted in 16%. Thirteen percent of patients had a positive antinuclear antibody $\geq$1:160, while16% had a positive rheumatoid factor. Only one patient tested positive for the SSA antibody and none were positive for SSB.

The above findings indicate that more than half the women that we saw with silicone breast implants had a Sjogrens-like syndrome. The sensation of dry eyes and dry mouth with other complaints such as Raynaud's phenomenon, alopecia and arthralgias were highly suggestive clinically of a connective tissue disease and particularly Sjogrens Syndrome. The histology which revealed mononuclear cell infiltrates also corresponded well with Sjogrens. More detailed analysis of the infiltrating cell phenotype however revealed a marked difference between the implant patients and classic Sjogrens. The number of monocyte/macrophages and the number of cells expressing Class II antigens was significantly different in patients compared with healthy controls.

The clinical picture of mucosal dryness, the monocyte/macrophage cellular infiltrates in the salivary glands coupled with the lack of SSA, SSB or Rheumatoid factor in sera in the implant patients form the picture of a unique process. Although these patients have features of connective tissue disease the resemblance may only be superficial. This may help explain the paucity of connective tissue disease cases found so far in some epidemiology studies of women with implants (Sanchez 1993). The mechanism for the salivary gland cell infiltrates needs to be elucidated. Preliminary studies using x-ray microanalysis to assay for the presence of silicone in the glands have so far been negative.

References

Chisholm DM, Mason DK (1968) Labial gland biopsy in Sjogrens disease. J Clin Path 21:656-660

Freundlich B, Altman C, Sandorfi N, Greenberg M, Tomaszewski J (1994) A profile of symptomatic patients with silicone breast implants: a Sjogrens-like syndrome. Seminars Arthritis Rheum 24:44-53

Hsu SM, Raine l, Fanger H (1981) A comparative study of the peroxidase-antiperoxidase method and an avidin-biotin complex method for studying polypeptide hormones with radioimmunoassay antibodies. Am J Clin Pathol 75:734-738

Kumagai Y, Abe C, Shiokowa Y:Scleroderma after cosmetic surgery. (1979) Arthritis Rheum 22:532-537

Kumagai Y, Shiokowa Y, Medsger T, Rodnan G (1984) Clinical spectrum of connective disease after cosmetic surgery. Arthritis Rheum 27:1-12

Lindhal G, Hedfors E, Klareskog L et al (1985) Epithelial HLA-DR expression and T-lymphocyte subsets in salivary glands in Sjogrens syndrome. Clin Exp Immun 61:475-482

Moutsopoulous HM, Hooks JJ, Chan CC et al (1986) HLA-DR expression by labial gland tissue in Sjogrens syndrome. Ann Rheum Dis 45:677-683

Sanchez-Guerrero J, Schur P, Sergent JS, et al (1994) Silicone breast implants and rheumatic disease. Arthritis Rheum 37:158-168

Novel Anti-Silicone Surface-Associated Antigen Antibodies (Anti-SSAA(x)) May Help Differentiate Symptomatic Patients with Silicone Breast Implants from Patients with Classical Rheumatological Disease

N. Kossovsky,[1] D. Conway,[2] R. Kossowsky and D. Petrovich
[1]Department of Pathology, UCLA School of Medicine, Los Angeles, California; [2]Information and Operations Management Department, School of Business Administration, University of Southern California, Los Angeles, California; and SBI Laboratories, Forbes Med-Tech Center, 1401 Forbes Ave, Pittsburgh Pennsylvania

Abstract

The frequency of novel autoreactive antibodies to silicone surface associated antigens (anti-SSAA(x)) was measured in healthy control patients, symptomatic patients with breast implants, asymptomatic patients with breast implants, and control patients with classical rheumatological diseases. The frequencies of elevated anti-SSAA(x) antibodies in 310 symptomatic breast implant patients were 17.4% anti-SSAA(fn), 12.9% anti-SSAA(col1), and 7.4% anti-SSAA(col3) and 7.1% anti-SSAA(fbgn) [Normal (n=173) = 0.6% for all four tests] ($p<.005$). In 11 asymptomatic breast implant patients, the frequencies of elevated values for the same anti-SSAA's were 0%, 9%, 0%, and 0% respectively, while in 50 patients with rheumatoid arthritis, the frequencies were 4%, 0%, 6% and 2% respectively. The anti-SSAA(x) profile for symptomatic patients with breast implants was different than the profile for control healthy patients ($p<.005$ on all eight tests) but differed significantly by two measures, anti-SSAA(fbgn) and anti-SSAA(col3), from the profile for the 19 patients with systemic lupus erythematosus. We conclude that anti-SSAA(x) antibodies levels in symptomatic patients with breast implants are elevated, that the antibodies are associated with symptoms, and that they differ both qualitatively and quantitatively from healthy controls, asymptomatic patients with breast implants, and symptomatic patients with classical rheumatological diseases.

---

* Disclosure: Over the past fourteen years, the first named author has provided and has received moneys for expert testimony on behalf of plaintiffs, defendants and the United States government in matters associated with breast implants, silicone, and biomaterials. In addition, the first named author and the last two authors have a financial interest in the commercial entity, SBI Laboratories, that offers the Detecsil Anti-SSAA(x) Test Battery. The second author is an Associate Professor of Statistics who has neither a financial interest in the commercialization of the test nor any other conflicting interest.

Introduction

Silicone is a hydrophobic immune adjuvant similar to the prototypical hydrophobic adjuvant developed by Freund. It is primarily effective in a microemulsion or dispersion formulation in which the net surface area of the hydrophobic moiety is maximized. Because the tissues surrounding silicone breast implants contain dispersed silicone in droplet form, we have previously suggested (NK) that silicone adjuvantizes the proteins in those tissues to form autovaccinating antigens [1]. Among the proteins hypothesized to bind to silicone and form antigens are elements of the inflammatory cascade including fibrinogen, fibronectin, collagen III and collagen I [2]. The antibodies hypothesized to be elicited by these silicone surface associated proteins would be directed against the epitopes presented by the autovaccinating antigens in the context of their association with the surfaces of the silicone droplets. These hypothesized autoreactive antibodies have been termed "anti-silicone surface associated antigen antibodies" (anti SSAA(x)).

We have previously shown in a pilot study involving approximately 250 patients with breast implants that antibodies to silicone surface associated fibronectin (anti-SSAA(fn)) and to silicone surface associated fibrinogen (anti-SSAA(fbgn) were elevated in a fraction of that population.[3] We have also shown that the presence of elevated anti-SSAA(fn) in these patients was associated clinically with fevers in the absence of local chest pain.[4]

In this study, an improved detection method for anti-SSAA(x) antibodies was used to measure a broader range of antibodies in a more robust test population. The tool, known commercially as the anti-SSAA(x) Test Battery, was used to measure antibodies captured by six antigens and well as two control surfaces. The purpose of this study was to address the following three questions:

- as a follow-up to the pilot study, are the levels of anti-SSAA(x) antibodies different in patients with breast implants relative to healthy control patients?
- to address the pathogenicity of the antibodies, are the levels of anti-SSAA(x) antibodies different in symptomatic patients with breast implants relative to asymptomatic patients with breast implants?
- to address the specificity of the antibodies, are the levels of anti-SSAA(x) antibodies different in symptomatic patients with breast implants relative to symptomatic patients with classical rheumatological diseases?

Last, we hypothesize that if anti-SSAA(x) antibodies levels in symptomatic patients with breast implants are elevated, if the antibodies are associated with symptoms, and if they differ both qualitatively and quantitatively from healthy controls, asymptomatic patients with breast implants, and symptomatic patients with classical rheumatological diseases, then anti-SSAA(x) antibodies levels may have clinical utility as a specific diagnostic marker.

Materials and Methods

Measurement of Anti-SSAA(x)

Using a modification of methods described previously [3], synthetic silicone surface-associated antigens (SSAA's) fabricated from the inflammatory proteins fibrinogen, fibronectin, collagen III and collagen I were used as surface immobilized ligands for routine solid-phase ELISA. Silicone surface-associated antigens were also fabricated from the non-inflammatory proteins insulin and myelin. Last, control surfaces consisting of unmodified silicone and unmodified polystyrene were also used. A total of 1365 serum samples were obtained from a broad range of sources and included healthy controls with no known silicone exposure and various human groups representing different degrees of silicone exposure and clinical symptomatology. Antibodies [anti-SSAA(x): anti-SSAA(fbgn), anti-SSAA(fn), anti-SSAA(col3), anti SSAA(col1), anti-SSAA(in) and anti-SSAA(my)] captured by the various synthetic antigens as well as those captured by the siliconized and unmodified polystyrene surfaces were quantified spectrophotometrically.

In detail, starting with a standard 96-well polystyrene ELISA plate (Dynatech, Chantilly, VA), zones were created on each plate to allow for the measurement of test values, positive controls, and negative controls. Wells to be filled with silicone-surface associated antigens (SSAAs) were prepared as follows: 300 μl of polydimethylsiloxane fluid, 100cs (Chemcentral, Pittsburgh, PA) were added to the wells and allowed to incubate at room temperature for 5 minutes to form a fine non covalently bonded film on the polystyrene surface. Excess silicone was removed by aspiration followed by 10 minutes of centrifugation at 250 x*g* with the plates in an inverted position. Silicone surface associated antigens (SSAAs) were created by filling the silicone-coated wells with 250 μl of one of seven solutions using a semi automated dispensing machine (Packard Multiprobe 104, Meriden, CT) with precision and reproducibility of volume of dispensed liquid certified by the manufacturer at better than 1%. All work was performed in a <Class 10,000 clean room. All reagents were from Sigma Chemicals, St. Louis, MO unless otherwise noted.

1. Fibronectin (Sigma #F-0895 - human) at a final concentration 8 μg/ml;
2. Myelin basic protein (Chemicon, Temecula, CA #AG42P - human), reconstituted in bicarbonate buffer and diluted in PBS to a final concentration of 0.8 μg/ml
3. Insulin (Sigma #I2643 - porcine) reconstituted in 10 mM HCl, and diluted in PBS to a concentration of 8 μg/ml
4. Fibrinogen (Sigma #4129 - human), reconstituted in HPLC-grade water and diluted in PBS to a final concentration of 8 μg/ml
5. Collagen I (Sigma #C3511 - calf), reconstituted in 0.5 M acetic acid and diluted in PBS to a final concentration of 8 μg/ml
6. Collagen III (Sigma #C4407 - calf), reconstituted in 0.5 M acetic acid and diluted in PBS to a final concentration of 8 μg/ml.
7. Phosphate buffered saline, only [silicone surface control].

After seven days of storage in the dark at 4°C, the plates were moved to a PLATO 3002 (Rosys, Wilmington, DE) automated washer pipetter/reader. The plates were emptied and washed three times with 10mM phosphate buffered saline, pH7.4 containing 0.05% w/v Tween 20 (PBS/Tween). To each well, 150 µl of a 1:100 dilution of human serum in 50mM Tris buffered saline, pH 8.0, were added to each well. Sera for analysis were obtained as noted below:

- 245 normal healthy female controls samples aged 25-50 yrs obtained from North American Biologicals, Inc., (NABI) Miami, FL and representing four geographic regions;
- 575 samples from well characterized patients with breast implants whose serum samples were submitted by collaborating physicians. Of these, 564 were symptomatic and 11 were asymptomatic;
- 457 samples from patients with breast implants whose serum samples were submitted by a variety of sources and about whom little else is known;
- 19 samples from patients without breast implants with signs and symptoms supporting American College of Rheumatology (ACR) criteria for scleroderma;
- 50 samples from patients without breast implants with signs and symptoms supporting ACR criteria for rheumatoid arthritis;
- 19 samples from patients without breast implants with signs and symptoms supporting ACR criteria for systemic lupus erythematosus.

After 120 minutes of serum incubation at 37°C, each well was again washed three times with PBS/Tween and then the amount of captured serum IgG was measured in triplicate following standard ELISA protocol with alkaline phosphatase conjugated to goat anti-Human IgG as the secondary antibody and p-nitrophenylphosphate (PNPP) serving as the substrate. Absorbance was measured at 405 nm.

ELISA controls consisted of solutions of human IgG stock concentrations buffered with BSA (positive) and empty wells (negative). Pass/No Pass criteria consisted of analyzing the variance in any triplicate sample measurement. Variances in excess of 25% resulted in a discard of the measurement and an automatic repetition of the assay.

Statistical Analysis

Graphical methods used to analyze the data revealed an upward shift of values for tests performed with an early lot of reference materials. The lot affected 70 samples from the normal reference group and 255 samples from the asymptomatic group. Because the 325 samples were analyzed with different lot materials, they are not strictly comparable with the remaining samples. They were removed from the analysis for repeat testing using the same lot of reference materials. Also, the 457 samples from patients with breast implants about whom little is known were excluded from the analysis. For this paper, the statistical analysis restricts attention to the remaining 583 of the original 1365 samples.

Graphical analysis of the test values for each group showed approximate normal distributions with few extreme values (outliers). The mean and median values of the tests within each group and the standard errors were computed with and without the extreme values and showed little change. The statistical significance of the observed differences among the groups were calculated in a pairwise manner using the conventional two-sample t-test (Analytical Tools, Excel 5.0, Microsoft, Redmond, WA) with a $p<.005$ set as the threshold for significance. For determination of positivity, the 99.5th percentile of the reference range calculated from the normally distributed reference population was set as the cutoff, and values in excess were interpreted as positive.

Results

A total of 583 samples were analyzed. The 175 reference samples were obtained from a commercial source and the donors were healthy females ages 25-50. The 309 symptomatic patients represented a population that is 44±11 (median 44) years old with an implant duration of 11±7 (median 12) years. Clinical data are not available for the 11 asymptomatic breast implant patients nor for the test subjects represented by the 88 samples obtained from individuals with various classical rheumatological diseases.

Both statistically significant ($p<.005$) quantitative and qualitative differences were seen among the various groups (**Table 1**). Quantitatively, the mean values obtained from the reference population differed significantly ($p<.000001$) from the mean values obtained from all implant patients (pooled) and from the mean values obtained from the symptomatic implant patients only. On the other hand, the mean values for the symptomatic patients differed significantly ($p<.005$) for only three measures from asymptomatic patients, for three measures from

Table 1. Statistically significant differences of antibody capture by the anti-SSAA(x) Test Battery ($p<.005$), pairwise comparisons, among the various populations.

	(fn)[b]	(my)	(in)	(fbgn)	(col1)	(col3)	sil	pst
Ref v Symp[a]	Y[c]	Y	Y	Y	Y	Y	Y	Y
Symp v Asymp	Y	-	Y	Y	-	-	-	-
Symp v RA	Y	-	-	-	Y	Y	-	-
Symp v Scl	Y	Y	Y	-	Y	-	Y	-
Symp v SLE	-	-	-	Y	-	Y	-	-

[a]Ref=reference population; Symp=symptomatic breast implant patient, Asymp=asymptomatic breast implant patient, RA=rheumatoid arthritis patient, Scl=scleroderma patient, SLE=systemic lupus erythematosus patient

[b]fn=anti-SSAA(fn), my=anti-SSAA(my), in=anti-SSAA(in), fbgn=anti-SSAA(fbgn), col1=anti-SSAA(col1), col3=anti-SSAA(col3), sil=silicone treated surface, only; and pst=untreated polystyrene

[c]Y=yes, there is a statistically significant difference between the groups at a $p<.005$

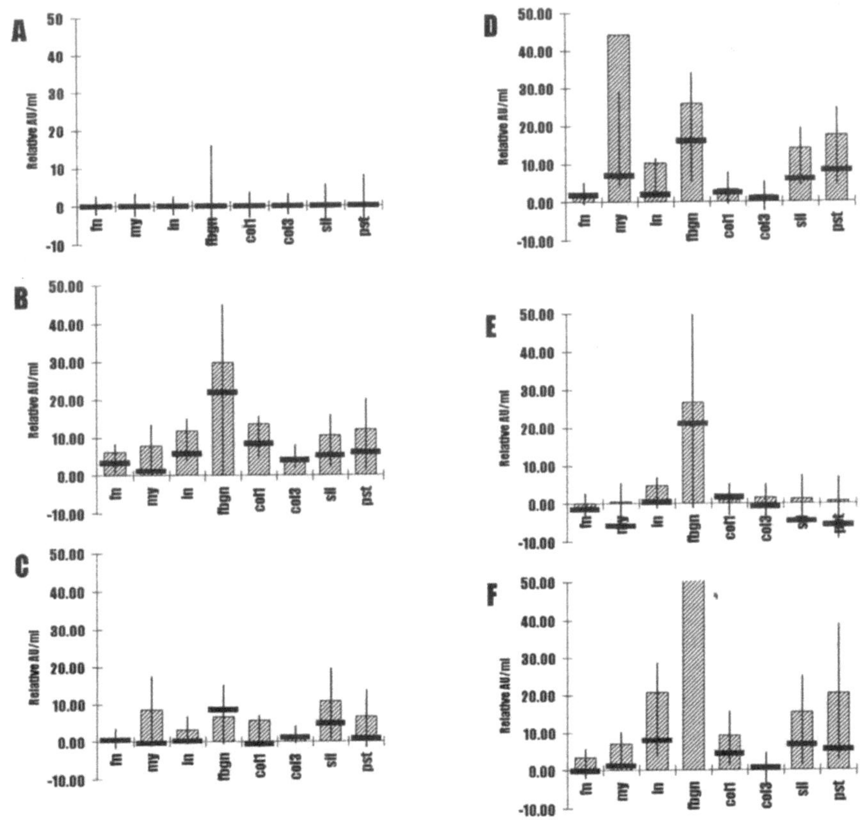

Fig. 1. The corrected mean, median and mid-quartile values obtained for the eight different assays (six anti-SSAA(x) and two surface controls, sil and pst. The hatched bars represent the mean values, the horizontal lines represent the median values, and the vertical bars represent the range of the mid quartiles.

fn=anti-SSAA(fn) [fibronectin], my=anti-SSAA(my) [myelin], in=anti-SSAA(in) [insulin], fbgn=anti-SSAA(fbgn) [fibrinogen], col1=anti-SSAA(col1) [collagen I], col3=anti-SSAA(col3) [collagen III], sil=silicone treated surface, only; and pst=untreated polystyrene.

(**A**) The Normal Reference Control population means differed from the (**B**) Symptomatic Implant population means for all eight parameters ($p<.005$). (**C**) The Asymptomatic Implanted population means differed from the Symptomatic Implant population means for anti-SSAA(fn), anti-SSAA(in) and anti-SSAA(fbgn); (**D**) Rheumatoid Arthritis population means differed from Symptomatic Implant population means for anti-SSAA(fn), anti-SSAA(col1) and anti-SSAA(col3); (**E**) Scleroderma populations means differed from Symptomatic Implant population means for anti-SSAA(fn), anti-SSAA(my), anti-SSAA(in), anti-SSAA(col1) and "anti-silicone;" and (**F**) Systemic Lupus Erythematosus populations means differed from Symptomatic Implant population means for anti-SSAA(fbgn) and anti-SSAA(col3).

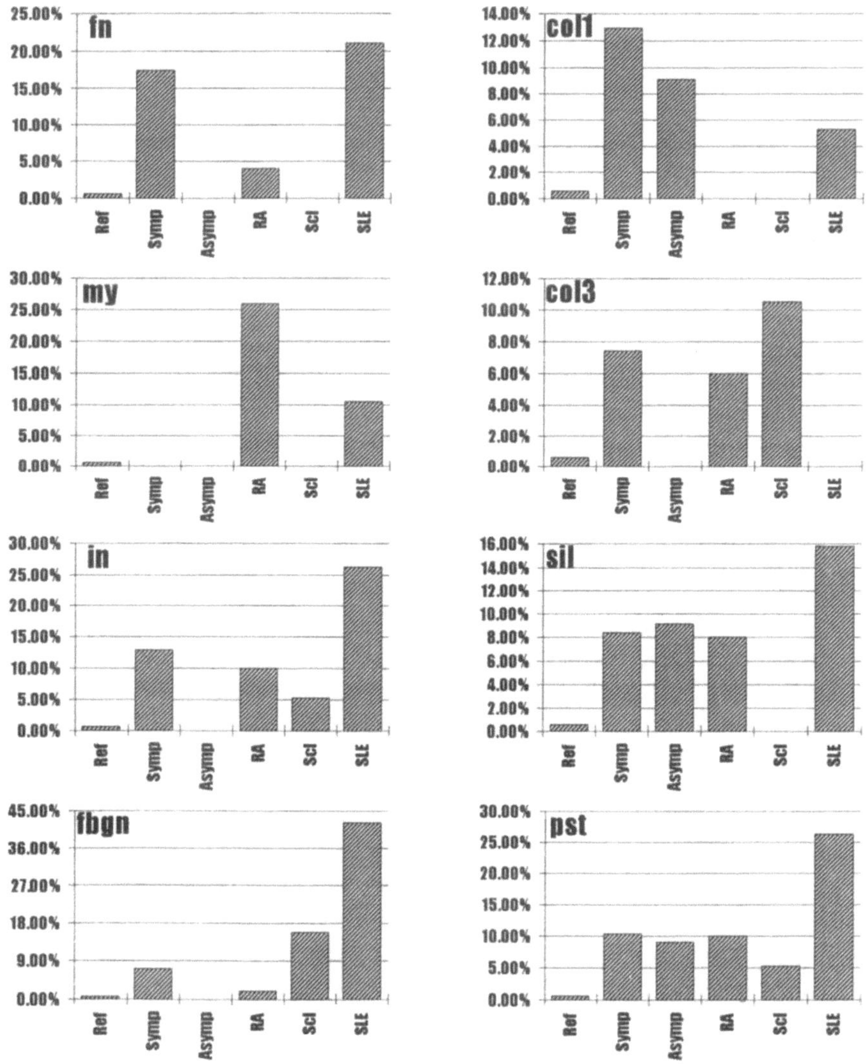

Fig 2. Frequency of positive values observed for the eight test anti-SSAA(x) Battery among the different populations, with a positive value defined as one exceeding the 99.5th percentile of the reference range ($p<.005$).
Ref=reference population; Symp=symptomatic breast implant population, Asymp=asymptomatic breast implant population, RA=rheumatoid arthritis population, Scl=scleroderma population, SLE=systemic lupus erythematosus population
fn=anti-SSAA(fn) [fibronectin], my=anti-SSAA(my) [myelin], in=anti-SSAA(in) [insulin], fbgn=anti-SSAA(fbgn) [fibrinogen], col1=anti-SSAA(col1) [collagen I], col3=anti-SSAA(col3) [collagen III], sil=silicone treated surface, only; and pst=untreated polystyrene.

patients with rheumatoid arthritis, for five measures from patients with scleroderma, and for only two measures from patients with systemic lupus erythematosus (**Fig. 1**).

Qualitatively, the frequency of test positivity, as defined by the frequency of values exceeding the 99.5th percentile of the reference population, differed among the various populations (**Fig. 2**). These differences produced distinctive profiles for the different test groups.

In the implant population as well as the control population, in general, there was little correlation between the values obtained among the six anti-SSAA(x) tests. Similarly, there was no correlation between age nor duration and any of the measured values. On the other hand, there was a strong correlation among the test values in the systemic lupus erythematosus population. Also, irrespective of the test group, there was a very strong correlation among the values obtained for sil and the values obtained for pst ($.90<r<.99$).

Discussion

Silicones, a family of polymers comprised of an alternating silicon-oxygen atom backbone, have served as the raw materials for the fabrication of a broad range of medical devices from breast implants to syringe lubricants. 5 Presumptively biocompatible, fundamental aspects of silicone surface activity and inflammatory activity in the biological environment have not been well studied, and many fundamental pathophysiological and clinical issues remain unresolved. [6]

About ten years ago, a rheumatologic syndrome observed in patients with a history of silicone exposure, primarily through silicone breast implants, was first proposed as possibly being a distinct clinicopathological entity causally related to silicone exposure. It has been variously named "silicone associated disease (SAD)", "silicone arthropathy," or "silicone adjuvant disease" and most recently, "silicone related disorder." [7 ,8] Neurological, neuromuscular and hematological components have been recently suggested as additional clinical features of the syndrome of silicone exposure. [9 ,10]

Further characterization of this syndrome, in the tradition of advances in medicine, [11] has been hampered by the current lack of a unique serological marker. Epidemiological studies designed to assess the potential risks of silicone-associated disease have been doubly hampered by the lack of both specific clinical features and serological markers that might constitute a working definition of silicone-associated disease. [12]

We have suggested that the pathogenesis of the silicone related disorders is one of autoimmunity initiated by chronic autovaccination with novel antigens that self assemble *in-vivo* as silicone encounters native macromolecules. [1] We have also suggested that among the proteins likely to encounter and be adjuvantized by silicone are fibrinogen and fibronectin - two of the surface active proteins that initiate the inflammatory cascade - and collagen III and collagen I - two of the proteins that are elements of the scarring that marks the end of inflammation. As evidence for the above model, we have shown previously the existence of antibodies directed against silicone surface associated fibronectin and silicone surface associated fibrinogen. [3]

The broader range of anti-SSAA(x) antibodies identified with the Detecsil Test, as the data show, may prove to be clinically useful with reference to helping to define the parameters of silicone associated disorders. The data presented herein show that the eight test anti-SSAA(x) battery is specific with significant ($p<.005$) differences noted between symptomatic breast implant patients and both healthy reference and classical rheumatological disease patient groups. The test battery also shows differences between symptomatic and asymptomatic breast implant patients.

Previous studies of patients with silicone breast implants have disclosed antibodies to novel antigens. For example, paralleling our demonstration in this communication of antibodies captured by surface associated (and therefore denatured) collagen I (anti-SSAA(col1)), Teuber et al. [13] demonstrated antibodies captured by heat denatured collagen I. Seventy self referred women with implants and no defined autoimmune disease and 45 normal women were studied. For the women with implants, antibodies to collagen I were present in 18 (26%), two had antibodies to native collagen I; 8 had antibodies to denatured collagen I only and 8 had to both native and denatured collagen I. Only one of 45 control patients had antibodies directed solely to denatured collagen I. By Western blotting, the sera of reactors identified several cyanogen-bromide digestions of collagen I but the reactivities of the implant sera differed significantly from those of the 15 SLE and 7 rheumatoid arthritis control patients. Perhaps, in view of our current work, the epitopes exhibited by the autovaccinating silicone-collagen I complexes in the breast implant patients differ from the epitopes associated with autoimmunity in the SLE and RA patients.

Tennenbaum [14] reported that 106 of 200 patients experiencing silicone implant complications produced serum antibodies that reacted with partially polymerized polyacrylamide on an immuno blot assay. Patient sera were 17 times more likely to react to this novel antigen than normal blood donor sera. In addition, 27% of patients with scleroderma produced antibodies to partially polymerized polyacrylamide. Similarly, Wolf, *et. al.*[15] reported that patients with implants demonstrated a statistically significant elevation in antibodies binding directly to the polymer, silicone. While our data similarly show elevated antibody capture by two polymer surfaces - silicone and polystyrene - the high correlation between the two suggests a lack of specificity.

It is apparent that the clinical challenge of silicone associated disorders will be advanced significantly as the parameters become better defined. Antibody assays in general, and the anti-SSAA(x) Test Battery whose results are presented in this communication, may help define those parameters. Future studies on the eight test anti-SSAA(x) battery consist of the development of a classification model that will define the diagnostic discriminating power of the complete assay.

References

1 Kossovsky N and Freiman CJ: Silicone breast implant pathology: Clinical data and immunologic consequences. *Arch Path Lab Med* 1994; 118:686-693.

2 Farber E. *Textbook of Pathology*, WB Saunders, New York, 1994.

3 Kossovsky N, Zeidler M, Chun G, Nugyen A, Rajguru S, Papasian N, Gelman A, Sponsler E: Surface dependent antigens identified by high binding avidity of serum antibodies in a subpopulation of patients with breast prostheses. *J of Appl Biomat.*, 1993, 4::281-288.

4 Kossovsky N, Gornbein JA, Zeidler M, Stassi J, Chun G, Papasian N, Nguyen A, Ly K, Rajguru S: Self reported signs and symptoms in breast implant patients with novel antibodies to silicone-surface-adsorbed antigens (anti-SSAA). *J Appl Biomat* 1995 IN PRESS

5 Kossovsky N, Heggers JP, Robson MC. The bioreactivity of silicone. In: Williams DF, Ed. *CRC Critical Reviews in Biocompatibility*. Boca Raton: CRC Press; 1987: 3:53-85.

6 Council on Scientific Affairs, American Medical Association. Silicone gel breast implants. *JAMA* 1993; 270:2602-2606.

7 Sergott TJ, Limoli JP, Baldwin CM, Laub DR: Human adjuvant disease, Possible autoimmune disease after silicone implantation. *Plast. Reconstr. Surg.* 1986; 78: 104-114.

8 Weiner SR and Paulus HE. Chronic arthropathy occuring after augmentation mammaplasty. *Plast Reconstr Surg* 1986; 77:185-192.

9 Grisolia JS, Herndon R, Ostermeyer-Shoaib B, Lezak M, Prange R, and Boksenbaum S. Spectrum of atypical neurology disease and cognitive disorders panels. Presented at the Silicone Related Disorders Study Group Workshop, New Orleans, 21-22 April 1995.

10 Silverman S, Berenson J, Silver D, Vescio R and Persselin J. Multiple myeloma. Two case histories and the incidence of increased immunoglobulin and monoclonal gammopathy in women with silicone breast implants. Presented at the NCI/NIH Workshop on the Immunology of Silicones, Bethesda, 13-14 March 1995.

11 Bernstein, RA: Humoral autoimmunity in systemic rheumatic disease. A review. *J Roy Coll Phys* (London) 1990; 24:18-25.

12 Gabriel SE, O'Fallon WM, Kuland LT, Beard CM, Woods JE, Melton LJ: Risk of connective tissue diseases and other disorders after breast implantation. *N Engl J Med* 1994; 330:1697-1702.

13 Teuber SS, Rowley MJ, Yoshida SH, Ansari AA, Gershwin ME: Anti-collagen antibodies are found in women with silicone breast implants. *Autoimmunity* 1993; 6:367-377.

14 Tennenbaum SA, Cuellar ML, Citera G, Silveira LH, Garry RF and Espinoza LR. Presented at the annual meeting of American College of Rheumatology, San Antonio, TX, November, 1993. Abstract published in *Arthritis & Rheumatism* 1993;36:S118,A123.

15 Wolf, LE, Lappe, M, Peterson, RD, Ezrailson, EG: Human immune response to polydimethylsiloxane (silicone). Screening studies in a breast implant population. *FASEB J*, 1993; 7:1265-1268

The authors wish to acknowledge the physicians who have helped provide many of the samples analyzed: Drs. A. Brawer, R. Fadal, B. Freundlich, G. Solomon, and A. Metzger and R. Morris of the Rheumatology and Diagnostic Laboratory. We also thank P. Glackin and B. Brandegee for their support.

Laboratory Studies in Breast Implant Patients: ANA Positivity, Gammaglobulin Levels, and Other Autoantibodies

R.I. Lewy MD FACP and E. Ezrailson, PhD
Baylor College of Medicine and University of Texas Health Science Center at Houston (Dr Lewy)* and Emerald Biomedical Sciences. Inc, The Woodlands, Texas (Dr Ezrailson)**

Introduction

SILICONE induced connective tissue disease has been anecdotally but heavily documented over the past 20 years soon beginning after the introduction of the substance for prosthetic use [1-16].Other syndromes reported include synovitis, adenopathy, splenomegaly, systemic sclerosis, granuloma formation, and possible carcinogenesis.

Antinuclear antibodies (ANA) are a family of autoantibodies characteristic of connective tissue disorders, although antibodies to antigens outside the nucleus are also known to be associated with rheumatic disease [17] These antigens are responsible for transcription and translation of proteins. The "ANA" test is useful for screening for Systemic Lupus Erythematosus and Scleroderma, but less so for Polymyositis/Dermatomyositis. The test is semiquantitative and has other technical deficiencies: rodent substrates may be deficient in Ro/SSA [18].

Five percent of healthy individuals may be positive and the frequency of positives rises above the age of 55 [19-21]. Drugs may trigger ANA production in susceptible individuals, and problems such as thyroid disease, chronic infections, and malignancy may trigger ANA production [22-24]. The ANA test can be further characterized when positive, though only a few cellular proteins (30 of 10,000) become targets of autoantibody production. ELISA techniques are more sensitive than Immunodiffusion techniques.However, this leads to higher detection rates of these antibodies in normals. Only DNA antibodies have been truly related to pathogenesis [19,25].

Using a HEP-2 system, de Vlam and colleagues found titers of 1:80 or less positive in 42/485 normal blood donor volunteers, though a total of 62 were positive at some level, 23 of the IGG type, which is more disease related. Only one had weak component activity (DNA) [26]. Guilbert [27] found naturally occurring autoantibodies to exist. Segal [28] found experimental lupus in mice was associated with less severity with increased aging due to DNA antibodies.

Silicone breast implant recipients are often found to experience rheumatic symptoms. The literature on the subject includes references to scleroderma [29-

---

Disclosures.

* Dr Lewy is President of Breast Implant Research, Inc of Houston Texas, and has both been deposed and testified in trial on breast implant related matters.

** Dr Ezrailson developed the Silicone Antibody Reactivity Assay (SARA™)

31], Sjogren's syndrome, and elevated levels of ANA, rheumatoid factors and other serological abnormalities have been described.

In other studies several authors [32-38] have detected the time-dependent development of either positive ANA tests or frank rheumatologic disease. These studies have been limited due to small numbers of patients, lack of a uniform database, or lack of consistent examination of each patient. Other studies [39-41] have purported that no such serological or clinical correlation even exists.

We report here the results of three closely related studies designed to evaluate a series of breast implant recipients. The first study attempts to determine if the likelihood of a positive ANA is a function of duration of implant exposure after controlling for various confounding factors able to also cause a rising likelihood of a positive ANA in such a series such as age. A second study was undertaken to determine if hypergammaglobulinemia would be seen in patients who were tested consecutively in view of evidence that humoral immunity as well as cell mediated immunity are affected by silicone exposure. Finally, the frequency of other autoantibodies were also examined.

Statistical Methods and Data Analysis

All Studies

Accrual was consecutive for this case series and represented patients who were self-referred, physician-referred, or referred from other sources, such as attornies or individuals responding to newspaper advertisements from legal committees soliciting medical evaluations for classification of breast implant recipients for reasons of injury claim settlement. No external control group was employed as the intent of the study was firstly to compare variables within the entire group tested, and the literature on positive test rates in studies where normal volunteers were utilized is adequate to assess relative risk. All patients were examined by one of two physicians (RIL or G. Armen) using a standardized protocol and questionnaire. This uniform questionnaire was prepared and administered to derive information regarding type of implant, duration of implant exposure, patient age, as well as other variables. The testing was performed by a commercial testing laboratory (Roche Biomedical Labs, Burlington, NC) that adheres to standards of quality control and assurance mandated by Federal law and every subject in this series had such an analysis performed. Specifically, testing was not restricted to degree or presence of what were suspected to be symptoms as previously described by other authors of connective tissue disease, neurological disease, or hypergammaglobulinemia, age, geographic considerations, duration of implant, manufacturer of implant or type of implant. No selection was made regarding medication history, number or previous surgeries, or source of referral.

Antinuclear antibodies

We evaluated the consecutive testing results from 3380 patients who were all examined by one of two physicians.The study attempted to confirm the excess presence of ANA occurrence in this group, as well as infer a possible causal relationship from evaluation of duration of implant use. Further, we attempted to rule out the alternative explanation that ANA development in this group was due to aging alone.The standard ANA test was conducted on blood specimens using the Hep-2 substrate by a commercial testing laboratory that adheres to standards fo quality control and assurance mandated by Federal law. The three thousand three hundred and eighty patients were tested consecutively without any selection process.

In Figure 1, the data were grouped according to titer class mark and the population percentages calculated for each group. While no statistical analysis was conducted on these preliminary data, the figure suggests that two populations may exist, one which responds almost immediately to implants and one that responds slowly over a long period of time. Since the failure rate for gel filled implants increases with age, this parameter may play a role in the response found in the second population.

The exposure duration effect on positive ANA was tested while controlling for the effect of age. Since a patient's exposure to implant duration and aging occur simultaneously, special methods are required for both the calculation of rates and for separating the effect of aging from exposure duration. To simultaneously account for implant duration and age in the rate calculations, a dynamic time exposure classification scheme was used. This scheme appropriately included a patient in all rate denominators for which she contributed both aging and exposure time, analogous to how survival analysis handles the single time variable case [42].

To separate the effect of aging from implant exposure duration (and control for age), stratification by age was used. The exposure duration effect on positive ANA rates is statistically tested using a chi-square trend test, both within each age interval as well as with a single summary test across all age intervals [43]. The overall incidence of positive ANA was compared to a fixed historical control incidence using a one-sample binomial test. All P values reported are for a two-tailed comparison.

Gammaglobulins

We undertook a review of total gammaglobulin levels in 2,721 consecutive women with breast implants, searching for evidence of monoclonal or polyclonal gammopathy which might indicate B-cell proliferation. The patients' average age was 45.23 $\pm$ 11.48 years, and the average duration of implantation was 141.51 $\pm$ 70.79 months.

Results

Antinuclear antibodies

Our study showed that ANA positivity increased with increasing implant exposure, while excluding age as an explanation. As displayed in Figure 1, the rates for ANA of 1:40 or greater increased with increased implant duration for every age interval in which the implant exposure occurred ($P<0.05$ for every age interval). The summary statistical comparison across all age intervals demonstrates that ANA positivity is a function of duration of implant use independent of age ($P<0.001$).

The overall incidence of ANA of 1:40 or greater was 22 percent. Our incidence compared to a historical control with an incidence of 5 percent results in a relative risk of 4.4, demonstrating an increased risk for positive ANA in breast implant patients ($P<0.001$). Figures 2-4 show the months of implant exposure in the group studied, the age distribution of the group and the distribution of the ANA results.

Gammaglobulins

Total gammaglobulin levels were then recalled as indicated in Figure 5. The mean was 3.02 ± 0.39 grams/dl. No apparent tendency toward elevated gammaglobulin levels was seen on preliminary inspection in the overall group, although the possibility of a subset of patients with a significant gammopathy certainly exists and may be related to silicone exposure or other factors. To explore this further, statistical analysis was performed which showed a significant correlation between the likelihood of a positive ANA and the total gammaglobulin level ($p<0.043$). Therefore the relative risk of a positive ANA was 7.7 in the hypergammaglobulinemia group.

Only a weak statistical correlation was seen between total gammaglobulin levels and the likelihood of positive neuroantibodies, specifically antibodies to Ganglioside GM1. Only three patients demonstrated elevated total gammaglobulins, while the same number demonstrated decreased total gammaglobulin levels.

Total gammaglobulin levels did not correlate with age of the patient at the time of testing or the duration of implantation as measured by linear regression, but this method fails to assess the time dependence of risk properly.

Other autoantibodies and clinical correlates

Four thousand three hundred and ten consecutive women with silicone,saline or polyurethane breast implants were uniformly studied regarding symptoms, gynecologic history, results of imaging of the brain and skeleton, thyroid status, and presence of autoantibodies. Despite an average age of 44.85

years ± 11.24. 28 % were receiving estrogen replacement, and 19% had had partial and 35% complete hysterectomies. Symptoms in decreasing order were fatigue (83%), joint pains and muscle pains (83%),chest or breast pain (81%), burning of the extremities or axillae (80%), numbness (80%), mood disturbances (72%), memory loss(68%) and insomnia (68%) and sicca symptoms (44%). Rupture or reoperation occurred in 48%. Thyroid insufficiency was seen in 10.38% based on elevated TSH levels. Autoantibodies were to myelin basic protein (84 % occurrence, IgG mean 72.83 ± 61.38, 38.46 % occurrence IgM mean 54.64 ± 38.49, 81 % occurrence IgA mean 25.38 ± 21.55), GM1 antibodies averaged 26.1 ± 40.81 (39.12% elevated above normal range) , Sulfatide antibodies were 24.52 ± 15.81(39% elevated above normal range, smooth muscle and parietal cell (49% and 19% occurrence, means 11.48 ±21.77 and 7.37 ± 49.03 respectively), and microsomal antibodies (17%, mean 67.18 ± 322.67). Thyroglobulin antibodies were found in 33.73%, and double-stranded DNA antibodies in 17.13%. The creatine phosphokinase was elevated in 18.84%.

A total group use of silicone implants of 455,316 months (37,943 implant-years) was evaluated. Some patients had both parietal cell antibodies and symptoms compatible with pernicious anemia though B12 levels were usually normal. Another pattern not surprisingly was the presence of functional hypothyroidism in patients with thyroglobulin or microsomal antibodies. Patients with Raynaud's phenomenon (15%) were usually older, had implants present for at least 15 years with few other major symptoms. Women had a broad range of implant use (139.97 ± 69.87 months) while the total period of exposure for the group was 37,943 implant-years. Seven percent of patients had initial treatment for fibrocystic disease, while 8% had mastectomies for breast cancer. Seventeen specific symptom responses were obtained from each patient. The individual use of prescribed estrogens whether or not concurrent with partial or total hysterectomy or spontaneous menopause were noted.

Evidence of thyroid insufficiency by TRH stimulation testing was found in 40% of those tested, a rate higher than by elevated TSH alone. Many patients had multiple serological findings of autoantibodies (usually antinuclear but less frequently anti smooth muscle, anti parietal cell, antithyroglobulin, anti-GM1 and anti microsomal). B12 levels were obtained, but few were abnormal, so no association with an antiparietal antibody was apparent. Evidence of liver disease, kidney disease, heart, pulmonary, gastrointestinal or blood disease was not common. Anemia was seen in few patients, surprising considering their age but consistent with their hysterectomy status. Fifty five percent of patient tests showed antibodies to myelin of some class.

Figures 6-11 display results of thyroid stimulating hormone, thyroglobulin antibody, DNA antibody, serum creatine phosphokinase, GM1 antibody and Sulfatide antibodies. The values are similar to those reported by Solomon in his series [67] with the exception of the incidence of GM1 antibodies, which are higher, and the absence of consecutive testing by serum protein electrophoresis and quantitative immunoglobins in the present report. Finally, Table 1 demonstrates quantitative symptoms and Table 2 shows quantitative antibody and related data.

Discussion

Antinuclear antibodies

While these data are preliminary and will require further additions to establish clear relationships, the mean time for developing a positive ANA was significantly greater than the group that remained negative suggesting that exposure to the implant increases the chances of developing a positive ANA with time. The mechanism for developing antinuclear antibodies must also be elucidated by actually isolating the DNA adducts that contain polydimethysiloxane (PDMS). Kossovsky [44] and others have suggested that denaturation due to silicone exposure may resemble lupus in that there is a loss of "self" tolerance due to the adjuvant activity of silicone. As Garrido has shown [45] that the PDMS is demethylated, we propose an extrahepatic metabolic pathway characteristic of peroxisomes found in macrophages. Since it is well known that these cells engulf silicone gel, it is likely that the PDMS is oxidized in peroxisomes.

While the ANA is not diagnostic of specific rheumatic disease, the excessive positive levels noted in this study and their exclusion due to aging suggest a possible adjuvant-induced breakdown of immune tolerance, or possibly a denaturation effect. In fact, autoimmune disease may arise due to the function of the immune system to react at birth to microbial stress proteins and their homology with host stress proteins [46-47] especially in chronic inflammatory arthritis. The cellular immune system may also be stimulated by stress protein epitopes, as has been seen in adjuvant-induced arthritis. Evidence for this last mechanism comes from studies with autoreactive T cells triggered by Mycobacterial antigens causing chronic arthritis,that synovial fluid T cells from rheumatoid arthritis patients proliferate in response to mycobacterial extracts, that T cells with $\gamma\delta$ receptors have special reactivity to mycobacterial antigens, and the discovery that patients with systemic autoimmune disease develop autoantibodies to stress proteins such as conserved peptides of hsp60 [48]. More recently the role of oxidative denaturation of silicones and the effects of that process on the immune system have received attention [49-51] as well as the role of superantigen activation related to infection [52-54],and still more recently the interplay of the HLA antigen system to these other factors has been appreciated [55-57].

The lack of emergence of a serological profile identical to Systemic Lupus Erythematosus is hardly surprising in this entity, as it is likely "drug-induced." Profiles of autoantibodies in patients have been described [33] with the ANA ranging from 7% to 68% being found. Bridges also found that if only ANA positive symptomatic patients were studied, the ANA rate by immunofluorescence was less often positive than in classical connective tissue disease. But Western blot testing revealed an additional 10% positive who were ANA negative. Scleroderma- like disease was associated with centromere and PM-Scl specificity, while lupus-like or undifferentiated disease with B'/B polypeptide.

Antibodies to high molecular weight protein have been seen by Western blot in 50% of silicone breast implant patients.

Systemic Lupus Erythematosus is known to have differing clinical and serological features consistent with a drug-induced autoimmune illness, and silicone's identification as a drug is well established in the literature [58]. While a cellular immunity defect has also been reported by Smalley and colleagues [59] and others [60] a humoral component seems to be present as well. Potter [61] and colleagues have shown experimentally that silicone gel is associated with plasmacytoma formation in genetically susceptible mice.

The elevated ANA rates in this group when compared to historical controls and shown by an increased relative risk, taken together with documented adjuvant activity of the silicone itself in certain experimental settings [62] and other studies demonstrating altered humoral immunity as cited above, may define women with silicone breast implants as a group at risk for seropositive rheumatic disease of an atypical variety. Elsewhere we and others have also reported widespread neurological symptomatology [63-65] so it can be said that the illness is not confined to the connective tissue system alone. Further, similar illnesses such as Chronic Fatigue Syndrome are easily excluded by the usual absence of fevers, pharyngitis, adenopathy, lymphocytosis, and hepatitis [66] . While fibromyalgia may be more difficult to exclude, Solomon [67] has noted that there appear to be fewer trigger points and other differential laboratory findings have been found [68-71].

Gammaglobulins

We conclude that the clinical illness experienced by many Breast Implant recipients resembles certain "native" illnesses in where gammopathies are seen. The group we examined was diverse, and some of the implant recipients suffered from neurological rather than rheumatological illness, while some were asymptomatic. However, the history of silicone exposure per se does not seem to produce a systematic overproduction of total gammaglobulins in all breast implant recipients. Further testing will be required to determine the presence of monoclonal gammopathies in these patients where no elevation of total gammaglobulin occurs, light chain disease is prevalent, or deficiency or excess of sub-fractions of gammaglobulin may be seen. Further study by immunoelectrophoresis and quantitative immunoglobin measurements is needed to determine if the observed increased likelihood of a positive ANA in the patients with higher gammaglobulin levels represents a clonal process, such as a monoclonal gammopathy of unknown significance (MGUS), or a polyclonal reactive pattern consistent of Systemic Lupus Erythematosus.

In conclusion, autoimmunity in silicone breast implant patients appears to be common, involves several arms of the immune system.The ANA test therefore is most useful in diagnosis of Human Adjuvant Disease in silicone breast implant patients beginning some time after implantation, probably 5 or more years according to our data and that of others. Its negativity does not exclude Human Adjuvant Disease at the time of initial evaluation or at a later time. Testing of the cellular immune system seems more accurate than testing the humoral immune system, perhaps related to etiologic transplantation factors.

Summary and Conclusions

Silicone polymers when used in augmentation prosthesis in breast surgery have been associated in the medical literature with various systemic clinical manifestations and abnormal laboratory testing suggestive of an atypical autoimmune disease. The most frequently cited abnormal test result is the antinuclear antibody . The literature regarding this test is reviewed in general, and then specific previous studies analyzed. The present study then compares the rate of positive antinuclear antibody tests in a case series of 3380 breast implant recipients with historical normal controls, and finds a six-fold increase in relative risk of a positive test. Analysis of the data show that this increased tendency is at least partially a function of duration of implant exposure to a significant degree ($p<0.001$), and the same data shows it is not patient age related. Possible explanations of this phenomenon are discussed, including animal studies suggesting that silicone serves as an adjuvant, and therefore might have an effect on immune tolerance in the subject population.

Acknowledgements

The assistance of Gregg Stoddard, Ph.D., Sally Marriott, M.P.H., and Emily Nedell, M.L.S. in the preparation of this manuscript and analysis of the data are greatly appreciated.

References

1. Brown, JB, Fryer MP, David A. (1960).Study and use of synthetic materials such as silicone and teflon as subcutaneous protheses. Plastic and Reconstruct Surg. 26:264-27.
2. Endo LP, Edwards NL, Longley S, Cormann LC, Panush RS. (1987).Silicone and rheumatic diseases. Semin Arthritis Rheum 17:112-118.
3. Fock KM, Feng PH, Tey B.(1984). Autoimmune disease developing after augmentation mammoplasty: report of 3 cases. J Rheumatol 11:98-100.
4. Goldblum RM, Pelley RP, O'Donnell AA, Pyron D, Heggers JP (1992). Antibodies to silicone elastomers and reactions to ventribuloperitoneal shunts. Lancet ; 340:510-513.
5. Heggers JP, Kossovsky N, Parson RW, Robson MC, Pelley RC, Talmage RJ.(1983). Biocompatibility of silicone implants. Ann Plastic Surg 11:38-45
6. Kaiser W, Biesenback, Stuby U, Grafinger P, Zazgornik J (1990). Human adjuvant disease: remission of silicone-induced autoimmune disease after explanation of breast augmentation. Ann Rheum Dis 49:937-938.

7. Kossovsky N, Heggers JP, Robson MC. (1987).Experimental demonstration of the immunogenicity of silicone-protein complexes. J Biomed Mater Res 21:1125-33.

8.Okano V, Nishikai M, Sato A. (1984).Scleroderma, primary biliary cirrhosis and Sjogren's syndrome after cosmetic breast augmentation with silicone injection: a case report of possible human adjuvant disease. Ann Rheum Dis 43:520-1.

9. Peimer CA, Medige J, Eckert BS, Wright JR, Howard CS (1986). Reactive synovitis after silicone arthroplasty. H Hand Surg IIA:624-38.

10.Sergott TJ, Limoli JP, Baldwin CM Jr, Laub DR.(1986). Human adjuvant disease, possible autoimmune disease after silicone implantation: a review of the literature, case studies, and speculation for the future. Plast Reconstr Surg 78:104-14

11.Silverstein MJ, Handel N, Gamagami P, Gierson ED, Furmanski M, Collins AR, Epstein M, Cohlan BF.(1992). Breast cancer diagnosis and prognosis in women following augmentation with silicone gel-filled prostheses. Eur J Cancer 1992; 28~635- 640

12. Spiera H. (1988).Scleroderma after silicone augmentation mammoplasty. JAMA 260:236-8.

13. Van Nunen SA, Gatenby PA, Basten A.(1983). Post-mammoplasty connective tissue disease. Arthritis Rheum 25:294-7.

14. Varga J, Jimenez SA. (1990).Augmentation mammoplasty and scleroderma. Is there an association? Arch Dermatol 126:1220-1221

15. Varga J, Schumacher HR, Jimenez SA. (1989).Systemic sclerosis after augmentation mammoplasty with silicone implants. Ann Intern Med 111:377-83.

16. Yoshida K.(1973). Post mammoplasty disorder as an adjuvant disease of man. Shikoku Acta Med 29:318-32.

17.Sontheimer RD, McCauliffe DP,et al. (1992) Antinuclear Antibodies: Clinical Correlations and Biological Significance. Adv Dermat .7:3-52

18.Lipscomb MF, Cope LD, Stephens GL, et al.(1984) Comparison of substrates for the Detection of Antinuclear Antibodies in Normals and In Patients with Connective Tissue Disease and Other Diseases. Diagn Immunol 2:181-187.

19. Anderson P.(1977). Correlation of amooth muscle and nuclear antibodies in normal subjects. Clin Exp Med 27:74-77.

20. Borak J, Vasey F, Lauter S et al.(1979). Immunofluorescence Assay for Antinuclear Factor: A Non-specific Test in Hospitalized Patients. Can Med J 121:1372-1374.

21. Shu S, Nidengard RJ, Hale WL et al (1975).Incidence and titers of Antinuclear Antismooth muscle and other autoantibodies in blood donors. J Lab Clin Med 86;259-265.

22. Carsons S.(1988).Newer laboratory parameters for the diagnosis of rheumatic disease. Am J Med 85(4A): 34-8

23. Shiel WC, Jason M.(1989) The Diagnostic Association of Patients with Antinuclear Antibodies Referred to a Community Rheumatologist. J Rheumatol. 91:249-255.

24. Smeenk RJ, van den Brink HG, Brinkman K, Termaat RM, Berden JH, Swaak AJ.(1991) Anti-dsDNA: choice of assay in relation to clinical value. Rheumatol Int 11(3): 101-7.
25. Tan EM.(1989).Antinuclear antibodies: diagnostic markers for autoimmune diseases and probes for cell biology. Adv Immunol 93-151.
26. De Vlam, K, De Keyser F, Verbruggen M. Et al .(1993).Detection and Identification of Antinuclear Antibodies in the Serum of Normal Blood Donors. Cliinical and Experimental Rheumatology 11:393-397.
27. Guilbert B, Dighiero G, Avrameas S. (1982).Naturally Occurring Antibodies Against Nine Common Antigens in Human Sera. J Immunol 128:2279-2287.
28. Segal R, Globerson A, Singer H et al.(1992) The Influence of Aging on the Induction and Manifestations of Experimental Systemic Lupus Erythematosus. J Clin Immunol. 12:5.341-346.
29. Spiera H, Kerr LD.(1993).Scleroderma following silicone implantation: a cumulative experience of 11 cases. J Rheumatol 20(6): 958-61.
30. Sahn EE, Garen PD, Silver RM, Maize JC.(1990).Scleroderma following augmentation mammoplasty. Report of a case and review of the literature [see comments] Arch Dermatol 126(9): 1198-202.
31. Gutierrez FJ, Espinoza LR.(1990).Progressive systemic sclerosis complicated by severe hypertension: reversal after silicone implant removal. Am J Med 89(3): 390-2.
32. Press RI, Peebles CL, Kumagai Y, Ochs RL, Tan EM.(1992).Antinuclear autoantibodies in women with silicone breast implants. Lancet 340(8831): 1304-7.
33. Bridges AJ.(1994)Autoantibodies in patients with silicone implants. Semin Arthritis Rheum 24(1 Sup54-60): 54-60.
34. Bridges AJ, Conley C, Wang G, Burns DE, Vasey FB.(1993).A clinical and immunologic evaluation of women with silicone breast implants and symptoms of rheumatic disease [see comments] Ann Intern Med 118(12): 29-36.
35. Claman H,.Robertson AD. (1994).Antinuclear Antibodies and Breast Implants. West J Med.160:225-228.
36. Coleman, EA, Lemon SJ, Rudick J et al.(1994).Rheumatic Disease Among 1167 Women Reporting Local Implant and Systemic Problems After Breast Implant Surgery. Journal of Women's Health. 3 (3): 165-177.
37. Wolf LE, Lappe M, Peterson RD, Ezrailson EG.(1993).Human immune response to polydimethylsiloxane (silicone): screening studies in a breast Implant population. FASEB J 7(13): 1265-8.
38. Teuber SS, Rowley MJ, Yoshida SH, Ansari AA, Gershwin ME.(1993).Anti-collagen autoantibodies are found in women with silicone breast implants. J Autoimmun 6(3): 367-77.
39. Schusterman MA, Kroll SS, Reece GP, Miller MJ, Ainslie N, Halabi S, Balch CM.(1993).Incidence of autoimmune disease in patients after breast reconstruction with silicone gel implants versus autogenous tissue: a preliminary report. Ann Plast Surg 31(1): 1-6.

40. Gabriel S, O'Fallon WM, Kurland L et al. (1994). Risk of Connective Tissue Diseases and Other Disorders After Breast Implantation. Nejm 330(24):1697-1702.
41. Chang YH. (1993). Adjuvanticity and arthritogenicity of silicone. Plast Reconstr Surg 92(3): 469-73.
42. Clayton D and Hills M. (1993). Statistical Methods in Epidemiology. New York, Oxford Press. 53-62.
43. Brestow NE, Day NE. (1980). Statistical Methods in Cancer Research. Vol 1- the analysis of case-control studies. IARC Scientific Publications No 32. Lyon, International Agency for Research on Cancer, 146-154.
44. Kossovsky N, Zeidler M, Chun G et al. (1993). Surface Dependent Antigens Identified by High Binding Avidity of Serum Antibodies in a Subpopulation of Patients with Breast Prostheses. J of Appl. Biomat 4:281-288.
45. Garrido L, Pfeiderer B, Papisov M et al. (1993). In vivo degradation of silicones. Magn Res Med 29(6):839-843.
46. Swaak AJ, Huysen V, Nossent JC, Smeenk RJ. (1990). Antinuclear antibody profiles in relation to specific disease manifestations of systemic lupus erythematosus. Clin Rheumatol 9(1 Sup82-94): 82-94.
47. Winfield JB, Jarjour WN. (1991). Stress Proteins, Autoimmunity and Autoimmune Disease. Curr Top Microbiol Immunol 167:161-189.
48. Weiss NL, Phillips MR, Sadock VA et al. (1990). False positive seroreactivity to Borrelia burgdorferi in rheumatic disease: the value of immunoblot analysis. Clinical Research 38:277A.
49. Yoshida SH, Teuber SS, Gerrman JB et al. (1994). Immunotoxicity of Silicone: Implications of Oxidant Balance Towards Adjuvant Activity. Fd Chem Toxic. 32: 1089-1100.
50. Yoshida SH, German JB, Fletcher MP et al. (1994). The toxic oil syndrome: a perspective on immunotoxicological mechanisms. Regulatory Toxicology and Pharmacology 19:60-79.
51. Heggers JP. (1994). Immunogenic Potential of Silicones and Subsequent Clinical Implications. Problems in General Surgery. 11:(2):June, 1994.
52. Lappe MA. (1993). Silicone-Reactive Disorder: A New Autoimmune Disease Caused by Immunostimulation and Superantigens. 1993. Medical Hypotheses 41:348-352.
53. Drake CG, Kotzin BL. (1992). Superantigens: biology, immunology and potential role in disease. J Clin Immunol 12:149-162.
54. Quinlan T, Spivack S, Mossman BT. (1994). Regulation of Antioxidant Enzymes in Lung after Oxidant Activity. Environmental Health Perspectives 102:79-87, 1994.
55. Morse J, Spiera H. (1992). Autoimmune Diseases, Immunoglobulin isotypes, and lymphocyte subsets in 30 females with breast augmentation mammoplasty. J Rheum:S65:185.
56. Barun WF. (1992). HLA molecules in autoimmune diseases. Clin Biochem 25:187-191.
57. Fox RI, Ho-Il Kang. (1992). Genetic and Environmental Factors in Systemic Sclerosis. Curr Opin in Rheum 4:875-861.

58. Pilbrant A and Strindberg B. (1975). Pharmacokinetics of 2,6-cis-Diphenylhexamethylcyclotetrasiloxane in Man. Acta Pharm et Tox 36:suppl 3, 139-145.
59. Smalley DL, Puckett DH, Osborne SH et al. (1994). Immunologic Stimulation of Lymphocytes in Silicone Gel Breast Implant Patients. Abstract 7th Annual Meeting of the Association of Medical Laboratory Immunologists, Boston, Mass. July 14.
60. Ojo-Amaize E A, Conte V, Lin H et al. (1994). Silicone-Specific Blood Lymphocyte Response in Women with Silicone Breast Implants. Clin Diag. Lab Immunol: 1 (6):698-695.
61. Potter M, Morrison S, Wiener F, et al. (1994). Induction of Plasmacytomas with Silicone Gel in Genetically Susceptible Strains of Mice. J Nat Canc Inst 86(14):1058-1065.
62. Naim JO, Lanzafame RJ, van Oss CJ. (1993). Adjuvant effect of silicone-gel on antibody formation in rats. Immunol Invest 22(2): 151-61
63. Shoaib B, Patten BM and Calkins DS. (1994). Adjuvant Breast Disease. An Evaluation of 100 Symptomatic Women with Breast Implants or Silicone Fluid Injections. Keio J Med 43(2):79-87.
64. Lewy, R.I. (1994). Auto immune Markers and Imaging Abnormalities in Silicone Breast Implant Users. Clinical Research, 42(2), 275A.
65. Lewy, R.I. (1994). Autoimmune Disease and Collagen Dermal Implants. Annals of Internal Medicine, 120(6), 524-525.
66. Komaroff AL. (1988). Chronic fatigue syndromes: relationship to chronic viral infections. J Virol Methods 21(1-4): 3-10
67. Solomon GA. (1994). Clinical and Laboratory Profile of Symptomatic Women with Silicone Breast Implants. Sem Arth Rheum 24(1) Suppl 29-37.
68. Freundlich B, Altman C, Sandorf N et al. (1994). A Profile of Symptomatic Patients with Silicone Breast Implants: A Sjogren's-like Syndrome. Sem Arth Rheum 24(1) Suppl 44-53.
69. Borenstein D et al. (1994). Siliconosis: A Spectrum of Illness. Sem Arth Rheum 24(1) Suppl 1-7.
70. Vasey FB, Havice DL, Bocanegra TS et al. (1994). Clinical Findings in Symptomatic Women with Silicone Breast Implants. Sem Arth Rheum 24(1) Suppl 22-28.
71. Lewy RI. (1995) Antinuclear Antibodies, Lipid Disturbances and Central Nervous System Imaging Abnormalities in Silicone Breast Implant Users. Journal of Investigative Medicine 43:333A.

Figure 1. ANA Positivity Over Length Of Implant Exposure Among Women With Silicone Breast Implants (N=3,349)

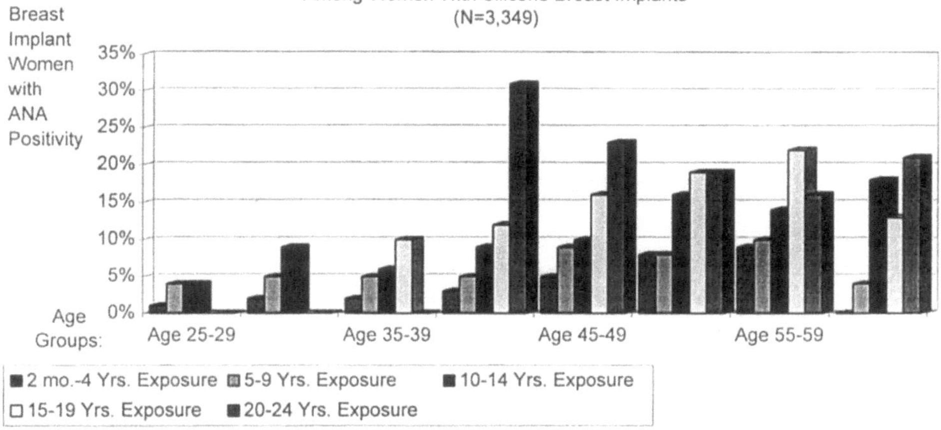

Figure 2. Duration of Exposure Among Women With Silicone Breast Implants (Median = 136 Months, Mean = 141.5 Months, SD = ± 69.2 Months) (N=3,349)

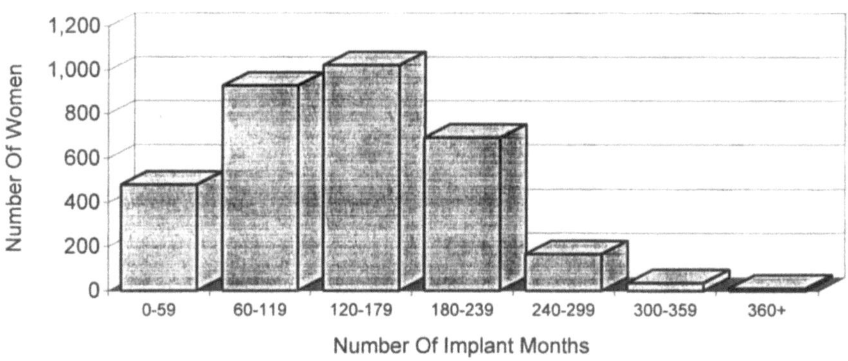

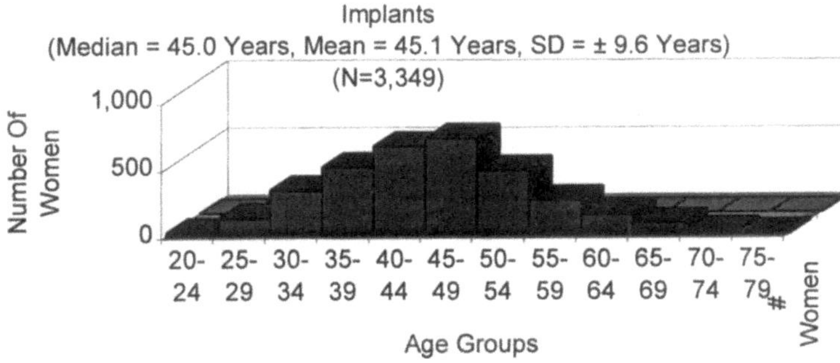

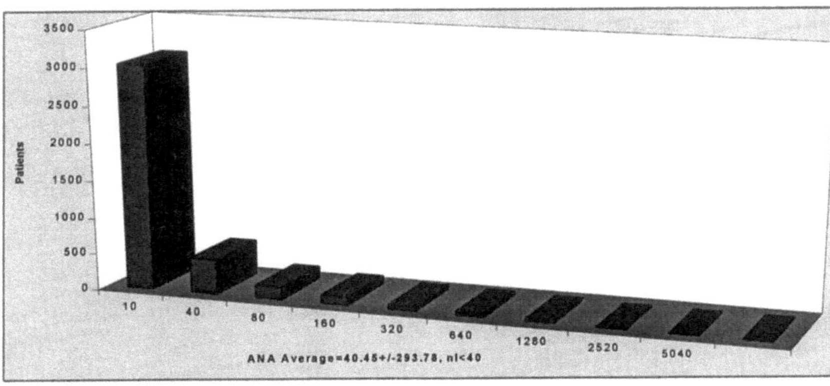

Figure 4. ANA Titers in Group Studied expressed independently of duration of implant exposure. The mean is a titer of slightly more than 1:40 (40.45 ± 293.78).

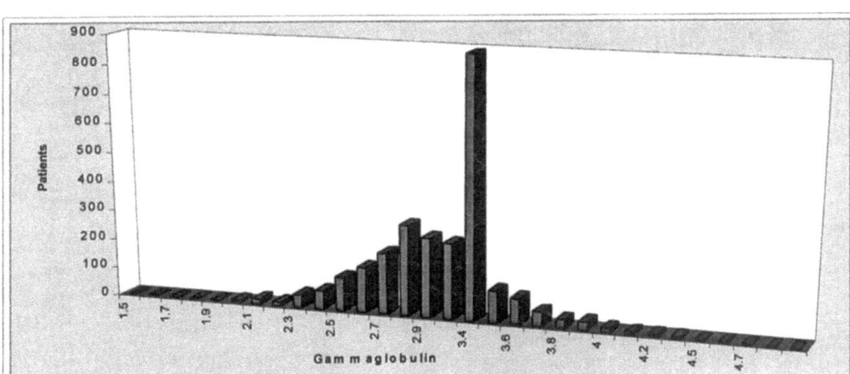

Figure 5. Total Gammaglobulin Levels.The normal range is 2.0 to 4.5 grams per deciliter. The Average Gammaglobulin level was 3.02 ± 0.39 grams per deciliter.

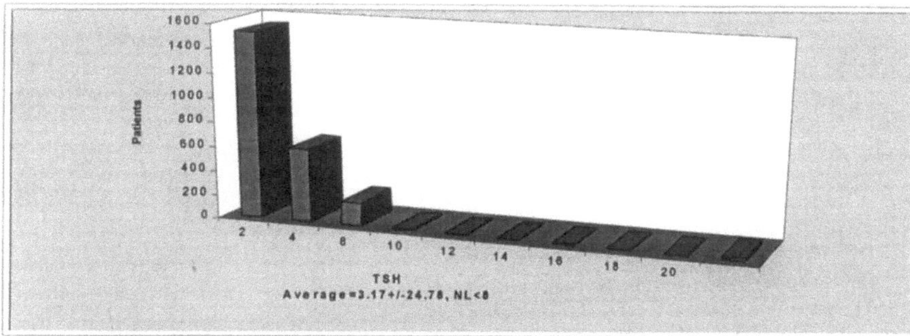

Figure 6. Thyroid stimulating hormone levels in a series of 4310 breast implant recipients.

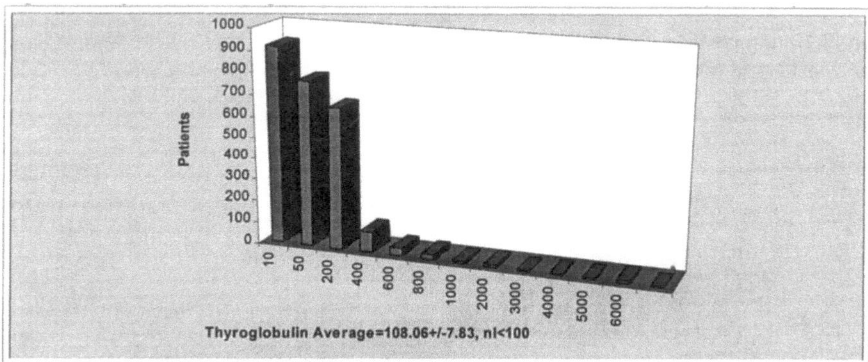

Figure 7. Thyroglobulin antibody levels in a series of 4310 breast implant recipients. The mean was mildly elevated.

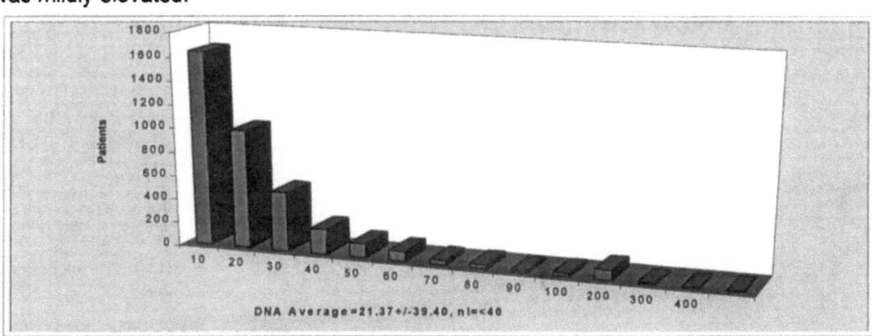

Figure 8. ds-DNA antibody levels in a series of 4310 breast implant recipients. The mean was in the normal range.

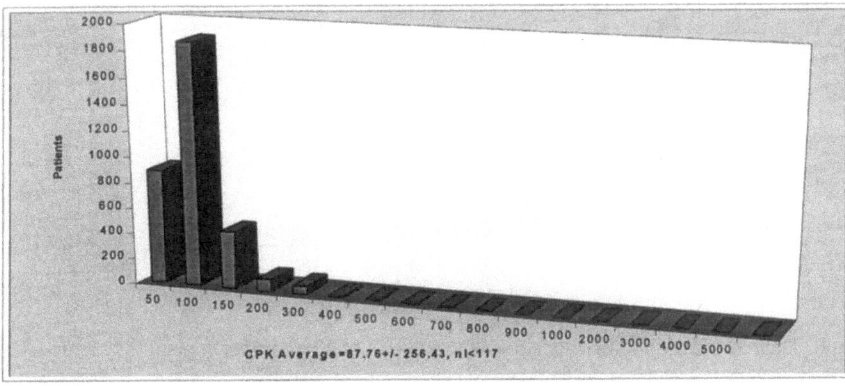

Figure 9. Serum creatine phosphokinase levels in a series of 4310 breast implant recipients. The mean was normal with a large standard deviation.

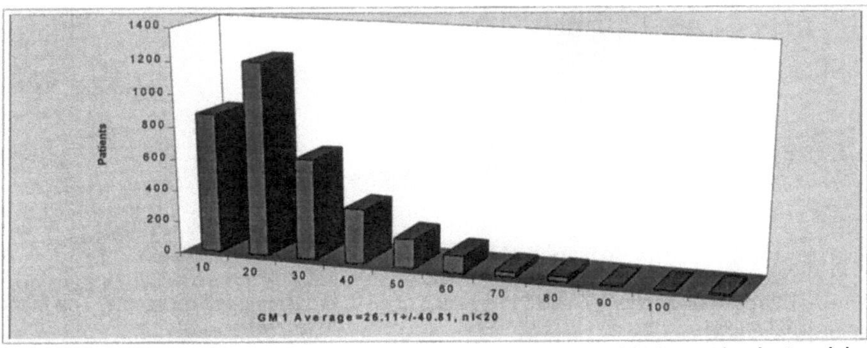

Figure 10. Serum antibody levels against GM1 neuroantibody in 4310 breast implant recipients. The mean is moderately elevated.

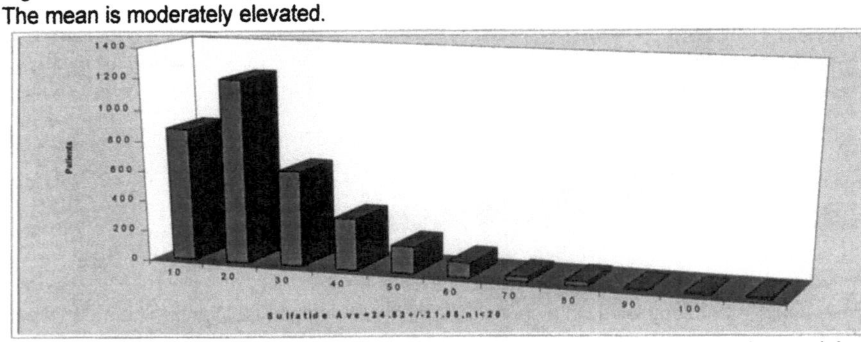

Figure 11. Serum Sulfatide neuroantibody levels in a series of 4310 breast implant recipients. The mean is moderately elevated.

SYMPTOM										
head ache	eye pain	cystitis	vision problems	raynaud	dysphagia	chest pain	tachy cardia	tic	lymph nodes	
43%	25%	28%	33%	11%	40%	81%	20%	22%		32%
rash	mood change	fatigue	insomnia	numbness	sweats	joint pain	pruritis	burning	memory loss	
30%	72%	84%	68%	80%	24%	83%	25%	88%	66%	

Table 1. Symptoms in 4310 breast implant recipients. Twenty were specifically asked for using a uniform questionnaire and standardized interview.

Measurement	% Abnormal	Abnormal/Total tests
Thyroid Stimulating Hormone (elevated)	10.38	246/2369
Antinuclear Antibody	22.13	861/3890
Thyroglobulin Antibody	33.73	858/2544
DNA Antibody(DS)	17.13	648/3781
Creatine Phosphokinase	18.84	643/3412
GM1 Antibody	39.12	1336/3415

Table 2. Autoantibodies, Hypothyroidism and CPK Levels in a series of 4,310 breast implant recipients.

MGUS, Myeloma, Plasmacytoma

Is the Risk of Multiple Myeloma Increased in Patients with Silicone Implants?

G. J. K. Tricot, M.D., Ph.D., S. Naucke, R.N., L. Vaught, B.A., D. Vesole, M.D., Ph.D., S. Jagannath, M.D. and B. Barlogie, M.D., Ph.D.

University of Arkansas for Medical Sciences
Arkansas Cancer Research Center
4301 West Markham, Slot 508
Little Rock, AR 72205

Clonal expansion and selection mediated by antigen stimulation has been hypothesized to contribute to the development of multiple myeloma (MM). Numerous case reports and epidemiologic surveys have linked chronic infections and inflammatory disorders to an increased incidence of MM[1,2]. Silicone implants have been associated with an increased incidence of auto-immune disorders. Much of the available information on the pathogenesis of plasma cell tumors comes from induction of peritoneal plasmacytomas by plastics and paraffin oils, such as pristane. This model does not appear to require carcinogens, transforming retroviruses or radiation. It relies upon genetic predisposition and natural mutations for the generation of the genetic changes in B cells leading to autonomous growth[3]. It is therefore conceivable that chronic antigen stimulation with silicone could lead to multiple myeloma in genetically predisposed individuals.

Between January 1992 and January 1995, a total of 324 new myeloma patients were seen: 210 males and 114 females. Ten of those patients (3%) had silicone implants: 9 females (breast implants) and 1 male (penile implant). The frequency in female patients was 7.9%. The reasons of silicone implants were augmentation in 9 and unknown in 1. The median time between the implants and the diagnosis of MM was 10 years with a range from 1 to 20 years. The median age at diagnosis was 44 years with a range from 39 to 61 years. One third of the patients had stage III disease according to the Durie-Salmon classification. A comparison between the 9 females with and the 105 without breast implants is provided in Table 1. All patients were entered on autotransplantation protocols with high dose cyclophosphamide to collect peripheral stem cells, followed by two autotransplants. The time to complete the entire treatment varied between 6 and 15

*Conflict of Interest Statement: There is no conflict of interest months. Patients were assessed for response 6 to 8 weeks after transplantation. As outlined in Table II, patients with implants were equally sensitive to standard chemotherapy. Although it might appear that implant patients fared worse after autotransplantation, it needs to be stressed that follow-up for the implant patients was

Table 1. SILICONE IMPLANTS AND MULTIPLE MYELOMA

	Silicone Implants (N=9)	Other Patients (N=105)	p Value
Age at Diagnosis	44 (39-61)	51 (27-72)	.8
Stage III	33%	53%	.4
Ig Isotype			
IgG	78%	53%	.3
IgA	11%	19%	
Other	11%	28%	
k / λ Ratio	1/1	2/1	.2
B2M	2.3 (1.2-10.5)	2.2 (0.9-17.1)	
CRP	0.3 (0.2-1.4)	0.3 (0.24-16.1)	
Creatinine	0.8 (0.6-1.7)	0.8 (0.3-2.0)	
Albumin	3.7 (2.5-5.5)	3.9 (2.0-4.7)	
LDH	174 (112-399)	135 (32-404)	
Calcium	101 (73-107)	93 (77-115)	

Table 2. SILICONE IMPLANTS AND MULTIPLE MYELOMA

Response to Treatment	Implants (N=9)	Other (N=105)
Standard Rx		
- Sensitive	67%	73%
- Resistant	33%	27%
Autotransplants		
- CR	22%	33%
- PR	33%	43%
- ED	0%	1%
- NR	45%	23%
Median Followup from Diag.	17 mos(1-119)	31 mos(9-134)

Table 3. SILICONE IMPLANTS AND MULTIPLE MYELOMA

Patient	Months from Implant to MM	Stage	Isotype	Age At Dx	Prior Resp	Max Resp	B2M	CRP	LDH	Creat	Alb	Hgb
JT**	1	II	KLC	67	Sens	PR	2.6	2.9	255	1 0	4 2	12.2
CC	4	II	IgGλ	44	Sens	NR	1 8	4	399	8	5 5	12 5
CS	4	II	IgGk	38	Ref	NR	2 7	3	134	.8	2.9	10.1
VG	5	III	KLC	61	Sens	PR	10.5	1 4	268	1.7	3 7	8.1
CM	6	I	IgGk	41	Sens	CR	1.5	.4	144	8	3.7	12.9
BC	14	II	IgGk	41	Sens	PR	3.6	3	119	6	4 2	9.8
HF	15	III	IgGλ	52	Sens	TE	3 9	2	246	1 1	3.5	8 1
PM	16	II	IgGλ	47	Ref	NR	1.2	.5	174	6	5 1	13.7
MN	19	III	IgAλ	51	Sens	CR	2 5	3	80	7	2.5	9 3
MM*	20	I	IgGλ	54	Ref	PR	2 8	1 6	165	7	3 7	11.2
Median	10 yr			44			2 3	3	174	.8	3.7	9.9

* Patient Expired 8-1-94
** Male
NOTE All Patients were Caucasian

shorter and 4/9 patients entered our studies less than 12 months ago. It is therefore likely that some of those patients will become partial or complete responders. Table III lists the characteristics of the 10 MM patients with silicone implants.

Our study cannot address the important question whether the incidence of MM is increased in MM patients. The 7.9% incidence of newly referred female MM patients may suggest such a correlation. However, only appropriate epidemiologic studies will provide the answer.

References:

1. Isobe T and Osserman EF. Pathologic conditions associated with plasma cell dyscrasias: a study of 806 cases. Ann. N. Y. Acad. Sci. 90:507-518, 1971.
2. Schafer AL and Miller JB. Association of IgA multiple myeloma with preexisting disease. Br. J. Haematol. 41:19-24, 1979.
3. Potter M. Perspectives on the origins of multiple myeloma and plasmacytomas in mice. Hematology/Oncology Clinics of North America 6:211-223, 1992.

Multiple Myeloma in Women with Silicone Breast Implants. Serum Immunoglobulin and Interleukin-6 Studies in Women at Risk.

L.L. Garland[1], O.F. Ballester[2], F.B. Vasey[5], K. Benson[3], L.C. Moscinski[3], M.J. Farmelo[2], M.J. Rodriguez[3] and D.P. Rapaport[4]

Divisions of Hematology and Oncology[1], Bone Marrow Transplantation[2] and Pathology[3], H. Lee Moffitt Cancer Center[4], Department of Internal Medicine[5], University of South Florida, Tampa, Florida.

Introduction

Multiple myeloma is a relatively rare malignancy, resulting from the neoplastic transformation of a B lymphocyte clone with terminal differentiation into plasma cells. With a median age at presentation of 64-69 years, it is uncommon before the age of 45. The incidence of multiple myeloma is significantly higher in men than women and in blacks than in whites [1, 2]. While its etiology is not known, some epidemiological studies have shown an increased rate of myeloma in persons with chronic inflammatory conditions including allergic disorders, rheumatoid arthritis and chronic bronchitis [2, 3]. These studies suggest a relationship between chronic antigenic stimulation, and the development of myeloma.

Intraperitoneal plasmacytomas can be induced in genetically susceptible strains of mice by the introduction into the peritoneum of materials that cause chronic inflammation. These materials include certain paraffin oils, solid plastics and as shown recently, silicone gel used for breast implantation in humans [4]. Studies in animals and humans have strongly supported the concept of implanted silicone materials as immune adjuvants [5,6].

We have attempted to identify women referred to our institution who were diagnosed with myeloma after exposure from silicone breast implants (SBI). We report here the clinical and laboratory characteristics, silicone exposure histories and measurement of serum anti-silicone antibodies in 5 such patients. Unexpectedly, three of the patients were young: 45 years or less at the time of diagnosis. In light of this finding, we attempted to define, on the basis of these cases, the incidence of myeloma in young silicone-exposed women in the state of Florida. This was then compared to the expected incidence of myeloma in women in the same age group.

Studies have indicated that the development of myeloma is preceded by a long latency period characterized by polyclonal B cell stimulation and the appearance of monoclonal gammopathies. Therefore, we evaluated the incidence of polyclonal and monoclonal gammopathies in a group of women with SBI but no underlying hematologic disorders. Serum levels of interleukin 6 (IL-6) were measured in this study group, because of the role of this cytokine as a mediator of inflammation and B lymphocyte responses.

Patients and Methods

All cases of women with multiple myeloma and SBI exposure referred to the H. Lee Moffitt Cancer Center for evaluation of their myelomas from November 1993 to January 1995 are included in this report. All had standard clinical and laboratory evaluations. Serum samples from all patients were assayed for anti-silicone antibodies using a previously described ELISA assay [6].

We utilized data from SEER (Surveillance, Epidemiology and Endpoints Registry), the Florida Cancer Data System (CDS) as well as census data for estimates of myeloma incidence [7, 8, 9]. Calculations of the silicone exposed population at risk were estimated from the national prevalence of SBI, a figure that has been referred to by previous studies but has not been formally published.

Frozen serum samples from 82 women with SBI who were seen at the Rheumatology Clinic at the University of South Florida from September 1991 to October 1993 were randomly selected for screening. In all samples serum protein electrophoresis, immunofixation and quantitation of total gammaglobulin concentration were performed by standard techniques. Serum IL-6 levels were measured with an ELISA assay (R&D systems, Minneapolis, MN). Data concerning patient's age, duration of implantation and whether or not implants were in place at the time of study were also collected. Serum samples from 41 healthy women were used as controls.

Results

Case Reports

Five women with SBI exposure and diagnosis of multiple myeloma were identified. All five were caucasian, all were diagnosed with myeloma between 1990 and 1993. Two of the patients had a preceding monoclonal gammopathy of undetermined significance (MGUS) identified 1 and 3 years prior to the diagnosis of myeloma. Table 1 presents age, clinical and laboratory data, and response to the therapeutic regimens given to each of the 5 patients.

Table 1. Clinical and Laboratory Characteristics: Myeloma and SBI

Patient	Age	Salmon-Durie Clinical Stage	Ig/Class subtype	Initial therapy	Response	Current Status of disease
1	38	IIIA	IgG-lambda	VAD	refractory disease	alive, with active disease
2	61	IIIA	IgG-kappa	VAD	partial remission	CR, post autologous transplant
3	45	IIIA	IgG-kappa	M2	partial remission	CR, post autologous transplant
4	43	IIIA	IgG-kappa	MP	refractory disease	PR, post autologous transplant
5	73	IIIA	IgG-kappa	MP	partial remission	alive, with active disease

*VAD = Vincristine, Adriamycin & Dexamethasone
M2 = Melphalan, Cyclophosphamide, BCNU, Vincristine & Prednisone
MP = Melphalan & Prednisone
CR = complete remission. PR = partial remission

As noted, all cases were IgG myelomas and presented with advanced stage. Duration of exposure to SBI, status of SBI at diagnosis of myeloma and implant status is shown in Table 2 below:

Table 2. SBI Exposure History: Myeloma and SBI

Patient	SBI duration (years)	SBI at diagnosis	Current status SBI	SBI at explanation
1	12	yes	explanted	gel leak
2	4	no	explanted	ruptured
3	12	yes	explanted	ruptured
4	14	yes	explanted	ruptured
5	2	yes	replaced	intact

Notably, the older women (patients #2 and #5) had relatively short exposure to SBI, but the young had silicone exposure of greater than one decade.

Samples tested for anti-silicone antibodies contained detectable myeloma protein in 4 of the 5 patients studied. Two patients had serum anti-silicone antibody levels above the reference range for healthy controls without SBI (0.4 - 0.9 O.D units). Interestingly, the sample with the highest anti-silicone activity (>1.5 O.D units) was observed in the only patient with no detectable myeloma protein at the time of study (patient was in complete remission post-transplant).

We estimated the number of women with SBI at risk for multiple myeloma in the age range 35-45 for the state of Florida as follows:

1) Total number of women in the US who have had SBI = 2 million women (estimated range 0.75 to 2 million, U.S., all ages)

2) Estimated number of women with SBI between the ages of 35-45 (using the age distribution of our study group of 82 women with SBI) = 40% of 2 million = 800,000 women

3) Because 3.6% of all women ages 35-45 live in Florida, the estimated number of women ages 35-45 with SBI in Florida = 3.6% of 800,000 = 28,800 women

Table 3 shows statistics describing the expected and observed number of cases of multiple myeloma in all women aged 35-45 in Florida. Also shown is the number of observed cases of myeloma over a 4 year period for women with SBI aged 35-45.

Table 3. Statistics for State of Florida: Myeloma and SBI

Age group 35-45	Population at risk	Expected cases myeloma per year*	Reported cases per year
All women	849,013**	2.5-6.7	6.9***
Women with SBI	28,800	0.09-0.23	0.75 (3 in 4 yr)

*SEER data
**Florida Census data
*** CDS data

Studies in women with SBI but no known hematological disorders

Median age for the 82 women in the study was 45 years with a range from 27 to 68. Figure 1 shows the age distribution of the study population. Women aged 35 to 45 represented 40% of the study population, while 17% of the patients were older than 55.

Median duration of implants was 12 years, with a range from 1.25 to 24 years (Figure 2). Only 14.6% of the study population had their SBI for 5 years or less. No significant differences in duration of implants was demonstrated in women younger than 45, when compared to those older. At the time of sampling, 30 women had their implants removed for a mean of 1.5 years.

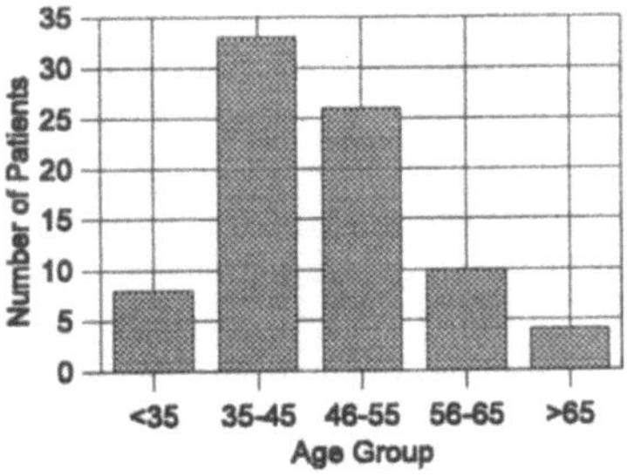

Fig 1. Distribution of age groups in the study population.

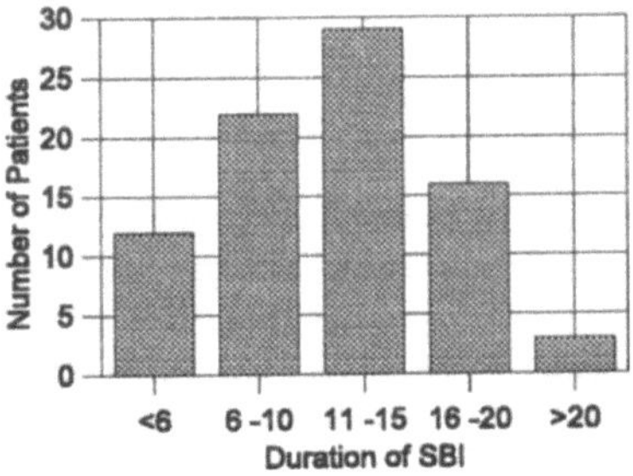

Fig 2. Distribution of implant duration (in years) in the study population.

Immunoglobulin Studies

In this study cohort, 30% of the patients had serum immunoglobulin concentrations (Ig) above the upper limit of normal for our laboratory's reference range (1.6 g/dL). As a group, younger women (45 years or less) had significantly higher Ig levels compared to older women ($p<0.005$) (Table 1). In the younger women group, 40% had elevated Ig levels compared to 15% of older patients ($p<0.01$).

No monoclonal gammopathies were noted on immunofixation studies. One patient, a 43 year old woman with SBI for 16 years, had a small oligoclonal IgG band. A second sample from this patient was evaluated 12 months after the initial study, demonstrating the persistence of the oligoclonal band.

Serum IL-6 Levels

As a group, women with SBI have serum IL-6 levels comparable to those of our healthy controls. There was a strong trend for a positive correlation between IL-6 levels and duration of implantation ($p=0.06$). This correlation was highly significant for women <45 of age ($p<0.01$), but not for older women. Similarly, the correlation was significant among women with their SBI still in place ($p=0.01$), but not for those women who had their implants removed. Among women age 45 or younger studied with their SBI in place (n=31), the correlation between serum IL-6 levels and duration of implantation was highly significant

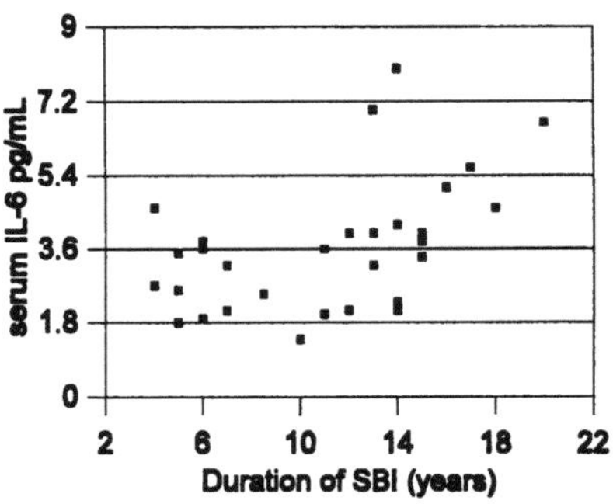

Fig 3. Correlation of serum IL-6 levels with duration of SBI in 31 women age 45 or younger and with implants in place.

(p=0.009) (Figure 3). No significant correlations were found between IL-6 levels and Ig concentrations in the group as a whole or in any of the subsets of patients.

Discussion

This report documents the occurrence of multiple myeloma in women with SBI. The clinical features of the disease in this small cohort of patients are similar to those of myeloma seen in the general population. Three of the 5 women reported here were 45 years of age or younger at the time of their diagnosis, a striking feature considering the rarity of myeloma among young caucasian women. In fact, these cases diagnosed during 1990 to 1993, may represent an excess of myeloma cases in women with SBI in the State of Florida. The estimated incidence of myeloma in young women with SBI appears to be at least 3 times that of the expected. This could be an underestimate, since it is based on figures using the highest estimate of women with SBI in the general population, and the number of myeloma cases included is limited to only those seen at our institution. However, our study sample is quite small and the trend toward higher observed than expected incidence of myeloma in these patients must be viewed in this context.

As previously reported, women with SBI frequently have increased Ig levels [10]. In our study, younger women (age 45 or less) had significantly higher levels of Ig than older women (age >45). An oligoclonal IgG band was found in a 42 year old patient. No monoclonal gammopathies were observed.

IL-6 is a multifunctional cytokine with an important mediator role in the inflammatory response, normal B cell differentiation (Ig production) and in the biology of multiple myeloma [11]. Serum IL-6 levels were not elevated in this cohort of patients. However, a correlation was found between IL-6 levels and duration of SBI. This correlation was significant only in younger women and in those with their implants in place, but not in older patients or in those who had their SBI removed.

Previous reports have documented that in healthy individuals Ig levels increase with age, as does the the incidence of monoclonal gammopathies [12]. Similarly, serum IL-6 levels are higher in older healthy individuals [13]. Our findings are of interest, therefore, as they represent the reverse of the expected patterns and taken together, may indicate a more intense inflammatory and/or B cell immune response to SBI in younger women.

As suggested by a recent editorial [14], a broader study with more significant statistical power is warranted to discern whether there is, or is not, a true association between silicone exposure and the development of multiple myeloma.

Acknowledgments

The Florida cancer incidence data used in this report has been derived from the Florida Cancer Data System.

Disclaimer

This work was supported solely by research grants from the H. Lee Moffitt Cancer Center and Research Institute. The authors have no professional affiliations with the silicone industry.

References

1. Riedel DA, Pottern LM. The epidemiology of Multiple Myeloma. Hematol Oncol Clin North Am 1992; 6:225-247.
2. Herrinton LJ, Weiss NS, Olshan AF. The epidemiology of myeloma. In Myeloma, Biology and Management. Malpas JS, Bergsagel DE and Kyle RA, editors. Oxford University Press, Oxford, England. Pages 127-168.
3. Isomaki HA, Hakulinen T, Joutsealahti U. Excess risk of lymphomas, leukemia and myeloma in patients with rheumatoid arthritis. J Chron Dis 1978; 31:691-696.
4. Potter M, Morrison S, Wiener F, Zhang XK, Miller FW. Induction of plasmacytomas with silicone gel in genetically susceptible strains of mice. J Natl Cancer Inst 1994; 86:1058-1065.
5. Naim JO, Lanzafame RJ, van Oss CJ. The adjuvant effect of silicone-gel on antibody formation in rats. Immunol Invest 1993; 22:151-161.
6. Wolf LE, Lappe M, Peterson RD, Ezrailson EG. Human immune response to polydimethylsiloxane (silicone): screening studies in a breast implant population. FASEB J 1993; 7:1265-1268.
7. SEER Cancer Statistical Review 1973-1990. Miller BA, Gloeckler Ries LA, Hankey BF, editors. NIH Publication No.93-2789: Section XVII.
8. The Florida Cancer Data System
9. U.S. Census Bureau
10. Bridges AJ, Conley C, Wang G, Burns DE, Vasey FB. A clinical and immunological evaluation of women with silicone breast implants and symptoms of rheumatic disease. Ann Intern Med 1993; 118:929-936.
11. Weber J. Interleukin-6: multifunctional cytokine. Biologic Therapy of Cancer Updates 1993; 3: 1-9.
12. Crawford J, Eye MK, Cohen HJ. Evaluation of monoclonal gammopathies in the "well" elderly. Am J Med 1987; 82:39-45.
13. Ershler WB. Interleukin-6: a cytokine for gerontologists. J Am Geriatrics Soc 1993; 41: 176-181.
14. Salmon SE, Kyle RA. Silicone gels, induction of plasma cell tumors, and genetic susceptibility in mice: a call for epidemiologic investigation of women with silicone breast implants. J Natl Cancer Inst 1994; 86:1040-1041.

Silicone Gel Implants and Monoclonal Gammopathies: Three Cases of Multiple Myeloma and the Prevalence of Multiple Myeloma and Monoclonal Gammopathy of Undetermined Significance

S. Silverman[1,3], R. Vescio[1,3], D. Silver[3], S. Renner[2], S. Weiner[3], and J. Berenson[1,3]
Departments of Medicine[1] and Pathology[2], Department of Veteran Affairs West Los Angeles, VA Medical Center and UCLA School of Medicine[3], Jonsson Comprehensive Cancer Center, Los Angeles, CA

Introduction

In 1994, Potter reported that plasmacytomas were inducible in susceptible BALB/C mice by the intraperitoneal injection of silicone gel [1]. These findings raised the possibility that long-term exposure to silicone gel in humans could result in plasma cell proliferation resulting in either monoclonal gammopathy of unknown significance (MGUS) or multiple myeloma (MM). We report three cases of MM in women with silicone gel breast implants (SGBIs) and preliminary data on the prevalence of increased immunoglobulins and MGUS in symptomatic women with breast implants.

The Prevalence of SGBI Among MM Patients at UCLA Medical Center

After chart review, we determined that 34 female patients were seen in the myeloma clinic at UCLA Medical Center with a diagnosis of MM within the past two years. Hospital charts were then reviewed and these patients were contacted to determine prior exposure to silicone gel implants. Two of these patients had received SGBIs for an estimated prevalence of 5.9% and their case histories are outlined below. In addition, a third patient was referred for evaluation from Oregon (Case #3). The time from SGBI to diagnosis of myeloma was 12, 14 and 36 years respectively (Table 1).

Table 1. Three cases of multiple myeloma in women with silicone gel breast implants

	Case 1	Case 2	Case 3
Patient Characteristics:			
Age at MM diagnosis	41	55	52
Current age	46	58	52
Si Implant Data:			
Reason for implant	cosmetic	cosmetic	cosmetic
Yrs (Si Implant to MM)	14	12	36
Number of sets	7 on left, 5 on right	2	2
Implant rupture	no	no	yes
Implant contracture	yes	yes	unknown
Postop complication	yes	yes	yes
Rheumatologic data:			
Rheumatic symptoms	fatigue, fever, photosensitivity, Raynaulds, sicca, arthralgia	arthralgia, myalgia, fatigue, fever, malar rash, sicca	arthralgia, fatigue sicca, irritable bowel
Neuro symptoms	dysesthesias		cognitive, neuropathy
ANA	negative	positive	positive
Myeloma-related:			
Monoclonal Protein*	nonsecretory	IgA kappa 1.2 gm/dL	IgG 1.0 gm/dL
Urine (24 hr protein)*	none	50 mg	450 mg
Stage (Durie-Salmon)	IA (?)	IIIA	IIIA
Bone disease*	yes	yes	yes
Hgb*	11.5	12.4	11.9
Calcium*	9.6	9.6	9.8

*- at diagnosis

Case 1: A 46 year old white female developed right low back pain accompanied by sciatica in September, 1989. She was found to have a large lytic lesion in the right sacrum. A biopsy revealed a B-cell tumor originally diagnosed as a large cell noncleaved lymphoma. A bone marrow biopsy and additional staging procedures revealed no other sites of disease. She was treated with VACOP-B chemotherapy which was changed to M-BACOD because of a lack of response. Postchemotherapy she received radiation therapy to the right sacroiliac area. She did well until August, 1992 when she developed left rib discomfort, and eventually was found to have destruction of the left fifth rib with an adjacent extrapleural density. A biopsy in April, 1993 revealed recurrence of the original tumor but a re-evaluation of this and the original biopsies was consistent with the diagnosis of MM rather than lymphoma. Further bone films demonstrated a new right femoral lytic lesion. Bone marrow was unremarkable. Serum and urine studies did not reveal a monoclonal protein, and the patient was diagnosed with nonsecretory myeloma. She was treated with high dose pulse dexamethasone therapy until September 1993 at which time she underwent an autologous peripheral blood stem cell transplant with a busulfan/cyclophosphamide conditioning regimen. She did well until August, 1994 when she was found to have increasing osteolytic disease in the right femur which required metal rod placement. Postoperatively, she underwent radiation therapy to this area as well as to the C-spine because of symptomatic disease. She has since begun pulse decadron therapy followed by radiation therapy to her left hip because of symptomatic disease in April, 1995. In 1975, the patient underwent placement of bilateral SGBIs and she required multiple repairs until 1985.

Case 2: A 58 year old white female was found to have an IgA kappa monoclonal gammopathy in June 1992 with a paraprotein level of 1.2 g/dL. Bone marrow showed 10% plasma cells with an unremarkable bone survey and she was diagnosed with MGUS. Her paraprotein gradually rose to 2.0 g/dL by November, 1994 so further staging was performed revealing 30% plasma cells on bone marrow biopsy and multiple osteolytic calvarial lesions on bone survey. She was diagnosed with MM and started on infusional VAD chemotherapy in February, 1995. This patient underwent bilateral SGBI surgery in 1980.

Case #3: A 52 year old white female developed sacral discomfort in January, 1994 and diffuse myalgias. She developed increasing sacral discomfort leading to bowel and bladder dysfunction. In November 1994, she was found to have a large presacral mass and underwent sacrectomy for a plasmacytoma. Further workup revealed an IgG lambda monoclonal gammopathy with paraprotein levels of 1.0 g/dL in the serum and 450 mg in a 24 hr urine collection. A skeletal survey revealed a pathologic fracture of the right humerus and an expansile right 8th rib lesion, and she was diagnosed with MM. She was treated with radiation therapy to these sites as well as the sacral area and also started on melphalan and prednisone chemotherapy. In 1958, the patient underwent SGBI surgery, which eventually required removal and replacement with new implants in 1976.

The Prevalence of Increased Immunoglobulins (Igs) in 630 SGBI Patients

We then studied the prevalence of increased Igs in 630 symptomatic women with SGBIs with a mean age of 47 years. The mean number of years since the first implant was 14 at the time of serum analysis. Ig levels were measured using a nephelometric technique (Table 2). There was no correlation between the level of Igs and patient age or mean number of years since first implant. In every case, there were a greater percentage of women with Ig subtype elevation in comparison to the number with subtype reduction. The differences between IgA elevation and reduction was less pronounced but this may be explainable by the 1-2% incidence of IgA deficiency in the general population (Table 3).

Table 2. Ig levels observed in 630 women with silicone gel implants

Ig Type	Mean Level (mg/dL)	Range (mg/dL)	Median (mg/dL)	Reference (mg/dL)
IgG	1153.0 ± 298	430-3760	1110	680-1445
IgA	200.1 ± 91	6-631	186	71-374
IgM	148.8 ± 76	4-689	136	40-248

The Prevalence of Monoclonal Gammopathy in 284 Sera

In order to determine the etiology of the elevated Igs found in these women, we obtained 284 random sera from the initial 630 patient cohort described above. Within this subgroup, 38% of the women had elevated Igs in contrast to the 23% incidence in the initial cohort. Our results were then compared to an age matched cohort from our medical center. We used agarose gel serum protein electrophoresis as our primary screening and analysis tool with immunoelectrophoresis being performed to confirm and characterize any suspicious monoclonal bands.

Table 3. Ig abnormalities in 630 women with silicone gel implants

Type	Elevation	Reduction
Abnormal Quantitative Igs	23% (142)	5.6% (35)
IgG	10.8% (68)	1.6% (10)
IgA	3.2% (20)	2.8% (18)
IgM	6.3% (40)	0.6% (4)
IgG and IgA	0.8% (5)	0.2% (1)
IgG and IgM	1.1 % (7)	0.2% (1)
IgA and IgM	0.2% (1)	0.2% (1)
IgG, IgM and IgA	0.2% (1)	0%

There were 4 sera that were positive for MGUS in the elevated Ig subset (n=108) for an estimated prevalence of 3.7 % in these women. There was 1 serum that was positive for MGUS in the non-Ig elevated subset (n=176) for an estimated prevalence of 0.6%. If we correct the prevalence of elevated Ig patients to the prevalence seen in the larger cohort, then we can estimate the total prevalence of MGUS in symptomatic women to be 1.3%. The majority (4/5) of the patients positive for MGUS had silicone exposure of greater than 10 years. The five patients positive for MGUS are described in Table 4.

Table 4. Description of the MGUS patients

Patient #	1	2	3	4	5
Age at Dx of MGUS	79	38	56	48	43
Yrs since SGBI	5	12	17	10	17
Reason for implant	Cosmetic	Cosmetic	Cosmetic	Cosmetic	Cosmetic
Ig isotype	IgG λ	IgG κ	IgM κ	IgG κ	IgG λ
Implant rupture	No	Yes	Unknown	Yes	No
Implant contracture	Yes	Yes	Yes	Yes	Yes
Follow-up at 1 yr	n/r*	disappeared†	no change	disappeared†	n/r*

n/r*- not repeated, †- disappeared following SGBI removal

Natural History of MGUS in Patients with Silicone Breast Implants

Of the five patients identified as having a monoclonal protein in 1994, we were able to recontact four of the patients (Patients 1 - 4). Patient #1 has been complaining of diffuse bony pain for the past few months and also has a reduction in the non-monoclonal Ig proteins, so she is currently being evaluated for malignant disease. Patient #2 had SGBI explantation one week after the initially tested serum was drawn in 4/94. A repeat serum sample obtained 11 months after explantation in 3/95 showed no residual monoclonal gammopathy. For Patient #3, the SGBIs had been previously revised to saline implants in 1993 prior to collection of her initial serum sample which showed the monoclonal gammopathy in 4/94. A repeat serum sample obtained on April, 1995 remained positive for MGUS. However, her increased alpha 2 and gamma fractions had disappeared. The initial serum sample from Patient #4 was also obtained in 4/94. Her implants were later revised from SGBIs to saline filled devices in 2/95. A repeat SPEP performed 4/95 showed resolution of the monoclonal gammopathy.

Prevalence Of Acute And Chronic Inflammation

Acute inflammation was present in 28.52% of the patients as judged by an elevated alpha 2 fraction without an elevated gamma fraction. Chronic inflammation was present in an additional 18.21% of the patients as determined by an elevated gamma fraction consistent with polyclonal gammopathy. Of the group with chronic inflammation, 64% also had evidence of acute inflammation as judged by a high alpha 2 fraction. No patient with evidence of inflammation had a decreased albumin fraction. Thus a total of 46.73% of our group of 284 symptomatic women had evidence of inflammation either chronic or acute. Monoclonal gammopathy as defined by a monoclonal band identified on SPEP and confirmed on IEP was present in 1.7%. A normal electrophoresis was observed in 35.05% (Figure 1).

Of the five patients with MGUS, 1 had elevated gamma fractions suggesting chronic inflammation, 1 had elevated alpha 2 suggesting acute inflammation and 1 had elevated alpha 2 and gamma suggesting both acute and chronic inflammation upon initial assessment.

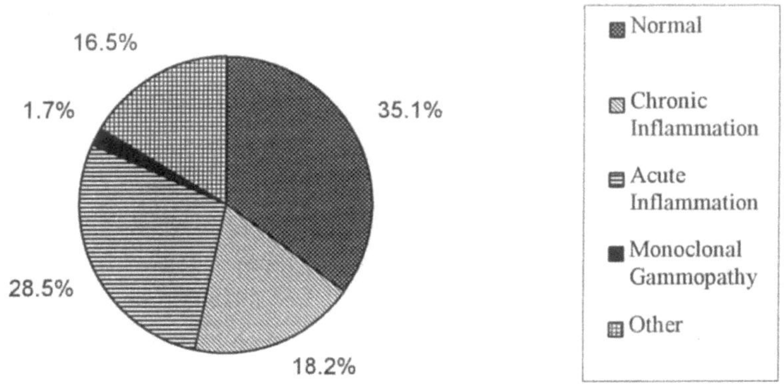

Fig. 1. Serum protein electrophoreses results from 284 women with silicone gel breast implants.

Discussion

The effects of silicone gel leakage from breast implants include immediate effects of the leakage or rupture into the surrounding tissue with fibrosis and capsular contracture [2]. Short term effects may include the development of fatigue, myalgias, arthralgias, sicca symptoms and cognitive defects [3,4,5]. Long term effects may include the B cell proliferative effects described in this manuscript including increased immunoglobulin, MGUS, and multiple myeloma. It is noteworthy that all three of our reported cases of multiple myeloma had ≥12 yrs of silicone exposure suggesting a long latency period. The mean silicone exposure of the MGUS patients was 12 years.

We found the prevalence of elevated immunoglobulins of 23% in a group of symptomatic women with breast implants. While this finding may be nonspecific, the finding of an increased prevalence of MGUS is disturbing. However, this finding may be biased by our sample, all of whom were symptomatic women. In order to determine causation, the prevalence of MGUS should be studied prospectively in a cohort of women who received silicone breast implants and who are enrolled irrespective of their symptoms and compared to age matched controls.

The presence of acute or chronic inflammation in approximately 46% of our patients suggests a possible relationship between MGUS and inflammation. In the 241 MGUS cases followed by Kyle, inflammatory diseases were found in 11% and connective tissue diseases in 6% [6].

If silicone is the antigenic or inflammatory stimulus for MGUS in these patients, then removal of the antigenic stimulus by explantation might be expected to eliminate the monoclonal protein. In the two patients who underwent either implant removal or revision to a saline filled device, the monoclonal gammopathy disappeared. Similar results are reported by Andersen [7] elsewhere in this volume who describes two other patients with transient monoclonal gammopathies. Transient monoclonal gammopathies, while uncommon, have been observed in association with other disease states such as HIV infection [8], and also following bone marrow transplantation primarily in patients with graft versus host disease [9]. T-cell dysfunction may play a role in this disorder.

After a median follow-up of 22 years, 24% of Kyle's MGUS patients (median age- 64 years) developed myeloma or other serious hematologic diseases at a median time to serious disease development of 10 years [10]. It is unknown whether a similar scenario will occur in MGUS patients with silicone implants due to the younger median age (45 years) and since the silicone gel may provide a chronic environment of antigenic stimulation. In our one patient who developed myeloma following MGUS, this progression occurred only two years from the diagnosis of MGUS.

Further studies of the paraproteins produced in women with silicone breast implants are needed to see if these paraproteins have characteristic features or are reactive to products within the implants. One such approach is to sequence the immunoglobulin heavy and light chain variable regions to determine similarities. One could also determine the three dimensional structure of the monoclonal antibody using computer modeling to determine antigen binding similarities. A third approach would be to express the antibody and to determine the reactivity to the chemical components present in the SGBIs.

Our data show evidence of acute and/or chronic inflammation in 46% of the sera studied of symptomatic women. These inflammatory states may eventually result in a higher incidence of MGUS and finally multiple myeloma [6]. Our study suggests that many of the symptomatic women referred to our practice have objective evidence of an underlying inflammatory disorder. Further studies are needed to characterize this condition.

References

1. Potter M, Morrison S, Wiener F, Zhang XK, Miller FW (1994).Induction of plasmacytomas in genetically susceptible strains of mice. J Natl Cancer Inst 86:1058-1065.
2. Stratmeyer ME (1991) ed. Silicone in medical devices, HHS Publication FDA 92-4249, Rockville Maryland, 330p.
3. Solomon G (1993) A clinical and laboratory profile of symptomatic women with silicone breast implants. Sem Arth Rheum 24 (1 Suppl 1) 29-37.
4. Borenstein D (1994) Siliconosis: A spectrum of illness. Sem Arth Rheum 24 (1 Suppl 1) 1-7.
5. Vasey FB, Havice DL, Bocanegra TS, Seleznick MJ, Bridgeford PH, Martinez-Osuna P and Espinoza L. (1994) Clinical findings in symptomatic women with silicone breast implants. Sem Arth Rheum 24 (1 Suppl 1) : 22-28.
6. Kyle RA (1994) Monoclonal gammopathy of undetermined significance Blood Rev 8:135-141.
7. Andersen elsewhere in this volume

8. Lefrere JJ. Debbia M, and Lambin P (1993) Prospective follow-up of monoclonal gammopathies in HIV-infected individuals. Brit J Haematology 84:151-155.
9. Mitus AJ. Stein R, Rappeport JM, Antin JH, Weinstein Hj, Alper A, and Smith BR (1989). Monoclonal and oligoclonal gammopathy after bone marrow transplantation. Blood 74: 2764-2768.
10. Kyle RA (1993). "Benign monoclonal gammopathy - after 20 to 35 years of followup. Mayo Clinic Proc 68:26-36.

Monoclonal Gammopathy of Undetermined Significance

R.A. Kyle
Consultant, Division of Hematology and Internal Medicine, Mayo Clinic and Mayo Foundation; Professor of Medicine and Laboratory Medicine, Mayo Medical School; Rochester, Minnesota

Monoclonal gammopathy of undetermined significance (MGUS) is characterized by the presence of a serum monoclonal protein (M-protein) less than 3 g/dL; fewer than 10 percent plasma cells in the bone marrow; no or only small amounts of M-protein (Bence Jones protein) in the urine; absence of lytic lesions, anemia, hypercalcemia, and renal insufficiency; and most importantly, stability of the M-protein and failure of development of other abnormalities. Detection of an M-protein is accomplished by electrophoresis on agarose or cellulose acetate followed by immunoelectrophoresis or immunofixation. The latter is more sensitive and is particularly useful when one is searching for a small M-protein (Kyle, 1994).

MGUS accounts for more than one-half of newly diagnosed patients with an M-protein. Multiple myeloma (MM), Waldenström's macroglobulinemia, primary amyloidosis, solitary or extramedullary plasmacytoma, lymphoma, and chronic lymphocytic leukemia must be considered in the differential diagnosis of a monoclonal gammopathy (Fig. 1). MGUS is found in approximately 3 percent of persons over 70 years of age in Sweden (Axelsson et al, 1966), in the United States (Kyle et al, 1972), and in France (Saleun et al, 1982). In Sweden, among 6,995 normal persons over 25 years of age the overall prevalence of an M-protein was 1 percent. In 1,200 patients 50 years or older who were residents of a small Minnesota community, 1.25 percent had an M-protein while 1.7 percent of adults greater than 50 years of age in Finistère, France had an M-protein. Thus, the prevalence of MGUS is considerable, so it is important to know whether the disorder will remain stable or will progress to a symptomatic plasma cell proliferative disorder such as MM, macroglobulinemia, or primary amyloidosis.

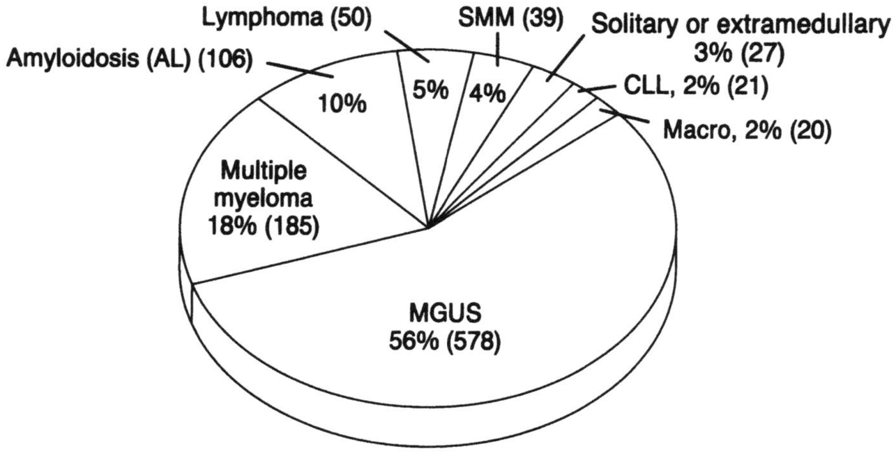

Fig. 1. Patients with monoclonal plasma cell disorders seen at Mayo Clinic in 1992. CLL, chronic lymphocytic leukemia; Macro, macroglobulinemia; MGUS, monoclonal gammopathy of undetermined significance; SMM, smoldering multiple myeloma.

Mayo Clinic Study

The medical records of all patients with a monoclonal gammopathy who were seen at the Mayo Clinic before January 1, 1971 were reviewed. Patients with MM, macroglobulinemia, amyloidosis, lymphoma, or related disorders were excluded; 241 patients remained for long-term follow up (Kyle, 1993).

Ninety-six percent of the 241 patients were more than 40 years of age. The median age was 64 years with one-third greater than 70 years of age. Males accounted for 58%. The presence of hepatomegaly or splenomegaly as well as anemia, thrombocytopenia, renal insufficiency, hypoalbuminemia, or hypercalcemia were the result of disorders unrelated to a plasma cell proliferative process. The heavy-chain type was IgG in 73 percent, IgA in 11 percent, IgM in 14 percent, and biclonal in 2 percent. The light chain was kappa (κ) in 62 percent and lambda (λ) in the remainder. The initial M-protein level ranged from 0.3 to 3.2 g/dL (median, 1.7 g/dL). The level of uninvolved or background immunoglobulins was reduced in 29 percent. Fifteen patients had a monoclonal light chain (Bence Jones protein), but the amount was small in most patients. The bone marrow contained 3 percent plasma cells (range, 1-10%) which were non-diagnostic in appearance. Approximately three-fourths of the patients had unrelated disorders such as cardiovascular or cerebrovascular disease, connective tissue disorders, inflammatory processes, and a variety of other conditions unrelated to the M-protein.

The 241 patients were classified into four groups after 24 to 38 years of follow up (Table 1).

Table 1. Course of 241 patients with monoclonal gammopathy of undetermined significance

Group	Description	No. of Patients at Follow-Up After 24-38 Years	
		No.	%
1	No substantial increase of serum or urine monoclonal protein (benign)	30	12
2	Monoclonal protein ≥ 3.0 g/dL but therapy not required	23	10
3	Died of unrelated causes	126	52
4	Developed myeloma, macroglobulinemia, amyloidosis, or related disease	62	26
Total		241	100

The patients in Group 1 are still at risk for development of malignant disease and continue to be followed. The M-protein disappeared in only two patients. Group 2 is composed of 23 patients in whom the serum M-protein increased to 3 g/dL or more but who did not require therapy for myeloma or macroglobulinemia. Only one patient is alive in this group and continues to be followed. More than one-half of patients (Group 3) died from unrelated diseases without recognition of a malignant plasma cell or lymphoproliferative process. As one might expect, cardiovascular and cerebrovascular diseases were the most common causes of death.

Sixty-two patients (26 percent) developed MM, macroglobulinemia, amyloidosis, or a malignant lymphoproliferative disorder during follow up. The actuarial rate of development of serious disease at 10 years was 16 percent, 33 percent at 20 years, and 40 percent at 25 years (Fig. 2). Actuarial development of serious disease in patients with IgG, IgA, and IgM gammopathies was not significantly different.

More than two-thirds of the 62 patients in Group 4 developed MM. The interval from the recognition of MGUS to the diagnosis of MM ranged from 2 to 29 years (Table 2).

Table 2. Development of myeloma or related diseases in 62 patients with monoclonal gammopathy of undetermined significance

			Interval to Diagnosis (yr)	
	No.	%	Median	Range
Multiple myeloma	42	68	10	2-29
Macroglobulinemia	7	11	8.5	4-20
Amyloidosis	8	13	9	6-19
Malignant lymphoproliferative disorders	5	8	10.5	6-22
Total	62	100		

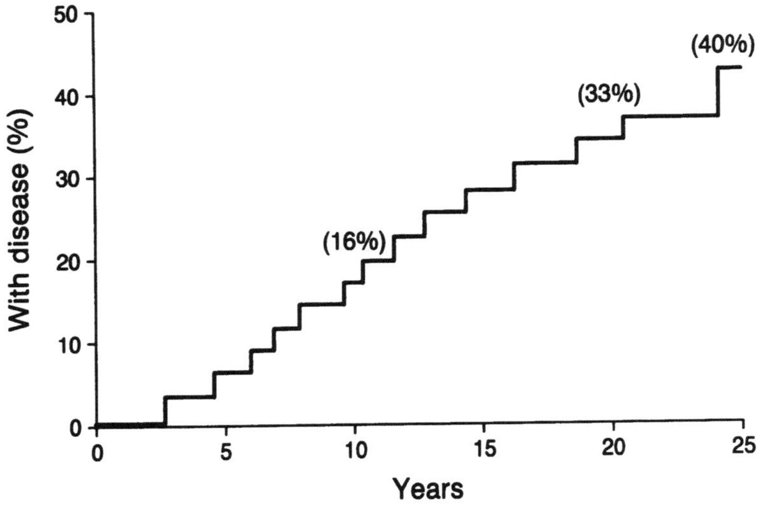

Fig. 2. Incidence of multiple myeloma, macroglobulinemia, amyloidosis, or lymphoproliferative disease after recognition of monoclonal protein.

The diagnosis of MM was made more than 20 years after the detection of a serum M-protein in seven patients. The median survival after diagnosis of MM was 33 months which is similar to that seen in the usual series of myeloma patients. Two of the patients are still alive. The development of myeloma varied from a gradual increase in the serum M-protein over many years to an abrupt onset in a matter of a few months. Macroglobulinemia of Waldenström occurred in seven patients. The median interval from the recognition of the M-protein to the diagnosis of macroglobulinemia was 8.5 years. Primary amyloidosis was recognized in eight patients 6 to 19 years after the diagnosis of MGUS (median, 9 years). Five patients developed a lymphoproliferative disorder 6 to 22 years after recognition of the M-protein. Three of the five patients had a malignant lymphoma. The course was aggressive in two while the third had a diffuse mixed lymphoma of the jejunum which was successfully resected. One patient developed chronic lymphocytic leukemia while the fifth patient had a malignant lymphoproliferative disorder resembling Waldenström's macroglobulinemia. The M-protein increased in only one of the five patients with a malignant lymphoproliferative process.

Results of Long-Term Follow-Up in Other Series

Seven (11 percent) of the 64 patients with an M-protein found in a survey of 6,995 persons had progression of their monoclonal gammopathy follow up for 20 years (Axelsson, 1986). In an Italian series of 313 patients with MGUS, 14 percent of 213 patients followed for 5 to 8 years and 18 percent of 100 patients with a follow up of 8 to 13 years developed malignant disease (Paladini et al, 1989).

Belisle et al. (1990) reported that 19 of 152 patients with BMG had progressive disease. In another series of 213 patients of apparently benign monoclonal gammopathy, the actuarial risk for development of malignant disease was 4.5 percent at 5 years, 15 percent at 10 years, and 26 percent at 15 years (Giraldo et al, 1991). Bladé reported that 10 percent of 128 patients had malignant transformation at a median of 56 months (Bladé et al, 1992).

Differentiation of MGUS from Myeloma or Macroglobulinemia

The differentiation of a patient with MGUS from one with myeloma may be difficult. The size of the serum M-protein is of some help in that higher levels (usually greater than 3 g/dL) are associated with a greater likelihood of myeloma or macroglobulinemia. In addition to the size of the M-protein, the hemoglobin value, percentage of bone marrow plasma cells, presence of hypercalcemia or renal insufficiency, larger amounts of monoclonal light chain in the urine (Bence Jones proteinuria), and the presence of lytic bone lesions are helpful. The presence of a serum M-protein greater than 3 g/dL usually indicates overt MM or macroglobulinemia, but some conditions such as smoldering multiple myeloma (SMM) exist (Kyle and Greipp, 1980). Patients with SMM are characterized by a serum M-protein level greater than 3 g/dL and more than 10 percent abnormal plasma cells in the bone marrow. They often have a reduction of uninvolved immunoglobulins in the serum and modest amounts of monoclonal light chain in the urine. These findings suggest the presence of MM, but anemia, renal insufficiency, and skeletal lesions do not develop, and the M-protein in the serum and urine, and the number of a bone marrow plasma cells remains stable. The proliferative rate of the plasma cells (plasma cell labeling index; PCLI) is low. These patients have a clinically benign monoclonal gammopathy, but it is not possible to make a definitive diagnosis of SMM when the patient is initially seen because most patients with this level of M-protein in the serum and those with more than 10 percent plasma cells in the bone marrow have symptomatic MM. Patients with SMM should not be treated unless laboratory abnormalities progress or symptoms of myeloma develop.

The presence of circulating plasma cells in the peripheral blood is a good indication of active MM. Peripheral blood plasma cells are detected in approximately 60 percent of patients with newly diagnosed symptomatic MM and in more than 90 percent of patients with refractory or relapsed myeloma (Witzig et al, 1992). The presence of circulating plasma cells in the peripheral blood is also helpful in determining which patients with SMM will progress. In a series of 57 patients with newly diagnosed SMM, 16 patients progressed to MM within 12 months. Sixty-three percent of those who progressed had an increase in peripheral blood plasma cells. In contrast, only 4 of 41 of those patients who remained stable had increased peripheral blood plasma cells. The median time to progression of myeloma was 9 months for patients with an increase in peripheral blood plasma cells and 2.5 years for those without an increase in peripheral blood plasma cells (Witzig et al, 1994).

It was not possible to determine whether our 241 patients presenting with MGUS would remain stable and benign or develop MM or a related disorder during long-term follow up (Kyle, 1993) (Fig. 3). The initial hemoglobin value, type and amount of serum M-protein, number and appearance of plasma cells in the bone marrow, levels of normal and uninvolved (background) immunoglobulins, age, sex, presence of organomegaly, presence of small amounts of monoclonal light chain in the urine, serum albumin level, and IgG subclass did not enable us to distinguish initially between patients with benign disease (Group 1) from those in whom a serious plasma cell proliferative process developed during follow up (Group 4). Thus, no single factor can differentiate a patient with benign monoclonal gammopathy (BMG) from one in whom a malignant plasma cell disorder will eventually develop.

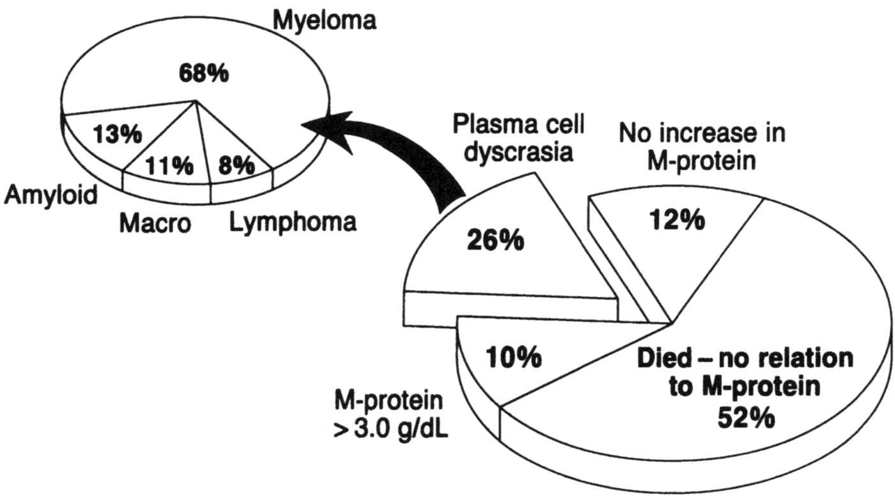

Fig. 3. Evolution of monoclonal gammopathies. Macro, macroglobulinemia; M-protein, monoclonal protein.

The serum M-protein must be measured periodically and a clinical evaluation conducted to determine whether serious disease has developed. In patients recently recognized with MGUS, protein electrophoresis should be repeated in 3 to 6 months (depending upon the size of the M-protein) and if the M-protein is stable, the test should be repeated in 6 to 12 months. If the M-protein remains stable and the patient appears to be well, electrophoresis and clinical evaluation should be performed annually thereafter. The patient should be told that malignancy occurs in only one-fourth of patients and that it often occurs only after a median follow up of 10 years. However, the physician should be aware that evolution from MGUS to MM can be abrupt and therefore, patients should be encouraged to seek medical evaluation if untoward symptoms develop (Kyle, 1993).

Possible Relationship of Silicone Breast Implants and Multiple Myeloma

Potter et al. (1994) reported that silicone gel injected intraperitoneally into plasmacytoma-susceptible mice produced a high frequency of intraperitoneal plasmacytomas. Murine plasmacytomas have some features in common with human plasma cell proliferative disorders such as MGUS, solitary plasmacytoma, MM, and primary amyloidosis. However, in contrast to human MM, murine plasmacytomas are usually extramedullary and rarely produce lytic lesions. In addition, extramedullary plasmacytomas are uncommon in humans and are generally less aggressive than is MM (Salmon and Kyle, 1994).

The SEER Group has estimated that in 1990, MM occurred in at least 3 of 100,000 persons in the population per year and that the sex-specific rates of MM were 2.5 cases per 100,000 women and 3.8 cases per 100,000 men (Miller et al, 1993). In Olmsted County, Minnesota, the annual incidence rate per 100,000 age-adjusted to the 1950 U.S. white population from 1978 through 1990 was 5.4 for males and 2.8 for females with an overall rate of 4.1 (Kyle et al, 1994). Since 1 to 2 million women in the U.S. have received silicone breast implants and most of these women range in age from the third to the eighth decade, an approximation of the number of multiple myeloma cases expended among implant recipients in the U.S. by each year by chance alone would be approximately 25 to 28 per million with implants; a larger number can be expected to have MGUS.

Gabriel et al. (1994) reported no association between breast implants and connective tissue diseases in 749 women who had received a breast implant in Olmsted County, Minnesota between January 1, 1964 and December 31, 1991. For each case, two women of the same age (within 3 years) in the same population who had not received a breast implant and who had had medical evaluation within 2 years of the date of the implantation of the case subject were selected as control subjects. At the time of the implant or corresponding index date for controls , the median age was 32 years; 9% were greater than 50 years, and 1 percent were ≥ 65 years of age. In 1993 when the study was completed, the median age was approximately 40 years for both women with implants and the controls. The breast implant patients were followed for 5,847 person-years from implantation (mean, 7.8 years per case subject) while the 1,498 control group were followed for 12,361 person-years (mean, 8.3 years per control subject).

All recognized patients with MGUS, MM, macroglobulinemia, primary amyloidosis, and related disorders seen at the Mayo Clinic since 1960 have been collected in a large data base. The patient identification numbers of this group of cases were matched with those of the 749 with breast implants and the 1,498 controls. None of the women with breast implants appear in the 1960 to 1992 Olmsted County data base for MGUS, MM, macroglobulinemia, primary amyloidosis, or a lymphoproliferative disorder associated with an M-protein. On the other hand, five of the controls had a monoclonal plasma cell proliferative disorder (one with multiple myeloma, 4 with MGUS). Of the four with MGUS, one developed multiple myeloma 13 years after MGUS was diagnosed while another had a monoclonal IgM kappa protein and a follicular small cleaved cell lymphoma. Three of the five controls were greater than 50 years of age.

This analysis fails to find an association of silicone breast implants with MGUS and MM. The higher frequency of MGUS and MM noted in the controls maybe due to chance; it seems unlikely that the silicone implants afford any protection from MGUS or MM. There may also be selection bias for the controls since subjects with a condition such as MGUS are more likely to be examined periodically and thereby more likely to be listed in the potential control pool. However, the same periodic examination frequency would also have applied to any silicone implanted patient who had a diagnosis of a monoclonal plasma cell proliferative disorder. Furthermore, the sample size is modest and no prospective serum measurements were done. Thus, there is no evidence in this group of patients with a silicone breast implant to suggest an association with MGUS or MM.

Since MGUS may be a precursor of MM, it would be of interest to determine the incidence of MGUS in patients greater than 50 years of age who have had a silicone breast implant for more than 15 to 20 years. The challenge will be to determine whether the incidence of MGUS or MM in women with breast implants will be greater than that expected in age-matched women who have not received silicone breast implants.

Acknowledgment

This work has been supported in part by Grant CA 62242 from the National Institutes of Health, Bethesda, Maryland.

References

Axelsson U (1986) A 20-year follow up study of 64 subjects with M-components. Acta Med 219:519-522

Axelsson U, Bachman R, Hällén J (1966) Frequency of pathological proteins (M-components) in 6,995 sera from an adult population. Acta Med Scand 179:235-247

Belisle LM, Case DC Jr & Neveux L (1990) Quantitation of risk of malignant transformation in patients with "benign" monoclonal gammopathy (BMG) (Abstract). Blood 76(Suppl 1):342a

Bladé J, Lopez-Guillermo A, Rozman C et al (1992) Malignant transformation and life expectancy in monoclonal gammopathy of undetermined significance. Br J Haematol 81:391-394

Gabriel SE, O'Fallon WM, Kurland LT, Beard CM, Woods JE, Melton III LJ (1994) Risk of connective-tissue diseases and other disorders after breast implantation. N Engl J Med 330:1697-1702

Giraldo MP, Rubio-Félix D, Perella M et al (1991) Aspectos clinicos, biológicos y evolutivos de 397 casos. Sangre 36:377-382

Kyle RA (1993) "Benign" monoclonal gammopathy--after 20 to 35 years of follow up. Mayo Clin Proc 68:26-36

Kyle RA (1994) The monoclonal gammopathies. Clin Chem 40:2154-2161

Kyle RA, : Finkelstein S, Elveback LR, Kurland LT (1972) Incidence of monoclonal proteins in a Minnesota community with a cluster of multiple myeloma. Blood 40:719-724

Kyle RA, Beard CM, O'Fallon WM, Kurland LT (1994) Incidence of multiple myeloma in Olmsted County, Minnesota: 1978 through 1990, with a review of the trend since 1945. J Clin Oncol 12:1577-1583

Kyle RA, Greipp PR (1980) Series on clinical testing. 3. The laboratory investigation of monoclonal gammopathies. Mayo Clin Proc 53:719-739

Miller BA, Ries LA, Hankey BF, et al (1993) SEER Cancer Statistics Review 1973-1990. NIH Publ No. 93-2789, Bethesda, Maryland: NCI

Paladini G, Fogher M, Mazzanti G et al (1989) Idiopathic monoclonal gammopathy: long-term study of 313 cases. Recent Prog 80:123-132

Potter M, Morrison S, Wiener F, Zhang XK, Miller FW (1994) Induction of plasmacytomas with silicone gel in genetically susceptible strains of mice. J Natl Cancer Inst 86:1058-1065

Saleun JP, Vicariot M, Deroff P (1982) Monoclonal gammopathies in the adult population of Finistère, France. J Clin Pathol 35:63-68

Salmon SE, Kyle RA (1994) Silicone gels, induction of plasma cell tumors, and genetic susceptibility in mice: a call for epidemiologic investigation of women with silicone breast implants. J Natl Cancer Inst 86:1042-1041

Witzig TE, Kyle RA & Greipp PR (1992) Circulating peripheral blood plasma cells in multiple myeloma. Curr Topics Microbiol Immunol 182:195-199

Witzig TE, Kyle RA, O'Fallon WM & Greipp PR (1994) Detection of peripheral blood plasma cells as a predictor of disease course in patients with smouldering multiple myeloma. Br J Haematol 87:266-272

The National Cancer Institute Silicone Implant/Multiple Myeloma Registry

C. S. Rabkin[1]*, S. Silverman[2], G. Tricot[3], L. L. Garland[4], O. Ballester[4], and M. Potter[5]

[1]Viral Epidemiology Branch, National Cancer Institute, Bethesda, MD 20892

[2]Department of Medicine, University of California, Los Angeles, CA 90211

[3]Developmental Therapeutics, University of Arkansas for Medical Sciences, Little Rock, AR 72205

[4]H. Lee Moffitt Cancer Center, University of South Florida College of Medicine, Tampa, FL 33612

[5]Laboratory of Genetics, National Cancer Institute, Bethesda, MD 20892

Following the initial report that the intraperitoneal injection of silicone gels leads to plasmacytoma formation in genetically susceptible strains of mice [1], clinical case-reports have appeared of multiple myeloma and monoclonal gammopathy of undetermined significance (MGUS) in people with silicone-implants. To characterize the cases identified to date, the National Cancer Institute has established a Silicone Implant/Multiple Myeloma Registry. The Registry also includes patients with MGUS and is not restricted to females, but only female patients with multiple myeloma are included in this report. Several individual series of cases have been reported earlier [2] (and see also other chapters in this volume), and some of these cases are also included herein.

Cases were defined as an occurrence of multiple myeloma in a silicone-implanted female. Eighteen cases in four medical practices have been identified to date. The patients' ages at diagnosis range from 38 to 75 years (mean 50, median 50), and all were white. The latency from initial silicone exposure to myeloma diagnosis ranges from 2 to 25 years (mean 12, median 14). Eighty percent of the myeloma proteins are IgG, and 50 percent have a λ light chain. Fifty-five percent of patients were clinically Stage III [3].

The reported cases were used to estimate the number of person-years at risk, under the assumption that there was no excess risk due to silicone exposure. Baseline age-specific rates of multiple myeloma for white females were obtained from the Surveillance, Epidemiology, and End Results (SEER) Program for 1987-91 [4]. The ratio of cases to SEER rate for a given age group therefore represents the point estimate for the number of person-years at risk. These estimates were converted to numbers of persons at risk, under the assumption that the average exposed woman had roughly 10 years at risk. Lower and upper 95% confidence limits on these estimates were calculated from the Poisson distribution [5].

---

*Dr. Rabkin attests that he has no financial interests related to silicone implants nor any participation in silicone-related litigation.

Table. Estimated Person-Years and Persons at Risk for Multiple Myeloma After Silicone Implantation

				Implied Population Size	
Age Group	Cases	SEER Rate*	Est. P-yr	Point Est.	(95% Confidence Limits)
35-39	1	0.3	330,000	33,000	(840 - 190,000)
40-44	6	0.7	860,000	86,000	(31,000 - 190,000)
45-49	2	2.5	80,000	8,000	(970 - 29,000)
50-54	5	4.1	122,000	12,200	(4,000 - 28,400)
55-59	2	5.8	34,000	3,400	(420 - 12,000)
60-64	1	10.2	9,800	980	(25 - 5,500)
65-69	0	14.7	0		
70-74	0	20.2	0		
75-79	1	27.2	3,700		

*Rate (per 100,0000) for white females, from the Surveillance, Epidemiology, and End Results (SEER) Program [4]

As shown in the Table, the 7 cases aged less than 45 years reflect an estimated 1,190,000 person-years at risk, if implanted women have the same risk as all women in SEER. This estimate therefore implies there have been 119,000 implanted women under age 45 (lower 95% confidence limit, 31,800). While it is plausible that this many people have accrued nationally since silicone implants were first used, one would have to assume that the Registry captured a high proportion of national cases of multiple myeloma in silicone-implanted women. If additional cases aged less than 45 years are identified, they may represent an excess over expected cases based on the estimated prevalence of silicone implants (approximately 1 million exposed women of all ages). Such an excess would indicate that the relative risk of multiple myeloma after silicone implantation is greater than 1.

These data suggest a possible excess risk among women aged less than 45 years, warranting further investigation. Further work will be needed to verify diagnoses as well as attempt to increase case-finding as the Registry continues to collect cases. More precise estimates of the at-risk population may indicate an excess risk for multiple myeloma among silicone-implanted women, but such an association is as yet unproven.

References

1. Potter M, Morrison S, Wiener F, Zhang XK, Miller FW (1994) Induction of plasmacytomas with silicone gel in genetically susceptible strains of mice. J Natl Cancer Inst 86:1058-1065
2. Ballester OF, Garland LL, Vasey FB, Ezrailson EG, Moscinski LC, Craddock L, Benson KP, Rapoport DP (1994) Multiple myeloma (MM) and monoclonal gammopathies (MG) in women with silicone breast implants. Blood 84:643a(Abstract)
3. Durie BGM, Salmon SE (1975) A clinical staging system for multiple myeloma. Correlation of measured myeloma cell mass with presenting clinical features, response to treatment, and survival. Cancer 36:842-852

4. Multiple myeloma. In: SEER Cancer Statistics Review, 1973-1991: Tables and Graphs (NIH Publication No. 94-2789), Ries LAG, Miller BA, Hankey BF, Kosary CL, Harras A, Edwards BK (eds) National Cancer Institute, Bethesda, Maryland, pp 300-312
5. Breslow NE, Day NE (1987) Confidence intervals for the SMR. In: Statistical methods in cancer research, vol. II—The design and analysis of cohort studies (IARC Scientific Publications No. 82), International Agency for Research on Cancer, Lyon, pp 69-72

The Epidemiology of Monoclonal Gammopathy of Unknown Significance: A Review

L.J. Herrinton
Division of Research, Kaiser Permanente, Oakland, CA 94611

The transient production of monoclonal components of immunoglobulins (M-components) occurs normally in response to trauma, particular drug treatments, and infection with specific antigens (Haas *et al.* 1990; Merlini and Aguzzi 1988). Chronic production can occur with malignancy (B cell, colon, prostate, and breast) and with rheumatoid arthritis, tuberculosis, cirrhosis, and several other chronic inflammatory and infectious processes (Merlini and Aguzzi 1988; Saleun *et al.* 1982). However, in approximately 60-90% of persons identified with elevated M-components in community-based surveys, the elevation is chronic and unexplained (Saleun *et al.* 1982; Axelsson *et al.* 1966; Kyle *et al.* 1972). These persons are given a diagnosis of monoclonal gammopathy of unknown significance (MGUS). Although MGUS is itself benign, it can evolve to amyloidosis, myeloma, or macroglobulinemia (Kyle 1993). To better understand the significance and consequences of MGUS, the author conducted a literature review. Two methodological issues that affect the interpretation of the literature are discussed first.

Methodological Issues

Differences among populations screened. The epidemiology of MGUS has been examined in (1) surveys of communities; (2) samples of blood donors and hospital and clinical patients unselected for serum proteins; and (3) hematology series in which patients were referred as a consequence of having elevated M-components determined in the course of their medical care. The prevalence pattern of MGUS is best observed from community surveys. The pattern noted in blood donors and readily observed groups of patients may not accurately reflect the pattern of MGUS in the population of interest because of factors related to peculiarities of the sample. Observations made on patients referred to hematology for protein electrophoresis are probably least representative because the patients may have signs or symptoms associated with plasma cell dyscrasia.

Differences among methods used to detect M-components. Electrophoresis on paper, cellulose acetate, and agarose gel, as well as immunofixation, have been used to screen for M-components. The former two methods are insensitive for light chains, IgA monoclonal proteins, and monoclonal proteins present at low concentrations (Kyle and Greipp 1988; Papadopoulos *et al.* 1982). The prevalence proportions observed in studies using paper and cellulose acetate electrophoresis were as much as 4-fold lower than those observed in studies using agarose gel or immunofixation (Schechter *et al.* 1990; Singh *et al.* 1990). However, only one study has directly compared the sensitivity of two methods: Using agarose gel electrophoresis as the gold standard, cellulose acetate identified M-components in only two of 30 affected persons, and the two that were detected had the darkest and widest banding on agarose (Papadopoulos *et al.* 1982).

Descriptive Epidemiology

In community-based surveys, the prevalence of MGUS increases with age and is 50-100% higher in men than in similarly-aged women (Table 1) (Axelsson *et al.* 1966, Kyle *et al.* 1972, Saleun *et al.* 1982). In addition, a French survey observed the prevalence to be 30% higher in farmers than in persons in other occupations after adjustment for age and sex (Table 1) (Saleun *et al.* 1982). From studies of unselected hospital and clinical populations, the prevalence has also been observed to be two-fold higher in blacks than whites (Schechter *et al.* 1990; Singh *et al.* 1990), and nearly four-fold higher in U.S. residents than in residents of Japan (Bowden *et al.* 1993). These trends are similar to those observed for myeloma (Herrinton *et al.* 1994).

Relationship of MGUS with Subsequent Risk of Myeloma and Macroglobulinemia

Progression of MGUS to myeloma and macroglobulinemia has been examined in a small community-based survey, in two studies of persons with MGUS detected during routine laboratory testing, and in five series of hematology patients referred for evaluation of serum and urine proteins.

The community-based survey was of 6,995 residents of the Värmland district of Sweden. Using paper electrophoresis, 61 persons were identified with MGUS who were initially free of myeloma; of these, two went on to develop myeloma during an average follow-up period of 15 years (Axelsson 1986). Considering the mean age (64 years) and the sex distribution (56% male) of the MGUS patients, together with the published age- and sex-specific incidence rates of myeloma in the general population (annual rates per 100,000: men, 14.5; women, 10.2) (Ries *et al.* 1994), the present author estimated the number of expected cases to be 0.11 (Table 2). It can therefore be concluded that the MGUS patients had approximately 20-fold increased risk of myeloma. Because the study was small, involving only two incident cases of myeloma, the estimated association between MGUS and subsequent myeloma risk is imprecise. It should also be borne in mind that an insensitive laboratory method was used; therefore, it is likely that only large M-components--or smaller components present at large concentration--were originally detected. If the concentration of M-component is important in predicting subsequent risk of myeloma, then one would expect this study to overstate the relationship between MGUS and myeloma risk relative to what would be observed using the more sensitive methods in use today. The strength of the study is that the sample was representative of the underlying population.

At the University of Barcelona, patients with MGUS identified during routine laboratory testing with cellulose acetate were observed during follow-up to be at approximately 150-fold increased risk of myeloma and macroglobulinemia (no. of cancers = 11) (Blade *et al.* 1992). The authors of the study remarked that the higher rate of progression noted in their study relative to Axelsson's (1986) probably resulted from differences in the populations surveyed as evidenced by the higher median concentration of M-component observed (19 g/l by Blade *et al* relative to 0.4 g/l by Axelsson). Among blood donors identified with MGUS during routine testing at a French transfusion center, the relative risk of myeloma was roughly 300 (no. of cancers = 1) (Fine *et al.* 1979).

Studies of hematology patients have given further evidence for an increased risk of myeloma and macroglobulinemia following detection of MGUS. At the Mayo Clinic, 47 patients have been diagnosed with myeloma or macroglobulinemia among 241 patients with MGUS who were followed for an average of 11.6 years (Kyle 1993). This number is roughly 130-fold higher than expected. Because the number of malignancies was relatively large, it was possible to examine changes in the rate over the follow-up period--it was essentially constant. Similar estimates of the relative risk have been observed in studies conducted in Maine (Manthorne *et al.* 1988), Italy (Ucci *et al.* 1993), and Israel (Carter and Tatarsky 1980), while a second Israeli study gave evidence for a relative risk of 20 (Pick *et al.* 1977).

Estimates of the rate of malignant transformation of MGUS that are based on samples of hematology patients, blood donors, and unselected hospital patients may be biased by factors related to health status and referral patterns. Among hematology patients, the indications for protein electrophoresis cannot be well characterized. For these reasons, the information provided by these studies is not generalizeable to community settings and may not be generalizeable to other clinical settings in which there are different physician practices.

Recommendations

Information concerning both the prevalence of MGUS and the rate of malignant transformation to myeloma and macroglobulinemia is available from the population-based study of Axelsson and coworkers. Given that the magnitude of the relative risk is 20 following the identification of MGUS (Axelsson 1986) and that the prevalence of MGUS in persons aged 50 years and older is 1.5% (Axelsson *et al.* 1966), we can estimate the population attributable risk percent (Kleinbaum *et al.* 1982), i.e., the proportion of myeloma in the general population that is preceded by MGUS, to be about 25%. This estimate is imprecise, being based on only two malignancies, and assumes screening for MGUS using insensitive laboratory methods. The magnitude of the association between MGUS and risk of myeloma and macroglobulinemia should be further evaluated in a population-based study with large numbers of cancer patients. In addition, the importance of M-component concentration as well as the time-dependency of the relationship should be evaluated .

Accepting MGUS as a marker of increased risk of malignancy, the prevalence of MGUS should be further characterized in relation to basic demographic features such as race, country of residence, and country of origin. Sensitive laboratory techniques (agarose gel electrophoresis and, when practical, immunoelectrophoresis) should be used. It is further recommended that pesticide exposure, occupation, and other putative risk factors for myeloma be evaluated in relation to the occurrence of MGUS.

References

Axelsson U (1986) A 20-year follow-up study of 64 subjects with M-components. Acta Med Scand 219:519-22.

Axelsson U, Bachmann R, Hallen J (1966) Frequency of pathological proteins (M-components) in 6,995 sera from an adult population. Acta Med Scand 179:235-247.

Blade J, Lopez-Guillermo A, Rozman C, Cervantes F, Salgado C, Aguilar JL, Vives-Corrons JL, Montserrat E (1992) Malignant transformation and life expectancy in monoclonal gammopathy of undetermined significance. Br J Haematol 81;391-394.

Bowden M, Crawford J, Cohen HJ, Noyama O (1993) A comparative study of monoclonal gammopathies and immunoglobulin levels in Japanese and United States elderly. J Am Geriatr Soc 41:11-14.

Carter A, Tatarsky I (1980) The physiopathological significance of benign monoclonal gammopathy: a study of 64 cases. Br J Haematol 46:565-574.

Fine JM, Lambin P, Leroux P (1972) Frequency of monoclonal gammopathy ('M components') in 13,400 sera from blood donors. Vox Sang 23:336-343.

Fine JM, Lambin P, Muller JY (1979) The evolution of asymptomatic monoclonal gammopathies. Acta Med Scand 205:339-341.

Haas H, Anders S, Bornkamm G, Mannweiler E, Schmitz H, Radl J, Schlaak M. (1990) Do infections induce monoclonal immunoglobulin components? Clin Exp Immunol 81:435-440.

Herrinton LJ, Weiss NS, Olshan AF (1994) Epidemiology of myeloma. In: Malpas JS, Bergsagel DE, and Kyle RA (eds) Myeloma: biology and management. Oxford Medical, Oxford, pp 127-168.

Kleinbaum DG, Kupper LL, Morgenstern H (1982) Epidemiologic research. Lifetime Learning, Belmont, CA, p 161.

Kyle RA (1993) "Benign" monoclonal gammopathy--after 20 to 35 years of follow-up. Mayo Clin Proc 68:26-36.

Kyle RA, Greipp PA (1988) Plasma cell dyscrasias: current status. CRC Crit Rev Oncol Hematol 8:93-152.

Kyle RA, Finkelstein S, Elveback LR, Kurland LT (1972) Incidence of monoclonal proteins in a Minnesota community with a cluster of multiple myeloma. Blood 40:719-724.

Manthorne LA, Dudley RW, Case CD, Turgeon WP, Ritchie RF (1988) A longitudinal study of monoclonal gammopathy of undetermined signficance (MGUS). Clin Res 36:414A.

Merlini G, Aguzzi F (1988) The laboratory investigation of monoclonal components. Haematol 73:79-85.

Papadopoulos NM, Elin RJ, Wilson DM (1982) Incidence of γ-globulin banding in a healthy population by high-resolution electrophoresis. Clin Chem 28:707-708.

Pick AI, Shoenfeld Y, Skvaril F, Schreibman S, Frohlichman R, Weiss H, Pinkhas J. (1977) Asymptomatic (benign) monoclonal gammopathy--a study of 100 patients. Ann Clin Lab Sci 7;335-343.

Ries LAG, Miller BA, Hankey BF, Kosary CL, Harras A, Edwards BK (eds) (1994) SEER cancer statistics review, 1973-1991: tables and graphs. National Cancer Institute, Bethesda, p 301.

Saleun JP, Vicariot M, Deroff P, Morin JF (1982) Monoclonal gammopathies in the adult population of Finistère, France. J Clin Pathol 35:63-68.

Schechter GP, Shoff N, Chan C, McManus CD, Hawley HP (1990) The frequency of monoclonal gammopathy of unknown significance in black and white veterans in a hospital population. In: Obrams GI and Potter M (eds) Epidemiology and biology of multiple myeloma. Springer-Verlag, New York, pp 83-85.

Singh J, Dudley AW, Kulig KA (1990) Increased incidence of monoclonal gammopathy of undetermined significance in blacks and its age-related differences with whites on the basis of a study of 397 men and one woman in a hospital setting. J Lab Clin Med 116:785-789.

Ucci G, Riccardi A, Luoni R, Ascari E (19993) Presenting features of monoclonal gammopathies: an analysis of 684 newly diagnosed cases. J Int Med 234:165-173.

Acknowledgement

The author is grateful to Drs. Gary D. Friedman and De-Kun Li for critical review.

Statement of Conflict of Interest

Kaiser Permanente operates a group medical practice, and some of its physicians have emplaced silicone gel implants. Dr. Herrinton has no conflict of interest beyond this affiliation.

Table 1. Prevalence of MGUS in relation to demographic factors

Study	Population	Electrophoresis	Characteristic	No. screened	Prevalence (%)*
Axelsson *et al.* 1966	Residents of the Värm-land district of Sweden, 1964	Paper (serum)	25-49 years	3,321	0.2
			50-59	1,631	1.1
			60-69	1,296	1.6
			70-79	611	1.6
			80-99	136	5.2
			Men	3,600	1.1
			Women	3,595	0.8
Kyle *et al.* 1972	Residents of Thief River Falls, Minnesota, 1969	Cellulose acetate (serum)	50-59 years	407	0.5
			60-69	368	0.3
			70-79	278	1.8
			Men	404	0.9
			Women	649	0.6
Saleun *et al.* 1982	Residents of Finistère, France, 1976-77	Cellulose acetate (serum and urine)	30-49 years	9,285	0.3
			50-59	5,898	0.7
			60-69	4,674	1.7
			70-79	720	2.8
			Men	15,100	1.4
			Women	15,179	0.7
			Agricultural	25,326	1.2
			Non-agricultural	4,953	0.9
Schechter *et al.* 1990	U.S. veterans, 1983-87, median age ≈ 60 years**	Cellulose acetate (serum)	Black	1,864	3.7
			White	857	1.7
Singh *et al.* 1990	U.S. veterans, median age ≈ 60 years	Immunofixation (serum)	Black	105	13.3
			White	231	7.7
Bowden *et al.* 1993	U.S. retirees, median age ≈ 85 years. Residents of Japan presenting for routine health check-ups, median age ≈ 70 years	Agarose gel (serum)	U.S.	111	7.5
			Japan	146	2.0

*Proportions may differ from those reported in the original studies because the present author directly standardized for age and sex using internal standards.
**Includes 535 patients who were referred for protein electrophoresis.

Table 2. Relation of MGUS with subsequent incidence of myeloma/macroglobulinemia

Study	Subjects	No. of patients with MGUS	Person-years	Observed number of cases	Expected number of cases*	Incidence rate (per 100/year)	Observed/expected
Axelsson 1986	Swedish residents identified during community screening with paper electrophoresis, 1964. Mean age = 64 yr, 56% ♂.	61	910	2	0.11	0.22	20
Blade *et al.* 1992	University of Barcelona patients identified during routine testing, 1970-90. Mean age = 61 yr, 51% ♂.	128	≈600	11	0.07	1.8	150
Fine *et al.* 1972, 1979	French blood donors. Mean age = 51 yr, 57% ♂.	12	73	1	0.003	3.8	300
Kyle 1993	Mayo Clinic patients, before 1971. Mean age = 64 yr, 51% ♂.	241	≈2,800	47	0.35	1.7	130
Manthorne *et al.* 1988	Patients presenting with MGUS, Foundation for Blood Research, Maine. Median age = 69 yr, 53% ♂.	113	≈340	8	0.06	3.6	130
Ucci *et al.* 1993	Patients screened for a clinical trial of myeloma treatment, University of Pavia, 1986-90. Median age = 62 yr, 55% ♂.	343	115	8	0.13	0.80	60
Carter and Tatarsky, 1980	Rambam Medical Center, Israel, hematology patients, 1967-77. Mean age = 60 yr, 41% ♂	64	300	4	0.04	1.3	100
Pick *et al.* 1977	Israeli hospital patients referred to an immunology clinic, mid 1970s, Mean age = 63 yr, 57% ♂.	100	≈400	1	0.05	0.25	20

*The expected number of cases is approximate. It was calculated by the present author using the mean or median age and the sex-distribution of the MGUS patients together with the age- and sex-specific incidence rates for myeloma among whites reported by Ries *et al.* (1994) for the geographic areas covered by the U.S. National Cancer Institute's Surveillance, Epidemiology, and End Results program (annual rates per 100,000: 50-54 years, men--4.9, women--4.1; 55-59 years, men--10.3, women--5.8; 60-64 years, men--14.5, women--10.2; 65-69 years, men--23.0, women--14.7).

Plasmacytoma Development in Mice Injected with Silicone Gels

M. Potter and S. Morrison
Laboratory of Genetics, DCBDC, National Cancer Institute, National Institutes of Health, Bethesda, MD 20892-4255 USA

Peritoneal plasmacytoma (PCT) development in mice depends upon the cooperative action of multiple factors: the genotype of the host (1-3); the deregulation of the transcription of c-myc usually by some form of chromosomal rearrangement of which translocation is the most common mechanism (4); induction of a chronic inflammatory tissue by an inducing agent; the special physiology of the peritoneal space (5,6); and an active immune system that is provided by rearing in a conventional environment (7). Each factor is required, but no single one is sufficient to transform a B-lymphocyte into an autonomously proliferating plasma cell. The factors are in themselves complex. Several genes have been located on chromosome 4 in the mouse that determine susceptibility or resistance to PCT induction by the paraffin oil pristane (2,6,10,14 tetramethylpentdecane) (2,3). Different kinds of chromosomal rearrangements can cause deregulation of *c-myc* [see (4) for review]. And relevant to the present meeting there appears to be no specificity in the materials that induce the chronic inflammation. Solid plastic objects (8), paraffin oils (9) and silicone gels (10) all appear to be effective and each induces a different form of chronic inflammation. However, as discussed below not all types of chronic inflammatory tissues provide effective microenvironments for PCT development. In this presentation an update on our studies on silicone gel induced PCT development in the highly induction susceptible BALB/c congenic strain of mice, BALB/cAnPt.DBA/2N-Idh1-Pep3 (C.D2-I/P) (3,10) is given. This strain has been selected for these studies as it gives a consistent high yield of PCTs with relatively short latent periods.

The authors have not been involved in litigations. All work was supported by the NIH. M.P. is on the Editorial Board of CTMI but receives no remuneration of any kind from Springer-Verlag.

Characteristics of the Intraperitoneal Silicone Gel

Silicone gels as plasmacytomagenic materials have unique features. First, small amounts of silicone gel are effective. We routinely administer three 0.1 ml injections of the gel on days 0, 60 and 120. The injected gel forms a single gelatinous mass that remains unattached to peritoneal surfaces for periods as long as 10 to 12 months. The gel mass consists largely, but not entirely, of silicone material. Examination of the extracted gel material under a dissecting microscope reveals that it has been invaded with spherical drops of aqueous material. These variably sized vacuoles contain amorphous debris and cells, suggesting the gel mass is imbibing and incorporating aqueous liquids. The gel mass does not seem to be the site where the PCTs form, as it is not adherent to mesothelial surfaces nor vascularized. Further, in fully developed PCTs the gel appears to be unattached and free in the peritoneal space. However, silicone liquids or particulates derived from the gel gain access to the peritoneal space either at the time of injection or break off gradually over many months. These small droplets become engaged by inflammatory cells, PMNLs, monocytes and macrophages and the complexes adhere to the mesothelial surfaces of the intestinal mesenteries. Mesothelium grows over the attached complexes, and vascularization from underlying blood vessels results in the formation of a long lasting reactive tissue. The vacuoles associated with the gel have highly refactile material at the interface between the tissue and the vacuole. After long periods of time the gel mass can in some mice deteriorate, and only strings of silicone material remain.

Histologically, the developing PCT occurs in the attached and organized silicone granuloma tissue. The early lesions are focal proliferations of atypical plasma cells (foci) which frequently resemble the plasma cells seen in fully developed primary tumors.

Histology of the Silicone Gel Granuloma

The early granulomas that form in the first 8-10 months in response to silicone gels have a highly inflammatory appearance characterized by relatively few vacuoles of silicone and the presence of many macrophages, epithelioid cells, multinucleated giant cells, fibroblasts, neutrophils, lymphocytes and other cell types surrounding the clear spaces containing silicone gel derived material (Fig. 1). After 10-12 months the silicone granuloma gradually begins to change, and the inflammatory granuloma is replaced by tissue that has many closely packed vacuoles of varying size and a relative paucity of interstitial inflammatory cells (Fig. 2). The reason why there is such a striking inflammatory response around the vacuoles of silicone gel related material is not yet known.

The silicone gel induced granuloma persists over a long period of many months in most mice, but there are striking changes in its histology. In later stages many of the vacuoles become surrounded by collagenous tissue (Fig. 3) and very late the remaining silicone granuloma found in the peritoneum has lost most of the inflammatory component and now more closely resembles the granuloma associated with silicone oils (see below). It is not certain that the inflammatory granuloma is transformed or replaced by inert foreign body granuloma or whether the inflammatory cells disappear leaving only the accumulated vacuoles. The transformation hypothesis is strengthened by the finding that interface material in these late vacuoles is highly refractile indicating the presence of silicone gel as the silicone oils do not have this refractility. It is also possible that in the early inflammatory granuloma materials such as low molecular weight cyclic compounds, e.g., D4 (octamethylcyclotetrasiloxane) are responsible for the inflammatory process and that these are progressively removed or degraded.

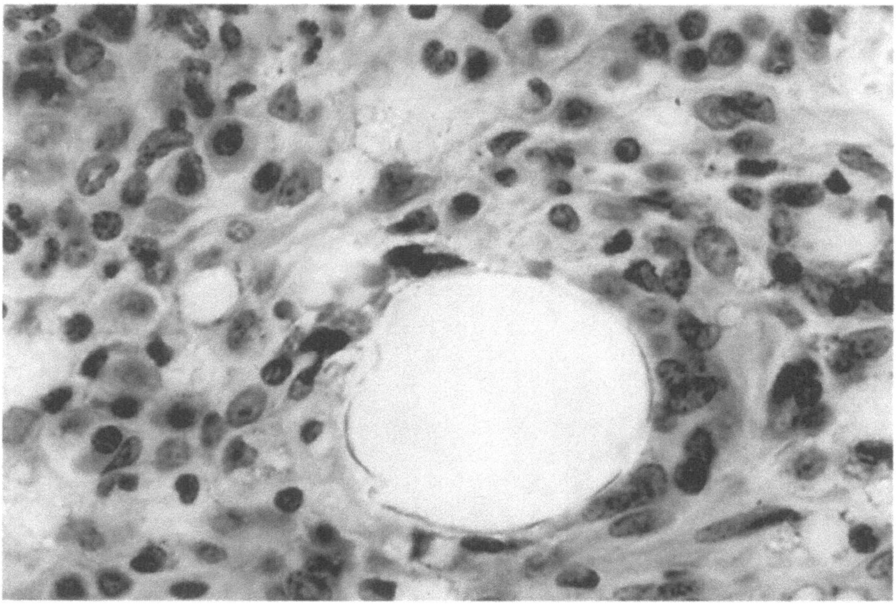

Fig. 1. Inflammatory silicone granuloma with a large vacuole lined with epithelial cells and developing giant cells, plasma cells, and other cell types surrounded by a collagenous tissue matrix.

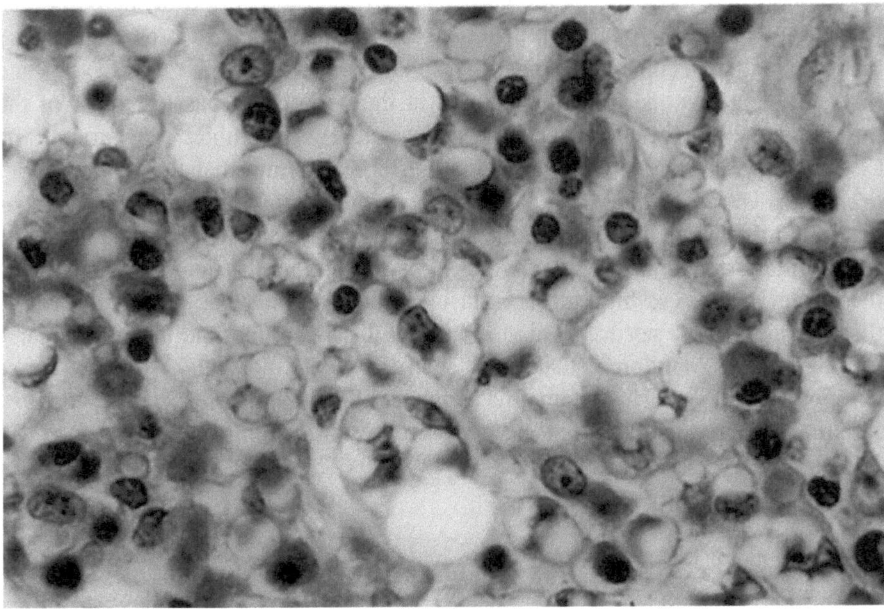

Fig. 2. Silicone granuloma in a mouse 6690 given 1000 centistoke DMPS 85 days previously. The silicone vacuoles are of variable size and are closely packed.

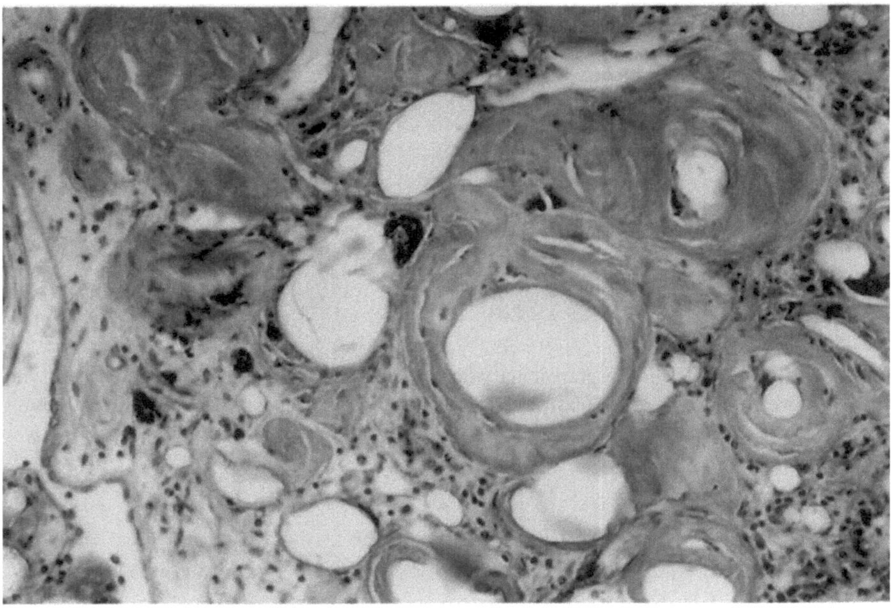

Fig. 3. Silicone granuloma from BALB/c mouse, 1-4-14, 441 days after a single injection of 0.4 ml silicone. The silicone vacuoles are surrounded by collagenous material. HauE, 100X

Plasmacytoma Development in Mice Injected Intraperitoneally with Silicone Gels

Two commercially obtained gels from mammary implants were used as sources of silicone gels. For convenience of discussion they are called Gel-1 and Gel-2, and their specifications have been described (10). A preliminary experiment was also carried out with a PEG015 gel prepared in our laboratory from liquid components A and B obtained from United Chemical Technologies, Bristol, PA. Different gel preparations evoke PCTs with different latent periods. We have continued to follow the induction curves with the two gels previously described (10) and particularly Gel-2 which at the time of the publication had only been in place for 260 days (Fig. 4). The mice implanted with Gel-2, however, have continued to develop PCTs, and currently the incidence of PCTs is between 60 and 70% for both Gel preparations; however, the latent periods are much longer for Gel-2 (Fig 4). Gel-1 was much like pristane giving a high incidence with a short latent period. The reason for the difference has not been established, but factors to be considered are the degree of cross-linking in the gel preparation or the length of time the gel sat in a glass container before being injected into the mice. Gel-1 may have been less cross-linked and, hence, released trapped liquids or liquids containing cross-linked silicones more readily. The liquids released from gels are chemically heterogeneous. An important biological point is that the injected gel maintained activity for an extended period of time, as many of the PCTs developed when the mice were between one and two years of age.

An important feature of the silicone gels is that they are well tolerated by the mice, produce few if any side effects, and many of the mice that do not succumb to early PCT development live to more advanced age. In contrast to pristane we can maintain mice for at least 2 years. This raises the important issue of the influence of aging on plasmacytomagenesis which cannot be studied as effectively in pristane-treated mice, as they develop secondary complications, i.e., ascites and extensive granuloma formation on the diaphram and in the peritoneal connective tissues that shorten the life span of the mice. Our earlier work did not reveal an influence of aging (11); however, Makinodan and his associates have presented evidence that pristane-injected old BALB/c mice are more prone than young mice to developing PCTs (12). The findings presented here raise the possibility that aging might be a factor in silicone gel peritoneal plasmacytomagenesis.

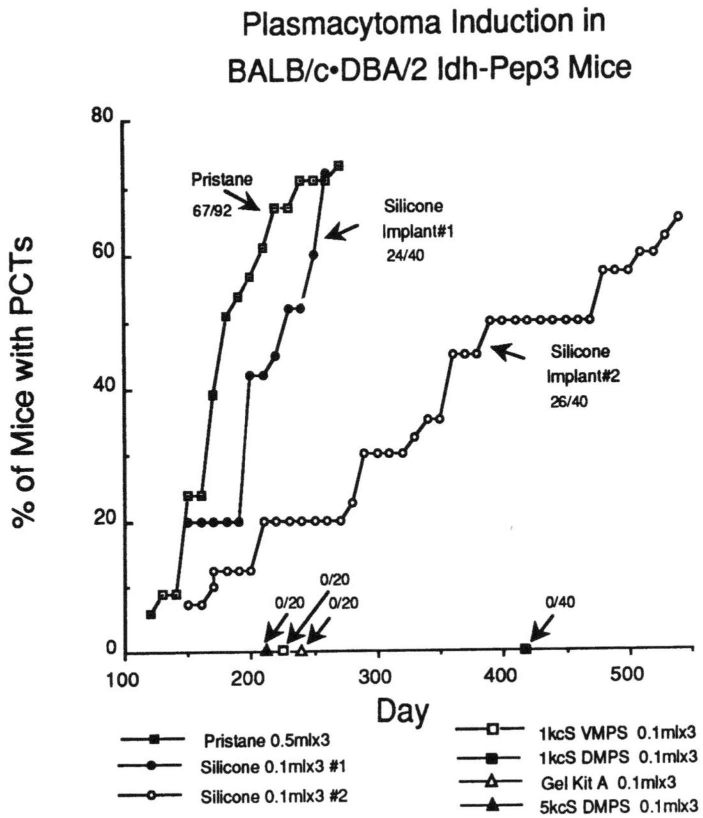

Fig. 4. Plasmacytoma development in mice injected with pristane, silicone gels and various silicone oils.

Failure Thus Far to Induce Plasmacytomas with Silicone Oils

Silicone oils such as 5,1000,or 12,500 centistoke (cs) dimethylpolysiloxanes (DMPS) are not plasmacytomagenic in C.D2-I/P mice. The 1000cs and 12,500 cs oils do not induce an inflammatory granuloma but rather a granuloma that contains large numbers of closely packed vacuoles of silicone oil and relatively much less interstitial reactive tissue. We have tested several other liquid silicones in the highly susceptible C.D2-I/P mice and have not yet obtained any PCTs. This has included: 1) the Gel Kit Part A liquid that is used to prepare the PEG015 gel and which contains DMPS, vinylmethylpolysiloxane with 1000 cs viscosity and platinic chloride, and 2) 1000cs vinylmethylpolysiloxane (also obtained from United Chemical Technologies). These materials were routinely injected with three doses of 0.1 ml or 0.2 ml each.

The highly effective paraffin oil pristane is usually given in 3 doses of 0.5 ml each. Since silicone gels proved to be effective when given in 0.1 ml doses, we used doses of 0.1 ml for pristane as well. We had not, however, previously tested pristane in three 0.1 ml doses and therefore have carried out one preliminary experiment with 0.1 ml doses of pristane and obtained a lower yield of PCTs of 40% in 364 days as compared to 60+% with 0.5 ml doses. When three 0.2 ml doses of pristane were given, however, the high yield of PCTs was obtained (60% in 248 days). Thus, comparable volumetric doses of pristane and silicone oils give a high incidence of PCTs for the pristane-treated mice and no PCTs in the same time periods for the silicone oils.

Plasma Cell Formation in the Silicone Granuloma

Plasma cell formation occurs in both the silicone gel and oil granuloma tissues in the form of scattered isolated plasma cells. Most of these resemble normal plasma cells by having relatively small nuclei and abundant cytoplasm. Pre-neoplastic plasma cells can be found in the silicone gel treated mice (Fig. 5). These appear in the form of aggregations of plasma cells. The colony sizes of these aggregates can vary from small clusters containing a few cells to relatively large foci with several hundred cells. The cells in some of these aggregates can be highly differentiated resembling the isolated scattered plasma cells, and these are considered to be plasmacytotic foci (Fig. 6). Other foci contain plasma cells with hyperchromatic with prominent densely staining nuclei (atypical foci, not shown). The atypical cells have larger nuclei and relatively less cytoplasm. These focal cells often resemble those seen in developed plasmacytomas. When atypical foci are found they are usually multiple, suggesting that cells in one focus can spread to new granuloma sites. In the advanced primary PCT much of the silicone granuloma is replaced by plasma cells. Some advanced PCTs are composed of large bizarre plasma cells. Morphological progression in silicone PCT formation is similar qualitatively to that seen with pristane (3) but may differ by having fewer numbers of atypical foci. This is currently under investigation.

Polyp Formation

Liquid, or at least transportable fragments, derived from the silicone gel mass, migrate into the peritoneal space, become engaged by macrophages or other cells, and after attachment to peritoneal surfaces form the silicone granuloma. The silicone granuloma forms on the intestinal mesenteries and in the omentum. Much of the granuloma tissue is organized in the form of mesothelial polyp-like

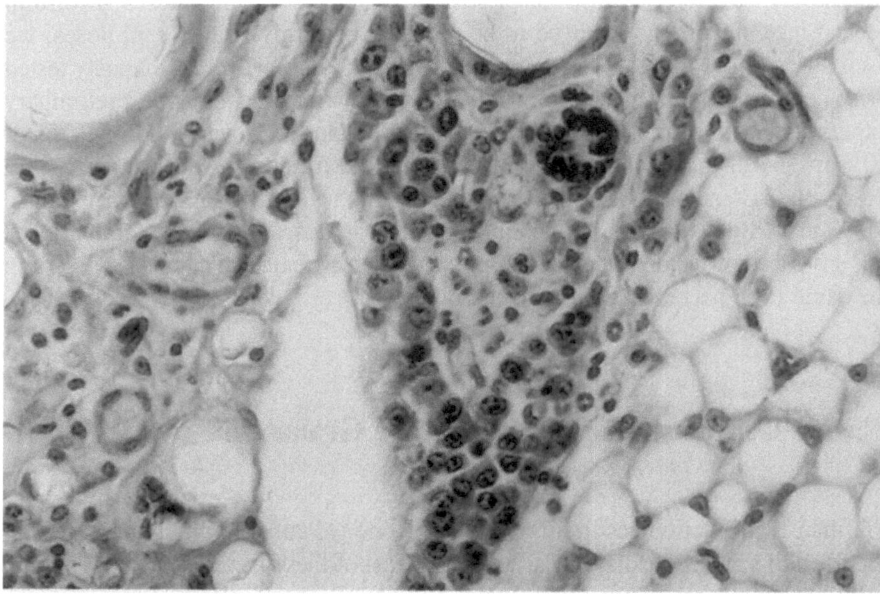

Fig. 5. Silicone granuloma attached to mesenteric fat (on left), silicone vacuole (lower right), with adjacent multi-nucleated giant cell. Intensely stained cells are plasma cells of various sizes. Some of the larger cells are typical of those seen in foci and early PCTs. Section from mouse 5249, 201 days post first injection with silicone gel. This mouse had 4 foci. 200X

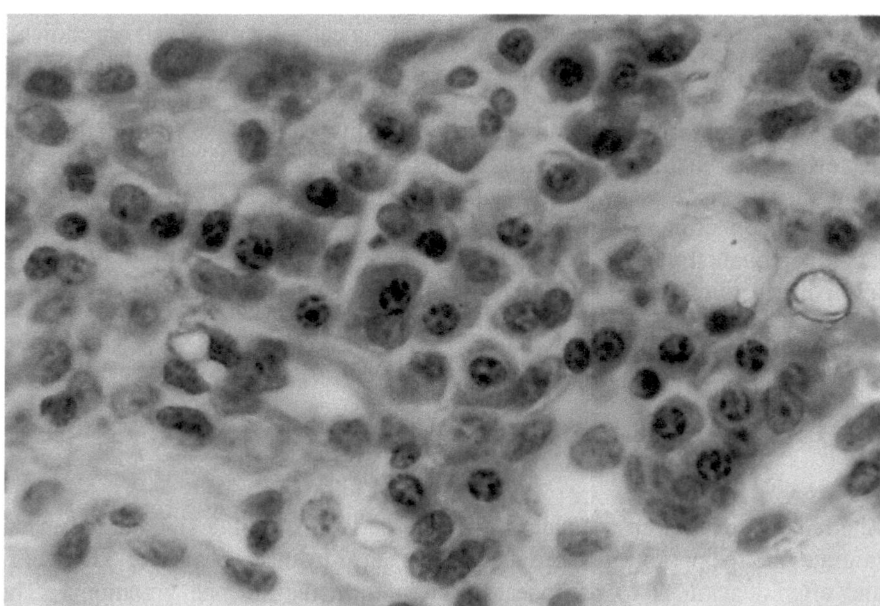

Fig. 6. Plasmacytotic aggregate from silicone granuloma in mouse 5372, 50 days post injection. Hand E stain. 200X. The plasma cells have small nuclei with condensed chromatin. A few silicone vacuoles with refractile contents are seen on the right.

structures that appear, developing first from mesothelial surfaces between the mesenteric fat pads and the serosal attachments of the gut. Under the dissecting microscope polyps with ellipsoidal bodies and long stalks can be seen moving in the liquid phase in freshly excised tissues. Mesothelial polyps have been described in association with the response to pristane (2,6,10,14 tetramethylpentadecane) (6) and also in mice that have been infected with *Schistosoma mansoni* (13); thus, they are not a unique response to silicone.

These interactions may cause tissue damage and/or the formation of immunogenic materials. This may induce B lymphocytes to immigrate into the granuloma. From previously described studies many years ago by Athanassaides and Speirs (14,15), it was shown that alum granulomas in the mouse were active sites of plasma cell formation. Later Holub (16) and Dux (17) described the development of plasma cells in milky spots in the omentum of immunized mice. Thus, in the peritoneum B cells can in the presence of antigen complete their terminal differentiation to plasma cells. This same process occurs in peritoneal granuloma tissues.

An important feature of silicone granuloma formation in the mouse peritoneum is that there are multiple separate sites where this tissue forms, i.e., there are multiple meosthelial polyps each with its own vascular system. Thus, silicone granuloma formation provides many opportunities for circulating B cells to enter the peritoneal connective tissues and interact with the inflammatory environment evoked by the silicones. Injection of silicone gels into the subcutaneous space results in the formation cystic structures that contain large vacuoles of the gel. Thus far, these do not appear to have the inflammatory granulomatous response as seen in the peritoneum. We have not seen PCTs in mice carrying the subcutaneous gels.

Genetics of PCT Formation

In general, other inbred strains of mice do not develop PCTs when silicone gels are introduced i.p. Specifically, DBA/2N, C57BL/6,C3H/HeN,and (BALB/c x DBA/2)F1 have not developed PCTs when injected i.p. with silicone gels. These strains of mice are also resistant to PCT induction by pristane [see (1) for references]. Using backcross (2) and congenic mice (3) derived from mating BALB/cAn and DBA/2N strains, several genetic loci have been found that contain genes that determine susceptibility or resistance to PCT induction by pristane. Neither the mode of action of these genes nor their identity has yet been determined.

An important characteristic of the peritoneal PCTs that are elicited by these procedures is that over 95% of them have some sort of chromosomal rearrangement that deregulates the transcription of the *c-myc* proto-oncogene (4). The most common of these rearrangements is the T(12;15) translocation in which an immunoglobulin switch region gene is inserted head to head into the 5' end of the *c-myc* gene (18). This dissociates the coding regions of *c-myc* (i.e., exons 2 and 3) from the normal regulatory sequences and places them under the control of new enhancers and promoters some of which are derived from the newly juxtaposed Ig genetic material. The regular involvement of Ig switch region sequences in the T(12;15) translocations strongly suggests that the formation of these translocations is related to the physiological process of immunglobulin heavy chain isotype switching and is incurred during this process. While we have not yet identified the genetic basis of susceptibility to PCT formation in BALB/c mice, the possibility that BALB/c mice have an increased proclivity to develop chromosomal rearrangements of *c-myc* and Ig switch region sequences must be considered.

Using sensitive nested PCR methodology, illegitimate rearangements involving Ig Switch Alpha region and *c-myc* in B cells can be detected as soon as 30 days after the first injection of pristane (19,20). This evidence suggests that the initial oncogenic event is deregulation of *c-myc* and raises the possibility that the process could occur in the lymphoid tissues outside the peritoneal cavity. However, the origin of the chromosomal rearrangement in the reactive paraffin oil granuloma or silicone gel granuloma has not been established. This question is currently being examined in the laboratory.

Summary

Silicone gels derived from commercially obtained implants induce plasmacytomas in 60-70% of highly susceptible BALB/cAn.DBA/2-Idh1-Pep3 congenic mice. In contrast, dimethylpolysiloxane (DMPS) silicone oils with viscosities of 5, 1000 and 12,500 cs fail to elicit these tumors. 1000 cs vinylmethylpolysiloxane is also inactive. Silicone gels, in contrast to the oils, induce a highly inflammatory silicone granuloma. Silicone gels contain chemical components not found in the oils. The chemical component responsible for inducing the permissive environment for plasmacytoma formation has not yet been identified. Silicone gels are well tolerated for long periods of time in mice without adverse effects other than plasmacytoma formation. The response to different gel preparations varies; some are associated with relatively rapid formation of plasmacytomas resembling that seen with pristane, while in others the plasmacytoma formation is extended nearly over a two year period.

References

1. Morse HC, III, Hartley JW, Potter M. (1980) Genetic considerations in plasmacytomas of BALB/c NZB and (BALB/c x NZB)F1 mice. In: Potter M (ed) Progress in myeloma. Biology of myeloma. Elsevier, North Holland, p. 263
2. Mock BA, Krall MM, Dosik JK. (1993) Genetic mapping of tumor susceptibility genes involved in mouse plasmacytomagenesis. Proc Natl Acad Sci USA 90:9499-9503
3. Potter M, Mushinski EB, Wax JS, Hartley J, Mock BA. (1994) Identification of two genes on chromosome 4 that determine resistance to plasmacytoma induction in mice. Cancer Res 54:969-975
4. Potter M, Wiener F. (1992) Plasmacytomagenesis in mice: model of neoplastic development dependent upon chromosomal translocations. Carcinogenesis 13:1681-1697
5. Leak LV, Potter M, Mayfield WJ. (1985) Response of the peritoneal mesothelium to the mineral oil, pristane. Curr Top Microbiol Immunol 122:221-233
6. Anderson AO, Wax JS, Potter M. (1985) Differences in the peritoneal response to pristane in BALB/cAnPt and BALB/cJ mice. Curr Top Microbiol Immunol 122:242-253
7. Byrd LG, McDonald AH, Gold LG, Potter M. (1991) Specific pathogen-free BALB/cAn mice are refractory to plasmacytoma induction by pristane. J Immunol 147:3632-3637
8. Merwin RM, Redmon LW. (1963) Induction of plasma cell tumors and sarcomas in mice by diffusion chambers placed in the peritoneal cavity. J Natl Cancer Inst 31:990-1007
9. Potter M, Boyce C. (1962) Induction of plasma cell neoplasms in strain BALB/c mice with mineral oil and mineral oil adjuvants. Nature 193:1086
10. Potter M, Morrison S, Wiener F, Miller FW. (1994) Induction of plasmacytomas with silicone gel in genetically susceptible strains of mice. J Natl Cancer Inst 86:1058-1065
11. Potter M, Wax JS. (1983) Peritoneal plasmacytomagenesis in mice: comparison of different pristane dose regimens. J Natl Cancer Inst 71:391-395
12. Sato K, Bloom ET, Hirokawa K, Makinodan T. (1986) Increased susceptibility of old mice to plasmacytoma induction. J Gerontol 41:24-29
13. Weinberg DF, Baldo-Correa E, Lenzi HL, Borojevic R. (1992) Schistosoma mansoni: peritoneal plasmacytogenesis and polypoid transformation of mesenteric milky spots in infected mice. Exp Parasitol 74:408-416
14. Athanassiades TJ, Speirs RS. (1968) Formation of antigen-induced granulomas containing plasma cells: a light and electron microscopic study. J Reticuloendothelial Soc 5:485-497
15. Athanassiades TJ, Speirs RS. (1972) Granuloma induction in the peritoneal cavity. A model for the study of inflammation and plasmacytopoiesis in nonlymphatic organs. J Reticuloendothelial Soc 11:60-76
16. Holub M, Polanova E. (1978) The response of omental lymphatics to antigen stimulation. Verlag T, Hgnot S (ed) Progress in lymphology, pp 264-267.
17. Dux K, Rouse RV, Kyewski B. (1986) Composition of the lymphoid cell populations from omental milky spots during the immune response in C57BL/Ka mice. Eur J Immunol 16:1029-1032
18. Shen-Ong GL, Keath EJ, Piccoli SP, Cole MD. (1982) Novel myc oncogene RNA from abortive immunoglobulin-gene recombination in mouse plasmacytomas. Cell 31:443-452
19. Janz S, Muller J, Shaughnessy J, Potter M. (1993) Detection of recombinations between c-myc and immunoglobulin switch alpha in murine plasma cell tumors and preneoplastic lesions by polymerase chain reaction. Proc Natl Acad Sci USA 90:7361-7365
20. Muller JR, Potter M, Janz S. (1994) Differences in the molecular structure of c-myc activating recombinations in murine plasmacytomas and precursor cells. Proc Natl Acad Sci USA 91:12066-12070

Epidemiology

The Association of Augmentation Mammoplasty with Connective Tissue Disease, Including Systematic Sclerosis (Scleroderma): A Meta-Analysis

M. C. Hochberg, M.D., M.P.H.[1,2,3] and D. L. Perlmutter, M.H.S.[4]
From the [1]Division of Rheumatology & Clinical Immunology, Department of Medicine, and [2]Department of Epidemiology and Preventive Medicine, University of Maryland School of Medicine, [3]Geriatrics (GRECC) Service, Veterans Affairs Medical Center at Baltimore, and [4]EPM Research Services, University of Maryland School of Medicine, Baltimore, MD.

The possible relationship between augmentation mammoplasty and definite connective tissue disease, particularly systemic sclerosis (scleroderma), has been the subject of many case reports and case series; these have been reviewed elsewhere in several review articles and editorials [1-9]. Several epidemiologic studies have been conducted to formally address the hypothesis that women who have undergone augmentation mammoplasty are at greater risk of developing connective tissue disease, particularly systemic sclerosis (scleroderma), than women who have not had this procedure performed [10-21]. Seven studies focused on the entire spectrum of rheumatic symptoms and/or connective tissue diseases [10,12-16,20], while three focused specifically on the potential association with systemic sclerosis [17-19] and one focused specifically on the potential association with rheumatoid arthritis [11]. Only one of these studies, however, demonstrated a statistically significant association between breast implants and the development of connective tissue disease, specifically systemic sclerosis [19]. The remaining studies had inadequate statistical power to demonstrate such an association because of either the low incidence rate of the connective tissue diseases or the relatively infrequent exposure of augmentation mammoplasty. We have recently conducted a case-control study of the association of augmentation mammoplasty with systemic sclerosis (scleroderma) [21], and in this paper combine our preliminary results with those from the previous epidemiologic studies which included data on specific diagnoses of connective tissue disease and had internal control and/or comparison groups, using the technique of meta-analysis.

Methods

Meta-analysis is a quantitative approach for systematically combining the results of previous research studies in order to arrive at a conclusion regarding a specific body of research [22]. Epidemiologic studies of the association of augmentation mammoplasty with connective tissue diseases were identified via a computerized Medline search covering the period 1988-1994, a search via review articles and editorials on the topic, a search of abstracts presented at the 1991-1994 meetings of the American College of Rheumatology and Society for Epidemiologic Research, as well as with discussions with investigators and colleagues in the field. This search identified twelve studies [10-21]; all studies were read by the primary author. Five studies were excluded from further consideration: two did not have an internal control or comparison group [10,19], two relied on self-reported data derived from mailed questionnaires only to determine disease status in women exposed to breast implants and control women who had undergone other cosmetic procedures [13,14], and one used as the comparison group women seen in a rheumatology practice with musculoskeletal symptoms who may have sought consultation because of complaints related to breast implants [20]. Thus, the meta-analysis included data from seven studies; two retrospective cohort studies [12,15], and five case-control studies [11,16-18,21].

The technique of Yusuf et. al. [23], as adapted for observational studies by Wald et. al. [24] was used for pooling of data. Briefly, for each study a 2x2 table containing cells for exposure to augmentation mammoplasty and presence or absence of connective tissue disease was calculated. The pooled logarithm of the odds ratio (OR) was calculated by summing the difference between the number of subjects observed and those expected to have undergone augmentation mammoplasty for each study divided by the sum of the individual variances of this value for each study. Confidence intervals (CI) for this pooled odds ratio were calculated from the sum of the individual variances. Finally, because the individual studies used adjustment for differences between exposed and non-exposed women or between cases and controls, the adjusted pooled odds ratio was also calculated.

Synopsis of Studies Included in Meta-analysis:

Prospective Studies:

Schusterman and colleagues determined the incidence of connective tissue diseases in 250 women who had undergone breast implantation after surgery for breast cancer and 353 women who had undergone reconstruction without implants after surgery for breast cancer between January 1986 and March 1992 [12]. Only one patient from each group developed an autoimmune disease, diagnosed by a rheumatologist, over 615.8 and 663.4 person-years of followup, respectively. Both diseases were considered mild and responded to treatment with low-dose corticosteroids. The relative risk estimated from these data was 1.08; not statistically significantly different from unity.

Gabriel and colleagues performed a retrospective cohort study of 749 women with breast implants and 1498 age-, sex-, and race-matched controls all of whom were residents of Olmsted County, MN [15]. Over a mean followup of 8 years, 5 women exposed to breast implants and 10 control women developed a definite connective tissue disease; the adjusted relative risk, derived from multivariate Cox proportional hazards models, was 1.10 (95% CI: 0.37, 3.23). None of the exposed or control women developed systemic sclerosis.

Case-Control Studies:

Dugowson and colleagues conducted a case-control study of 349 women with newly diagnosed rheumatoid arthritis and 1456 similarly aged control women living in King County, WA [11]. Data on history of breast implants were available for 300 (86%) cases. Only 1 (0.3%) case and 12 (0.8%) controls reported a history of breast implantation; the age-adjusted OR (95% CI) was 0.41 (0.05, 3.13).

Sanchez-Guerrero and colleagues performed a case-control study using data from the Nurse's Health Study [16]. They identified 448 women with definite connective tissue disease and compared the frequency of augmentation mammoplasty with silicone breast implants in these cases and 10 age-matched controls per case. Only five of the 448 cases had augmentation mammoplasty; the adjusted OR was 0.94 (95% CI: 0.37, 2.37). All five implanted cases had rheumatoid arthritis; none of the 20 cases of systemic sclerosis had undergone augmentation mammoplasty.

Englert and Brooks performed a case-control study of 215 women with systemic sclerosis and 289 age-matched control women living in Sydney, Australia [17]. Four cases and 5 controls reported augmentation mammoplasty; the OR, adjusted for socioeconomic status, was 0.89 (95% CI: 0.23, 3.41).

Burns performed a case-control study of 274 women with sytemic sclerosis and 1184 age-, and race-matched controls living in Michigan [18]. Two cases and 14 controls reported augmentation mammoplasty; the OR, adjusted for age, race and income, was 0.35 (95% CI: 0.05, 2.74).

Hochberg and colleagues performed a case-control study of the association of augmentation mammoplasty with systemic sclerosis; included in the meta-analysis are results based on preliminary data from 869 women with systemic sclerosis and 2051 age-, and race-matched controls [21]. Twelve (1.4%) cases and

23 (1.1%) controls reported augmentation mammoplasty: the age-, race-, and site-adjusted OR (95% CI) was 1.25 (0.62, 2.53).

Results of Meta-analysis

The number of subjects that had and had not undergone augmentation mammoplasty by presence or absence of connective tissue disease in each study, and the published relative risk or odds ratios and 95% confidence intervals of the individual studies are shown in Table 1. The pooled crude odds ratio for the association of augmentation mammoplasty with definite connective tissue disease was 1.07 (95% CI: 0.68, 1.68), and the pooled adjusted odds ratio was 1.03 (95% CI: 0.65, 1.62).

When the analysis was limited to the three case-control studies which specifically addressed the hypothesis relative to systemic sclerosis (scleroderma) [33,34,36], the pooled crude odds ratio was 1.07 (95% CI: 0.60, 1.89), and the pooled adjusted odds ratio was 1.04 (95% CI: 0.58, 1.88).

Table 1. A summary of results of observational studies of the association of augmentation mammoplasty with connective tissue disease.

	Implanted		Notimplanted		
Author [ref]	CTD	No CTD	CTD	No CTD	OR (95% CI)
Dugowson et al [11]	1	12	299	1444	0.41 (0.05, 3.13)
Schusterman et al [12][a]	1	249	1	352	1.08 (n/a)
Gabriel et al [15]	5	744	10	1488	1.10 (0.37, 3.23)
Sanchez-Guerrero et al [16]	5	44	443	4436	0.94 (0.37, 2.37)
Englert & Brooks [17]	4	5	211	284	0.89 (0.23, 3.41)
Burns [18]	2	14	272	1170	0.35 (0.05, 2.74)
Hochberg et al [21]	12	23	857	2038	1.25 (0.62, 2.53)
Pooled results: Crude					1.07 (0.68, 1.68)
Adjusted					1.03 (0.60, 1.62)

CI, confidence interval; CTD, connective tissue disease; OR, odds ratio

[a] OR estimated from person-years of followup of implanted and nonimplanted women; CI not given in paper.

Discussion

The conclusion from this meta-analysis is that there is no evidence of a significant association between augmentation mammoplasty and the development of definite connective tissue disease including systemic sclerosis (scleroderma).

Meta-analysis is a quantitative approach for systematically combining the results of previous research studies in order to arrive at a conclusion regarding a specific body of research; it is particularly useful when there are many individual studies that are either too small and lack adequate statistical power [37]. Such has occurred in this particular area of epidemiologic research because of the rarity of connective tissue diseases in general, and systemic sclerosis (scleroderma) in particular [25], and the uncommon practice of performing augmentation mammoplasty. Indeed, the prevalence of augmentation mammoplasty is estimated as between 8 and 10 per 1000 women aged 18 and above in the United States [26,27].

None of the individual studies included in the meta-analysis demonstrated a statistically significant association between augmentation mammoplasty and the development of connective tissue disease, including systemic sclerosis (scleroderma). Nonetheless, because of small sample size, a low incidence rate of development of connective tissue disease in both exposed and unexposed women, or a low frequency of exposure to augmentation mammoplasty in cases and controls, the point estimates of the relative risks or odds ratios were imprecise with wide confidence intervals. Indeed, the lower bound of the 95 percent confidence intervals ranged from 0.05 to 0.62, while the upper bound ranged from 2.37 to 3.41. Thus, the individual studies could not exclude either a protective effect or a causal association with up to a 3-fold increase in risk for development of connective tissue disease. The results of the meta-analysis, however, suggest that one cannot reject the null hypothesis that there is no association between augmentation mammoplasty with silicone breast implants and connective tissue disease, including systemic sclerosis. Furthermore, with 95 percent confidence, even if there was a causal association, the increased risk would be less than 2-fold greater than that among unexposed women.

This meta-analysis was unable to address the hypothesis that only implants complicated by rupture and leakage are associated with the subsequent development of connective tissue disease, including systemic sclerosis, as the individual studies failed to provide adequate data on this variable. Finally, this meta-analysis was also not designed to investigate the possible association of breast implantation with a "new and unique rheumatic syndrome" characterized by chronic fatigue, myalgia, arthralgia, cognitive dysfunction, sicca symptoms, rash and other neurologic disturbances [28], as no epidemiologic studies have been conducted concerning this putative association.

In conclusion, the results from this meta-analysis fail to demonstrate a significant association between augmentation mammoplasty with silicone breast implants and the development of definite connective tissue disease, including systemic sclerosis.

References

1. Kumagai Y, Shiokawa Y, Medsger TA Jr, Rodnan GP (1984) Clinical spectrum of connective tissue disease after cosmetic surgery: observations on eighteen patients and a review of the Japanese literature. Arthritis Rheum 27:1-12.
2. Endo LP, Edwards NL, Longley S, Corman LC, Panush RS (1987) Silicone and rheumatic diseases. Semin Arthritis Rheum 17:112-8.
3. Davis P (1993) Augmentation mammoplasty: beauty or the beast? [editorial]. J Rheumatol 20:927-8.
4. Hochberg MC (1993) Cosmetic surgical procedures and connective tissue disease: the Cleopatra syndrome revisited [editorial]. Ann Intern Med 118:981-3.
5. Sanchez-Guerrero J, Schur PH, Srgent JS, Liang MH (1994) Silicone breast implants and rheumatic disease: clinical, immunologic, and epidemiologic studies. Arthritis Rheum 37:158-68.
6. Spiera RF, Gibofsky A, Spiera H (1994) Silicone gel fiflled breast implants and connective tissue disease: an overview. J Rheumatol 21:239-45.
7. Hochberg MC (1994) Silicone breast implants and rheumatic disease [editorial]. Br J Rheumatol 33:601-2.
8. Edelman DA, Grant S, van Os WAA (1994) Autoimmune disease following the use of silicone gel-filled breast implants: a review of the clinical literature. Semin Arthritis Rheum 24:183-9.
9. Borenstein D, ed. (1994) A symposium on silicone-related disorders. Semin Arthritis Rheum 24(Suppl 1):1-60.
10. Weisman MH, Vecchione TR, Albert D, Moore LT, Mueller MR (1988) Connective-tissue disease following breast augmentation: a preliminary test of the human adjuvant disease hypothesis. Plast Reconstr Surg 82:626-30.
11. Dugowson CE, Daling J, Koepsell TD, Voigt L, Nelson JL (1992) Silicone breast implants and risk for rheumatoid arthritis [abstract]. Arthritis Rheum 35(9,Suppl):S66.
12. Schusterman MA, Kroll SS, Reece GP, et al. (1993) Incidence of autoimmune disease in patients after breast reconstruction with silicone gel implants versus autogenous tissue: a preliminary report. Ann Plast Surg 31:1-6.
13. Wells KE, Cruse CW, Baker JL Jr, et al. (1994) The health status of women following cosmetic surgery. Plast Reconstr Surg 93:907-12.
14. Giltay EJ, Bernelot Moens HJ, Riley AH, Tan RG (1994) Silicone breast prostheses and rheumatic symptoms: a retrospective followup study. Ann Rheum Dis 53:194-6.
15. Gabriel SE, O'Fallon WM, Kurland LT, Beard CM, Woods JE, Melton LJIII (1994) Risk of connective tissue diseases and other disorders after breast implantation. N Engl J Med 330:1697-1702.
16. Sanchez-Guerrero J, Karlson KW, Colditz GA, et al. (1994) Silicone breast implants and connective tissue disease [abstract]. Arthritis Rheum 37(9,Suppl):S282.
17. Englert HJ, Brooks P (1994) Scleroderma and augmentation mammoplasty - a causal relationship? Aust NZ J Med 24:74-80.
18. Burns CG (1994) The epidemiology of systemic sclerosis: a population-based case-control study. Ph.D. thesis. University of Michigan, Ann Arbor.

19. McLaughlin JK, Fraumeni JF Jr, Olsen J, Mellemkjaer L (1994) Re: breast implants, cancer, and systemic sclerosis [letter]. J Natl Cancer Inst 86:1424.
20. Goldman JA, Greenblatt J, Joines R, White L, Aylward B, Lamm SH (1995) Breast implants, rheumatoid arthritis, and connective tissue diseases in a clinical practice. J Clin Epidemiol in press.
21. Hochberg MC, Perlmutter DL, White B, et al. (1994) The association of augmentation mammoplasty with systemic sclerosis: results from a multi-center case-control study [abstract]. Arthritis Rheum 37(9,Suppl):S369.
22. Pettiti DB (1994) Meta-analysis, decision analysis, and cost-effectiveness analysis. Oxford, Oxford University Press.
23. Yusuf S, Peto R, Lewis J, Collins R, Sleight P (1985) Beta blockade during and after myocardial infarction: an overview of the randomized trials. Prog Cardiovasc Dis 27:335-71.
24. Wald NJ, Nanchahal K, Thompson SG, Cuckle HS (1986) Does breathing other peoples tobacco smoke cause lung cancer? Br Med J 293:1217-22.
25. Silman AJ, Hochberg MC (1994) Epidemiology of the Rheumatic Diseases. Oxford, Oxford University Press, 192-219.
26. Cook RR, Delongchamp RR, Woodbury MA, Perkins LL, Harrison MC (1995) The prevalence of women with breast implants in the United States - 1989. J Clin Epidemiol in press.
27. Gabriel SE, O'Fallon WM, Beard CM, Kurland LT, Woods JE, Melton LJ III (1995) Trends in the utilization of silicone breast implants, 1964-1991, and methodology for a population-based study of outcomes. J Clin Epidemiol in press.
28. Solomon G, Espinoza L, Silverman S (1994) Breast implants and connective-tissue diseases [letter]. N Engl J Med 331: 1231.

Acknowledgment

Supported in part by a grant from the Plastic Surgery Educational Foundation.

The Prevalence of Breast Implants Among Women in the United States

R.R. Cook, M.D. and L.L. Perkins, Ph.D.
Dow Corning Corporation, Midland, Michigan 48686-0994

Abstract

Estimates of the number of women with breast implants have varied from less than one million to over three million. Most of these appear to be extrapolations from either industry production figures or reports of surgical procedures. In late 1989 under contract to the Dow Corning Corporation, Market Facts, Inc. conducted a mail survey of 40,000 households selected to be representative of the population of the United States. They received responses from 70.7%. Based upon the data collected, 8.08 per 1,000 women in the United States reported ever having had some type of breast implant. Approximately 60% of the procedures had been done for cosmetic reasons. Most of the women were White (94.6%) and rates were highest in the South or West. Although younger women were more likely to have had implants for augmentation and older women for reconstruction presumptively following breast cancer surgery, the largest prevalences for either of the two procedures were in the 45 to 54 year old age group. Breast implant prevalence also increased in direct proportion to household income with the largest increases being related to cosmetic augmentation. Based upon the data collected in this survey, the total number of women in the United States in late 1989 who had ever had breast implants was estimated to be 815,700 (95% confidence interval: 715,757 - 924,729).

Introduction

According to Barton [1], the utilization of alloplastic materials in the body for contour enhancement and replacement of lost anatomical parts dates from the 16th century. Ivory, glass, paraffin and sponges made of various synthetics such as Ivalon, Etheron, Teflon, and polyurethane all have been used at one time or another with limited success.

Autogenous tissues have also been utilized [2]. The first recorded augmentation mammaplasty was done in 1895 when a lipoma was successfully transplanted to reconstruct a patient's breast after surgical removal of an adenoma.

Subsequently, others injected fat or used flaps of dermis-fat and dermis-fascia-fat. Even in those patients with sufficient transplantable tissues, these attempts have been complicated by fat necrosis, unpredictable absorption of the graft, and unsightly donor site scars.

Dissatisfied with previous biomaterials and procedures, in the early 1960s two surgeons at Baylor University worked with Dow Corning personnel to develop an implant composed of a smooth silicone elastomer shell filled with a soft silicone gel. Over the years, Dow Corning and other manufacturers made various design modifications, largely in an attempt to limit capsule formation around the implant and thereby limit the potential for painful and disfiguring capsular contracture. Barrier coats were added to reduce "silicone bleed", thought at one time to be the etiologic agent. For similar reasons, silicone gel was replaced in whole or in part with saline. In a parallel effort to eliminate contracture, Surgitek modified the surface morphology of their product through the application of polyurethane foam sheeting, the theoretical intent being to disrupt the orderly alignment of cells in the capsule. The relative success of the latter lead to "textured" implants by other manufacturers, devices in which the silicone elastomer itself was made less smooth. Reportedly this reduced contracture in both experimental and clinical settings [3].

Irrespective of the local complications, and until the temporary voluntary moratorium in early 1992, breast implantation was a relatively frequent surgical procedure. Based on a series of surveys conducted by the American Society of Plastic and Reconstructive Surgeons, Deapen et al [4] estimated the 1981 prevalence of breast implants in the United States at 1,000,000. Recently others have quoted numbers as high as 2,000,000 and one even up to 6,000,000 worldwide [5-6].

These figures stand in marked contrast to the results of a National Center for Health Statistics survey [7]. Based on data collected as part of the 1988 National Health Interview, the NCHS and FDA estimated there were 620,000 silicone implants at that time, of which approximately 90% were breast implants. Further, they calculated the implants were in a total of 304,000 (95% CI: 239,000 - 369,000) women. The authors of the government report cautioned that the discrepancy between their results and the oft quoted figure of one million may have been due to reporting errors.

Methods and Materials

To estimate the number of women in the United States who had ever had a breast implant of any type and for any reason, the Dow Corning Corporation contracted with a commercial survey firm, Market Facts, Inc., to conduct a mail survey. At the time, 1989, the survey company maintained a Consumer Mail Panel, a nationwide sample of about 270,000 households. Their data base included the following demographic information: number of residents, sex, age, race, household income, region and state. For the purposes of the implant survey, Market Facts selected 40,000 households from the panel balanced against the 1988 census data on key geodemographic variables.

In October 1989, these households were mailed a short questionnaire which asked whether anyone in household had ever had a breast implant, the year of the first implant, and the reasons for the implant -- basically cosmetic (augmentation) versus medical (reconstruction). To be eligible for our analyses, the household had to have a woman 15 years of age or older in residence. Additional details about the survey and the statistical analyses can be found in a paper that was published in the April 1995 issue of the *Journal for Clinical Epidemiology* [8].

Results

Of the 40,000 questionnaires, 28,264 (70.7%) were returned, a response rate comparable to other Market Facts surveys and approximately twice that found in comparable surveys based upon random digit dialing [9]. After quality control checks and adjustments for households in which there were two or more eligible women, the overall prevalence rate for women over the age of 14 who had ever had a breast implant was 8.08 per 1,000. This translates to 815,700 (95% CI: 715,757 - 924,729) women in late 1989 with these medical devices. Approximately 40% had their breast implants for reconstruction.

Among the implanted women, 94.6% were White. For that reason, even though the total figure of 815,700 is for women of all races, the figures in this report display the results for White women.

Fig. 1 presents the prevalence rates by age group for White women in 1989 who had implants for either medical (largely reconstruction) or cosmetic reasons. Overall, 63.5% were implanted for cosmetic augmentation, a finding that mirrored

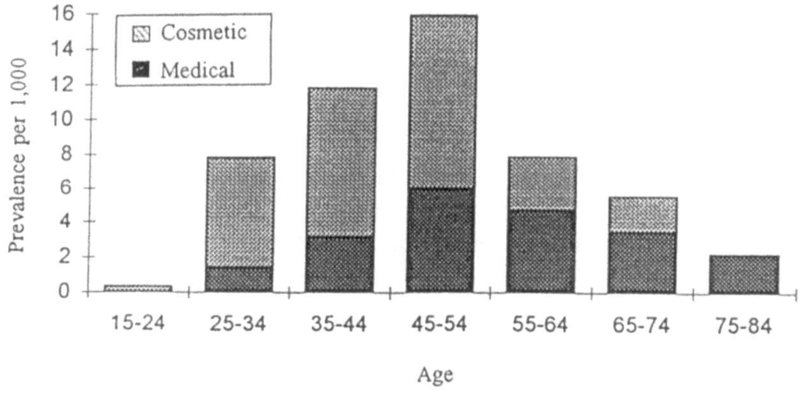

Fig. 1 Breast Implant Prevalence by Age Among US White Women, 1989.

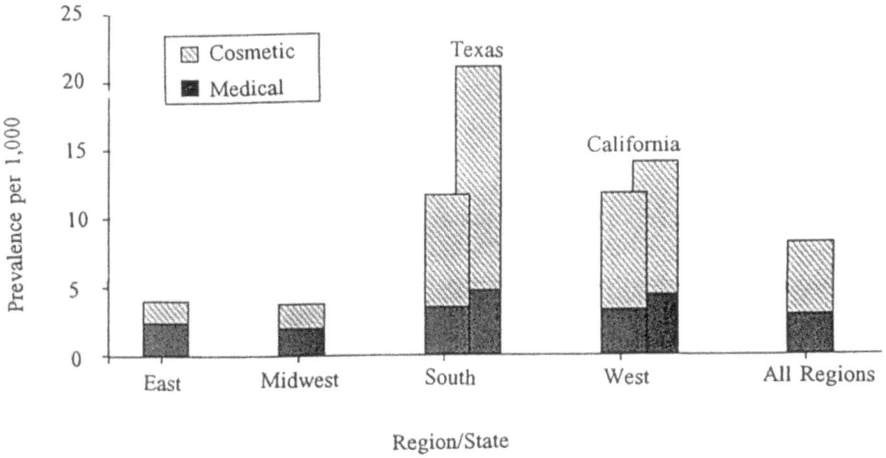

Fig. 2 Breast Implant Prevalence by Region and Selected States Among US White Women, 1989.

the 60:40 cosmetic:medical ratio found among women of all races. The total prevalence increased to a peak of 16.26 per thousand among White women in the age group 45 to 54. This was also the age group that reported the highest prevalences for the subcategories of cosmetic and medical. Furthermore, the relative prevalence of medical to cosmetic increased with age to the point where, in the oldest age group, effectively all were implanted for medical reasons. Conversely no medical procedures were reported in the 15 to 24 age group.

The cosmetic prevalence rates were directly correlated with household income (data not shown) and varied from a low of 1.57 (95% CI: 0.84 - 2.62) per thousand in households reporting incomes of less than $17,500 per year to a high of 13.84 (95% CI: 8.84 - 20.41) per thousand among those with incomes in excess of $75,000. In contrast, the medical rates appeared to be largely unrelated to household income with all income groups reporting prevalence rates in the low single digit figures. In view of the relatively large contribution cosmetic had to the overall rates, it is not surprising to note that the total rates were also strongly correlated to household income.

By region, the lowest rates were reported in the East and Midwest and the highest in the South and West (Fig. 2). In the regions with the lowest total rates, the prevalence rates for cosmetic purposes were lower than those for medical reasons. In the other regions and subregions, the cosmetic rates were 1.5 to over 4 times higher than those of medical.

The marked regional variations were consistent with the generally held clinical opinion of a sunbelt phenomenon. What was surprising was the observation that over 2% of the women in Texas had implants, a rate higher than that of California. Furthermore, women in the Mountain states -- Arizona, Colorado, Idaho, Montana, Nevada, New Mexico, Utah and Wyoming -- also had a higher prevalence (about 50% higher) than did women in the Pacific states of Oregon, Washington and California. Obviously those states with higher rates but smaller populations contributed fewer women to the total absolute number, i.e., the most women came from the more populous states irrespective of the prevalence per 1,000.

Discussion and Summary

Most of the previous estimates of the number of women with breast implants appear to have been extrapolations of data obtained from industry production figures or member surveys by the American Society of Plastic and Reconstructive Surgeons [10-14]. While each source provides valuable information, both must be used cautiously when estimating the prevalence of women with breast implants. Manufacturing records count devices and such counts often include numerous inventories along the distribution network. Surgeon surveys provide data on the frequency of procedures. In addition, numbers based upon both tend to be cumulative, that is they do not account for replacements, removals or other causes of attrition. Furthermore, some of the higher extrapolations may not have adjusted for the usual bilateral nature of the procedure. They also may have erroneously equated "breast implants" to "silicone gel breast implants", that is, they ignored the contributions by saline and urethane foam coated devices.

The only other survey that attempted to get direct estimates of the number of women with breast implants was conducted in 1988 by the National Center for Health Statistics. They concluded there were approximately 304,000 (95% CI: 239,000 - 369,000) women with these medical devices [7]. Part of the divergence between their figure and that derived from the Market Facts survey can be explained by the different years in which the surveys were conducted; but this is only a partial explanation. It is more likely that systematic differences between the questionnaires were accountable. For many women, "silicone breast implants" are a very specific type of breast implant, one with a silicone envelope filled with silicone gel. They do not consider either so-called saline or polyurethane coated breast implants to be "silicone" even though all three used a similar envelope constructed of silicone elastomer. In addition, women tend to differentiate between augmentation for cosmetic reasons and reconstruction secondary to surgical excision of the breast. The NCHS survey specifically asked about breast implants as a subcategory of silicone implants and as related to reconstruction. As a consequence, it probably underestimated the number of breast implants that had been used for augmentation and also those that had been constructed in part with materials other than silicone.

The results of both the NCHS and the Market Facts surveys support the long held clinical opinion that breast implants were more frequent in specific regions and augmentation in particular was a procedure preferred by White women in the higher income groups. Conversely, reconstruction was not income dependent. This difference probably reflects an insurance bias, i.e., reconstruction following breast cancer surgery often has been a compensable procedure. Cosmetic surgery has not, but rather appears to be a function of discretionary income.

Based upon the data obtained in the 1989 Market Facts survey, and estimating the number of women who received implants in 1990 and 1991 prior to the voluntary moratorium on the manufacture and distribution of silicone gel implants, the number of women who continued to get saline implants during and subsequent to the moratorium, and the limited number of women who received silicone gel breast implants after the moratorium was lifted by the FDA in mid-1992, the best estimate of U.S. women currently with or who ever had these medical devices is approximately one million.

References

1. Barton FE Jr (1983) Augmentation mammaplasty. Selected Readings Plast Surg 2:1-14.
2. Gerow FJ (1976) Breast Implants. In Georgiade NG (ed) Reconstructive breast surgery, CV Mosby Company, St. Louis, pp 31-67.
3. Clugston PA, Perry LC, Hammond DC, and Maxwell GP (1994) A rat model for capsular contracture: the effects of surface texturing. Ann Plast Surg 33:595-599.
4. Deapen DM, Pike MC, Casagrande JT, and Brody GS (1986) The relationship between breast cancer and augmentation mammaplasty: an epidemiologic study. Plast Recon Surg 77:361-367.
5. Mishra N (1988) Potential risks for silicone breast implants, Minutes of the November 22, 1988 General and Plastic Surgery Devices Panel meeting, Washington, DC.
6. Julliard AF (1994) Business for lawyers or surgeons? Proceedings of the VII International Symposium of Plastic and Aesthetic Surgery, October 14-15, 1994, Cannes, France.
7. Bright RA, Jeng LL, and Moore RM (1993) National survey of self-reported breast implants: 1988 estimates. J Long-Term Effects Med Implants 3(1):81-89.
8. Cook RR, Delongchamp RR, Woodbury M, Perkins LL, and Harrison MC (1995) The prevalence of women with breast implants in the United States - 1989. J Clin Epidemiol 48(4):519-526.
9. Anonymous (1995) Mail panels vs. general samples: how similar and how different? In *Research on Research*, a publication of Market Facts, Inc., Washington, DC.

10. Anonymous (1987) The soft tissue implant market. Theta Corporation Report 606, Middlefield, CT.
11. American Society of Plastic and Reconstructive Surgeons (1985) Plastic surgery procedures performed in 1984 and 1981 by ASPRS members, news release, Arlington Heights, IL.
12. American Society of Plastic and Reconstructive Surgeons (1987) Plastic surgery procedures performed in 1986 and 1984 by ASPRS members, news release, Arlington Heights, IL.
13. American Society of Plastic and Reconstructive Surgerons (undated) Estimated number of cosmetic surgery procedures performed by ASPRS members, fact sheet (for 1981 and 1988), Arlington Heights, IL.
14. American Society of Plastic and Reconstructive Surgeons (1989) Breast reconstruction on the rise, news release, Arlington Heights, IL.

Epidemiology of Autoimmune and Immunological Diseases in Association with Silicone Implants: Is There an Excess of Clinical Disease or Antibody Response in Population-based or Other "Controlled" Studies?

L. T. Kurland, MD, DrPH,[1] and H. A. Homburger, MD[2]*
From the [1]Department of Health Sciences Research, Section of Clinical Epidemiology and the [2]Department of Laboratory Medicine and Pathology, Division of Clinical Biochemistry and Immunology, Mayo Clinic and Mayo Foundation, Rochester, MN

Case reports, small case series and media coverage have led to the general perception that patients with silicone breast implants are at increased risk of connective tissue diseases or rheumatologic disorders. Our understanding of rheumatologic disorders would be enhanced if such an association could indeed be confirmed by controlled studies, but the reported associations of autoimmune diseases have been based on case reports which have had one or more of the deficiencies noted in table 1. Such case reports or case series provide no evidence of an excess of the specified rheumatologic diseases among implant subjects compared to expected incidence. Furthermore, case reports or case series have no denominators and cannot provide rates for comparison. Comparisons between exposed and nonexposed can best be done through a historical cohort study or through case-control analyses.

Table 1. Silicone breast implant associations with autoimmune diseases (rheumatological and neurological)

The published case reports or case series have one or more of these features:

- ◇ Poor or absent case definition
- ◇ Failure to apply conventional diagnostic criteria
- ◇ Lack of identification of type of implant
- ◇ Unknown status prior to implant
- ◇ Lack of consistent latent period
- ◇ Inconsistent effects on symptoms after removal of implant
- ◇ Some reports based on liquid injections (silicone and paraffin) in the '50s and '60s

* The authors of this paper are salaried employees and have no financial interest in the development, manufacture or distribution of silicone breast implants, nor have they served as expert witnesses or consultants in any litigation on the silicone breast implant issue. The mechanics of data collection and analysis for the Olmsted County, Minnesota, silicone breast implant study (references #1 and #2) were funded by Mayo Clinic, by the National Institutes of Health, and by the Educational Foundation of the Plastic Surgeons Association.

The first population-based historical cohort study of connective tissue disease in recipients of silicone breast implants and matched controls was that for the population of Olmsted County, Minnesota, by Gabriel et al. [1]. In that study of implant recipients and age-matched controls from the same community, there was no difference in the proportion with diagnosed connective tissue diseases or controls (5 of 749 implant recipients versus 10 of 1,498 controls). Data were provided not only for classical connective tissue diseases but also on each criterion necessary to make these diagnoses so that information on both incomplete and overlap connective tissue diseases was included. A detailed methodologic paper describes the assembly of the study population and a step-by-step accounting for each individual on the exposed cohort and the control group, from the original diagnostic computer listing to the final cohort comparison [2].

In addition to this negative study on silicone breast implants and connective tissue diseases, there have now been several case-control comparisons as shown in table 2 [3-8] or in the meta analysis that Dr. Hochberg has just presented. In none of these studies is there a significant increase of rheumatologic disorders.

There is an excellent, balanced review on this issue from the Medical Devices Agency of the British Department of Health [9] which concludes "that there is no evidence of an increased risk of connective tissue disease in patients who have had silicone gel breast implants and therefore no scientific case for changing practice or policy in the UK with respect to breast implantation."

There is also a description of a large (n=824) cohort study in Denmark [10] with no excess of connective tissue diseases of all forms combined. Two cases were confirmed to have systemic sclerosis, whereas 0.07 were expected. But in a subsequent review of the surgical records, one of these had breast reduction which was miscoded as breast augmentation. The finding for systemic sclerosis was no longer statistically significant ($p=0.07$) [11].

With respect to immunological studies performed on breast implant recipients, some authors report association of autoantibodies with the presence of disease [12], others describe an association of the level of antibodies and the severity of clinical disease [13], and still others report no association [14]. A problem in assessing these studies is selection or referral bias and quality control for clinical diagnosis. An immunological survey of exposed and controls in a delineated population is needed to assess whether silicone has an adjuvant effect and, if so, whether it has any clinical significance. In such a study, it would be desirable to focus on detecting antibodies of two types--antibodies known to be associated with autoimmune diseases (e.g., antinuclear antibodies) and antibodies to putative antigens of silicone or its metabolites. Tests for many autoantibodies, including antinuclear antibodies, are standardized and have well described associations with various autoimmune diseases, particularly the connective tissue diseases [15]. Antibodies to silicone are newly described, require independent verification and remain to be standardized [16].

Table 2. Summary of controlled studies examining the relationship between breast implants (BI) and connective tissue diseases(CTD)

Investigator	Study Design	Cases (exposed)	Controls (unexposed)	Outcome(s) Examined	Main Result	Conclusions
Gabriel et al. 1994 [1]	Historical cohort	749	1,498	CTD, AD	RR for any of diseases of interest **1.10 (CI 0.37-3.23)**	No association between BI and CTD and other disorders studied
Englert and Brooks 1994 [3]	Case-control	315	371	SS	Ratio of BI among cases **(1.59%)** and controls **(1.73%)**	Ratio of BI similar in cases and controls
Strom et al. 1994 [4]	Case-control	195	143	SLE	One **(0.8%)** SLE case and 0 **(0%)** controls reported having a BI **(p=0.57)**	No statistically significant association between BI and SLE
Dugowson et al. 1992 [5]	Case-control	349	1,456	RA	OR for history of BI **0.41 (CI 0.05-3.13)**	No increased risk demonstrated for RA among women with BI
Hochberg et al. 1994 [6]	Multi-center retrospective cohort	869	2,061	SS	OR for BI surgery **1.25 (CI 0.62-2.53)**	No significant causal relationship demonstrated between BI and development of SS
Sanchez-Guerrero et al. 1994 [7]	Nested case-control	121,700 (registered nurses)		CTD	448 CTD, 1,209 BI, 5 CTD (RA) & BI OR (CTD) **0.94 (CI 0.37-2.37)**, OR (RA) **1.46 (CI 0.58-3.69)**; 0 BI among: 123 SLE, 20 SS, 3 Sjögren's, 13 dermato/polymyositis, 2 mixed CTD	No statistically significant association found between BI and CTD
Burns and Schottenfeld et al. 1995 [8]	Case-control (preliminary results)	592	1,184	SS	OR for BI surgery **0.61 (CI 0.14-2.68)**	No statistically significant association found between BI and SS

AD = autoimmune diseases
BI = breast implants
CTD = connective tissue diseases
RA = rheumatoid arthritis
SS = systemic sclerosis (scleroderma)
SLE = systemic lupus erythematosus
RR = relative risk
OR = odds ratio
CI = 95% confidence interval

References

1. Gabriel SE, O'Fallon WM, Kurland LT, Woods JE, Beard CM, Melton LJ (1994) Risk of connective-tissue diseases and other disorders after breast implantation. N Engl J Med 330:1697-1702
2. Gabriel SE, O'Fallon WM, Beard CM, Kurland LT, Woods JE, Melton LJ (1995) Trends in the utilization of silicone breast implants, 1964-1991, and methodology for a population-based study of outcomes. J Clin Epidemiol 48:527-537
3. Englert HJ, Brooks P (1994) Scleroderma and augmentation mammoplasty--a causal relationship? Aust NZ J Med 24:74-80
4. Strom BL, Reidenberg MM, Freundlich B, Schinnar R (1994) Breast silicone implants and risk of systemic lupus erythematosus. J Clin Epidemiol 47:1211-1214
5. Dugowson CE, Daling J, Koepsell TD, Voigt L, Nelson JL (1992) Silicone breast implants and risk for rheumatoid-arthritis (abstract). Arthritis Rhem 35:S66
6. Sanchez-Guerrero J, Karlson EW, Colditz GA, Hankinson SE, Hunter DJ, Speizer FE, Liang MH (1994) Silicone breast implants (SBI) and connective tissue disease (CTD) (abstract). Arthritis Rheum 37(Suppl.):S282
7. Burns CG (1994) The epidemiology of systemic sclerosis: A population-based case-control study. [Dissertation submitted in partial fulfillment of the requirements of the degree of Doctor of Philosophy (Epidemiologic Science), University of Michigan]
8. Hochberg MC, Perlmutter DL, White B, Steen V, Medsger TA, Weisman M, Wigley FM (1994) The association of augmentation mammoplasty with systemic sclerosis: Results from a multi-center case-control study (abstract). Arthritis Rheum 37(Suppl.):S369
9. Gott DM, Tinkler JJB (1995) Silicone implants and connective tissue disease: Evaluation of evidence for an association between the implantation of silicones and connective tissue disease. Data published from the end of 1991 to July 1994. Medical Devices Agency, Department of Health of England and Wales, 14 Russell Square, London WC1B 5EP
10. McLaughlin JK, Fraumeni JF Jr, Olsen J, Mellemkjaer L (1994) Breast implants, cancer, and systemic sclerosis (letter). J Natl Cancer Inst 86:1424
11. McLaughlin JK, Olsen JH, Friis S, Mellemkjaer L, Fraumeni JF Jr. Re: Breast implants, cancer, and systemic sclerosis (letter). J Natl Cancer Inst 87:1415-1416
12. Vojdani A, Campbell A, Brautbar N (1992) Immune functional impairment in patients with clinical abnormalities and silicone breast implants. Toxicol Ind Health 8:415-429
13. Claman HN, Robertson AD (1994) Anitnuclear antibodies and brest implants. West J Med 160:225-228
14. Keystone E, Peters W, Snow K, Rubin L, Smith D (1993) Frequency of autoantibody detection in patients with silicone-gel implants (abstract). 57Th Annual Meeting American College of Rheumatology, San Antonio, Texas, November 8-11, p. S71
15. Tan EM (1982) Autoantibodies to nuclear antigens (ANA): Their immunobiology and medicine. Adv Immunol 33:167-240
16. Wolf LE, Lappe M, Peterson RD, Ezrailson EG (1993) Human immune response to polydimethylsiloxane (silicone): Screening studies in a breast implant population. FASEB J 7:1265-1268

Current Topics in Microbiology and Immunology

Volumes published since 1989 (and still available)

Vol. 168: **Mason, William S.; Seeger, Christoph (Eds.)**: Hepadnaviruses. Molecular Biology and Pathogenesis. 1991. 21 figs. X, 206 pp.
ISBN 3-540-53060-6

Vol. 169: **Kolakofsky, Daniel (Ed.)**: Bunyaviridae. 1991. 34 figs. X, 256 pp.
ISBN 3-540-53061-4

Vol. 170: **Compans, Richard W. (Ed.)**: Protein Traffic in Eukaryotic Cells. Selected Reviews. 1991. 14 figs. X, 186 pp.
ISBN 3-540-53631-0

Vol. 171: **Kung, Hsing-Jien; Vogt, Peter K. (Eds.)**: Retroviral Insertion and Oncogene Activation. 1991. 18 figs. X, 179 pp.
ISBN 3-540-53857-7

Vol. 172: **Chesebro, Bruce W. (Ed.)**: Transmissible Spongiform Encephalopathies. 1991. 48 figs. X, 288 pp.
ISBN 3-540-53883-6

Vol. 173: **Pfeffer, Klaus; Heeg, Klaus; Wagner, Hermann; Riethmüller, Gert (Eds.)**: Function and Specificity of γ/δ TCells. 1991. 41 figs. XII, 296 pp.
ISBN 3-540-53781-3

Vol. 174: **Fleischer, Bernhard; Sjögren, Hans Olov (Eds.)**: Superantigens. 1991. 13 figs. IX, 137 pp. ISBN 3-540-54205-1

Vol. 175: **Aktories, Klaus (Ed.)**: ADP-Ribosylating Toxins. 1992. 23 figs. IX, 148 pp.
ISBN 3-540-54598-0

Vol. 176: **Holland, John J. (Ed.)**: Genetic Diversity of RNA Viruses. 1992. 34 figs. IX, 226 pp. ISBN 3-540-54652-9

Vol. 177: **Müller-Sieburg, Christa; Torok-Storb, Beverly; Visser, Jan; Storb, Rainer (Eds.)**: Hematopoietic Stem Cells. 1992. 18 figs. XIII, 143 pp. ISBN 3-540-54531-X

Vol. 178: **Parker, Charles J. (Ed.)**: Membrane Defenses Against Attack by Complement and Perforins. 1992. 26 figs. VIII, 188 pp. ISBN 3-540-54653-7

Vol. 179: **Rouse, Barry T. (Ed.)**: Herpes Simplex Virus. 1992. 9 figs. X, 180 pp.
ISBN 3-540-55066-6

Vol. 180: **Sansonetti, P. J. (Ed.)**: Pathogenesis of Shigellosis. 1992. 15 figs. X, 143 pp.
ISBN 3-540-55058-5

Vol. 181: **Russell, Stephen W.; Gordon, Siamon (Eds.)**: Macrophage Biology and Activation. 1992. 42 figs. IX, 299 pp.
ISBN 3-540-55293-6

Vol. 182: **Potter, Michael; Melchers, Fritz (Eds.)**: Mechanisms in B-Cell Neoplasia. 1992. 188 figs. XX, 499 pp.
ISBN 3-540-55658-3

Vol. 183: **Dimmock, Nigel J.**: Neutralization of Animal Viruses. 1993. 10 figs. VII, 149 pp.
ISBN 3-540-56030-0

Vol. 184: **Dunon, Dominique; Mackay, Charles R.; Imhof, Beat A. (Eds.)**: Adhesion in Leukocyte Homing and Differentiation. 1993. 37 figs. IX, 260 pp.
ISBN 3-540-56756-9

Vol. 185: **Ramig, Robert F. (Ed.)**: Rotaviruses. 1994. 37 figs. X, 380 pp.
ISBN 3-540-56761-5

Vol. 186: **zur Hausen, Harald (Ed.)**: Human Pathogenic Papillomaviruses. 1994. 37 figs. XIII, 274 pp. ISBN 3-540-57193-0

Vol. 187: **Rupprecht, Charles E.; Dietzschold, Bernhard; Koprowski, Hilary (Eds.)**: Lyssaviruses. 1994. 50 figs. IX, 352 pp. ISBN 3-540-57194-9

Vol. 188: **Letvin, Norman L.; Desrosiers, Ronald C. (Eds.)**: Simian Immunodeficiency Virus. 1994. 37 figs. X, 240 pp. ISBN 3-540-57274-0

Vol. 189: **Oldstone, Michael B. A. (Ed.)**: Cytotoxic T-Lymphocytes in Human Viral and Malaria Infections. 1994. 37 figs. IX, 210 pp. ISBN 3-540-57259-7

Vol. 190: **Koprowski, Hilary; Lipkin, W. Ian (Eds.)**: Borna Disease. 1995. 33 figs. IX, 134 pp. ISBN 3-540-57388-7

Vol. 191: **ter Meulen, Volker; Billeter, Martin A. (Eds.)**: Measles Virus. 1995. 23 figs. IX, 196 pp. ISBN 3-540-57389-5

Vol. 192: **Dangl, Jeffrey L. (Ed.)**: Bacterial Pathogenesis of Plants and Animals. 1994. 41 figs. IX, 343 pp. ISBN 3-540-57391-7

Vol. 193: **Chen, Irvin S. Y.; Koprowski, Hilary; Srinivasan, Alagarsamy; Vogt, Peter K. (Eds.)**: Transacting Functions of Human Retroviruses. 1995. 49 figs. IX, 240 pp. ISBN 3-540-57901-X

Vol. 194: **Potter, Michael; Melchers, Fritz (Eds.)**: Mechanisms in B-cell Neoplasia. 1995. 152 figs. XXV, 458 pp. ISBN 3-540-58447-1

Vol. 195: **Montecucco, Cesare (Ed.)**: Clostridial Neurotoxins. 1995. 28 figs. XI., 278 pp. ISBN 3-540-58452-8

Vol. 196: **Koprowski, Hilary; Maeda, Hiroshi (Eds.)**: The Role of Nitric Oxide in Physiology and Pathophysiology. 1995. 21 figs. IX, 90 pp. ISBN 3-540-58214-2

Vol. 197: **Meyer, Peter (Ed.)**: Gene Silencing in Higher Plants and Related Phenomena in Other Eukaryotes. 1995. 17 figs. IX, 232 pp. ISBN 3-540-58236-3

Vol. 198: **Griffiths, Gillian M.; Tschopp, Jürg (Eds.)**: Pathways for Cytolysis. 1995. 45 figs. IX, 224 pp. ISBN 3-540-58725-X

Vol. 199/I: **Doerfler, Walter; Böhm, Petra (Eds.)**: The Molecular Repertoire of Adenoviruses I. 1995. 51 figs. XIII, 280 pp. ISBN 3-540-58828-0

Vol. 199/II: **Doerfler, Walter; Böhm, Petra (Eds.)**: The Molecular Repertoire of Adenoviruses II. 1995. 36 figs. XIII, 278 pp. ISBN 3-540-58829-9

Vol. 199/III: **Doerfler, Walter; Böhm, Petra (Eds.)**: The Molecular Repertoire of Adenoviruses III. 1995. 51 figs. XIV, 324 pp. ISBN 3-540-58987-2

Vol. 200: **Kroemer, Guido; Martinez-A., Carlos (Eds.)**: Apoptosis in Immunology. 1995. 14 figs. XI, 242 pp. ISBN 3-540-58756-X

Vol. 201: **Kosco-Vilbois, Marie H. (Ed.)**: An Antigen Depository of the Immune System: Follicular Dendritic Cells. 1995. 39 figs. IX, 209 pp. ISBN 3-540-59013-7

Vol. 202: **Oldstone, Michael B. A.; Vitković, Ljubiša (Eds.)**: HIV and Dementia. 1995. 40 figs. XIII, 279 pp. ISBN 3-540-59117-6

Vol. 203: **Sarnow, Peter (Ed.)**: Cap-Independent Translation. 1995. 31 figs. XI, 183 pp. ISBN 3-540-59121-4

Vol. 204: **Saedler, Heinz; Gierl, Alfons (Eds.)**: Transposable Elements. 1995. 42 figs. IX, 234 pp. ISBN 3-540-59342-X

Vol. 205: **Littman, Dan. R. (Ed.)**: The CD4 Molecule. 1995. 29 figs. XIV, 184 pp. ISBN 3-540-59344-6

Vol. 206: **Chisari, Francis V.; Oldstone, Michael B. A. (Eds.)**: Transgenic Models of Human Viral and Immunological Disease. 1995. 53 figs. XII, 350 pp. ISBN 3-540-59341-1

Vol. 207: **Prusiner, Stanley B. (Ed.)**: Prions Prions Prions. 1995. 42 figs. VI, 180 pp. ISBN 3-540-59343-8

Vol. 208: **Farnham, Peggy (Ed.)**: Transcriptional Control of Cell Growth. 1995. 17 figs. VIII, 250 pp. ISBN 3-540-60113-9

Vol. 209: **Miller, Virginia L. (Ed.)**: Bacterial Invasiveness. 1995. 16 figs. IX, 180 pp. ISBN 3-540-60065-5